Renal Diseases: Pathology, Diagnosis and Management

Renal Diseases: Pathology, Diagnosis and Management

Editor: Emma Farlow

FOSTER ACADEMICS
www.fosteracademics.com

www.fosteracademics.com

FOSTER ACADEMICS

Cataloging-in-Publication Data

Renal diseases : pathology, diagnosis and management / edited by Emma Farlow.
p. cm.
Includes bibliographical references and index.
ISBN 978-1-64646-575-0
1. Kidneys--Diseases. 2. Kidneys--Diseases--Diagnosis. 3. Kidneys--Diseases--Treatment. I. Farlow, Emma.
RC902 .K53 2023
616.61--dc23

Foster Academics,
118-35 Queens Blvd., Suite 400,
Forest Hills, NY 11375, USA

ISBN 978-1-64646-575-0 (Hardback)

Contents

Preface

The kidneys are a pair of bean-shaped organs located on either side of the spine, which filter blood in the human body. They are responsible for maintaining proper electrolyte levels, eliminating waste and regulating fluid balance in the body. The condition wherein the kidneys cannot filter the blood properly due to an injury is called renal disease or kidney disease. Renal diseases are classified into two categories, namely, acute kidney diseases and chronic kidney diseases. Kidneys can regenerate after an incident of acute kidney disease provided injury is not severe. In circumstances where the kidneys are not capable of producing new nephrons, and incidents of acute kidney disease occurs frequently, it can lead to chronic kidney disease and renal fibrosis. People who have diabetes, high blood pressure or heart disease, have a family history of kidney disease, or are over the age 60, are at a higher risk of chronic kidney disease. This book unravels the recent studies on renal diseases. Its extensive content provides the readers with a thorough understanding of these diseases, their pathology, diagnosis, and management.

Various studies have approached the subject by analyzing it with a single perspective, but the present book provides diverse methodologies and techniques to address this field. This book contains theories and applications needed for understanding the subject from different perspectives. The aim is to keep the readers informed about the progresses in the field; therefore, the contributions were carefully examined to compile novel researches by specialists from across the globe.

Indeed, the job of the editor is the most crucial and challenging in compiling all chapters into a single book. In the end, I would extend my sincere thanks to the chapter authors for their profound work. I am also thankful for the support provided by my family and colleagues during the compilation of this book.

Editor

1

Diagnostic Performance of Cyclophilin A in Cardiac Surgery-Associated Acute Kidney Injury

Cheng-Chia Lee [1,2,†], Chih-Hsiang Chang [1,2,†], Ya-Lien Cheng [1], George Kuo [1], Shao-Wei Chen [2,3], Yi-Jung Li [1,2], Yi-Ting Chen [4] and Ya-Chung Tian [1,*]

1 Kidney Research Center, Department of Nephrology, Chang Gung Memorial Hospital, College of Medicine, Chang Gung University, Taoyuan 333, Taiwan; chia7181@gmail.com (C.-C.L.); franwisandsun@gmail.com (C.-H.C.); yolien0205@gmail.com (Y.-L.C.); b92401107@gmail.com (G.K.); r5259@cgmh.org.tw (Y.-J.L.)

2 Graduate Institute of Clinical Medical Sciences, College of Medicine, Chang Gung University, Taoyuan 333, Taiwan; josephchen0939@gmail.com

3 Department of Cardiothoracic and Vascular Surgery, Chang Gung Memorial Hospital, Linkou branch, College of Medicine, Chang Gung University, Taoyuan 333, Taiwan

4 Department of Biomedical Sciences, College of Medicine, Chang Gung University, Taoyuan 333, Taiwan; ytchen@mail.cgu.edu.tw

* Correspondence: dryctian@adm.cgmh.org.tw.

† These authors contributed equally to this manuscript.

Abstract: Acute kidney injury (AKI) is associated with increased morbidity and mortality and is frequently encountered in cardiovascular surgical intensive care units (CVS-ICU). In this study, we aimed at investigating the utility of cyclophilin A (CypA) for the early detection of postoperative AKI in patients undergoing cardiac surgery. This was a prospective observational study conducted in a CVS-ICU of a tertiary care university hospital. All prospective clinical and laboratory data were evaluated as predictors of AKI. Serum and urine CypA, as well as urine neutrophil gelatinase-associated lipocalin (uNGAL), were examined within 6 h after cardiac surgery. The discriminative power for the prediction of AKI was evaluated using the area under the receiver operator characteristic curve (AUROC). We found that both serum CypA and urine CypA were significantly higher in the AKI group than in the non-AKI group. For discriminating AKI and dialysis-requiring AKI, serum CypA demonstrated acceptable AUROC values (0.689 and 0.738, respectively). The discrimination ability of urine CypA for predicting AKI was modest, but it was acceptable for predicting dialysis-requiring AKI (AUROC = 0.762). uNGAL best predicted the development of AKI, but its sensitivity was not good. A combination of serum CypA and uNGAL enhanced the overall performance for predicting the future development of AKI and dialysis-requiring AKI. Our results suggest that CypA is suitable as a biomarker for the early detection of postoperative AKI in CVS–ICU. However, it has better discriminating ability when combined with uNGAL for predicting AKI in CVS-ICU patients.

Keywords: cardiovascular surgical intensive care units; cardiac surgery; acute kidney injury; cyclophilin A; neutrophil gelatinase-associated lipocalin

---

1. Introduction

Acute kidney injury (AKI) is a severe complication after cardiac surgery and significantly affects morbidity and mortality [1,2]. Up to 15–40% of patients undergoing cardiac surgery develop AKI, with 1–6% requiring renal replacement therapy (RRT) [1–4]. The mortality rate in cardiac surgery patients with a severe, RRT-requiring AKI can be as high as 60% [3,4]. Even minor increases in serum creatinine (SCr) levels (that is, 20–25% from preoperative baseline) following cardiac surgery are associated with increased mortality [5,6]. AKI is associated with not only postoperative mortality but long-term complications, such as increased risks of myocardial infarction, heart failure, mediastinitis, and stroke [2,7–9]. Therefore, novel biomarkers that can predict the development and severity of AKI earlier after cardiac surgery are important tools in clinical practice.

Recently, a secreted molecule, cyclophilin A (CypA), was found to have a physiological and pathological role in cardiovascular diseases, including atherosclerosis, acute coronary syndrome, and aortic aneurysm [10–14]. Extracellular CypA has been found to promote either the development of atherosclerosis or the vulnerability of atherosclerotic plaques by enhancing vascular oxidative stress and inflammation [14]. CypA has also been shown to be a damage-associated molecular pattern molecule that can initiate and perpetuate the inflammatory response [15]. It can stimulate inflammatory cell recruitment and subsequent tissue injury through binding to membrane receptor CD147 [16]. Critically, Dear et al., by using a mouse model of sepsis based on cecal ligation and puncture, found that inhibition of CypA receptor CD147 attenuates sepsis-induced acute renal failure [17]. Furthermore, the increased secretion of CypA from human proximal tubular cells has been demonstrated after exposure to harmful insults, such as free radical treatment [18]. Thus, it is conceivable that urine CypA might be a potential early marker of kidney injury.

Our hypothesis was that serum CypA can be a crucial mediator leading to adverse outcomes in patients after cardiac surgery. Therefore, this study aimed to evaluate whether serum or urine CypA could be a potential marker to predict AKI after cardiac surgery.

2. Materials and Methods

2.1. Study Design

We conducted a prospective, observational study in the CVS-ICU at a tertiary care referral center in Taiwan between September 2015 and December 2016. Patients who received cardiac surgery were enrolled in this investigation. A total of 186 patients were included and divided into the AKI and non-AKI groups. Patients who had an estimated glomerular filtration rate (eGFR) < 30 mL/min/1.73 m^2, were receiving dialysis, were aged < 18 years, or reported any prior organ transplantation were excluded. To ensure early detection, only those who underwent cardiac surgery and were admitted to the CVS-ICU within 72 h were enrolled. Demographic data, clinical characteristics, and echocardiographic data were collected. Routine biochemistry test results, such as white blood cell, hemoglobin, creatinine (Cr), and alanine aminotransferase levels were measured by the central laboratory of Chang Gung Memorial Hospital. Based on the Kidney Disease Improving Global Outcomes (KDIGO) Clinical Practice Guidelines for Acute Kidney Injury, AKI was defined under either of the following criteria: increase in SCr by ≥0.3mg/dL within 48 h or increase in SCr to ≥1.5 times the baseline within 7 days. In addition, the severity of AKI was staged according to the KDIGO guidelines [19]. The study protocol was approved by the local Institutional Review Board (number 103-1993B).

2.2. Clinical Assessment

All the patients received standard medical therapy after cardiac surgery. The cardiac surgical details included coronary artery bypass grafting (CABG), valve surgery, and aortic surgery. Surgical risk was assessed using the European System for Cardiac Operative Risk Evaluation (EuroSCORE) II score [20]. To determine the predictive value of potential biomarkers for AKI, the primary outcome was the development of AKI within 7 days after cardiac surgery. To assess the prognostic utility of potential biomarkers, new-onset dialysis-requiring AKI and 90-day mortality were considered secondary outcomes. After hospital discharge, a 6-month follow-up examination was performed by reviewing the electronic medical records or using telephone interviews as needed.

2.3. *Sampling and Quantifying Urine Neutrophil Gelatinase-Associated Lipocalin (uNGAL) and Cyclophilin A (CypA)*

Urine samples were collected in sterile non-heparinized tubes immediately after cardiac surgery and then centrifuged at 5000× *g* for 30 min at 4 °C to remove cells and debris. The clarified supernatants were stored at −80 °C until analysis. CypA and uNGAL were measured by an enzyme-linked immunosorbent assay using kits purchased from Cusabio Biotech (Carlsbad, CA, USA) and R&D Systems (DLCN20; Minneapolis, MN, USA), respectively, according to the manufacturers' specifications.

2.4. *Statistical Analysis*

Continuous data, such as preoperative laboratory value, were expressed as means ± standard deviations. Since most biomarkers did not fit a normal distribution, we expressed them as median and interquartile range. Data of continuous variables for the AKI and non-AKI groups were compared using the Student's *t*-test or Mann–Whitney U test. Fisher's exact test was used to compare the categorical variables. The trends of uNGAL/Cr and serum CypA across chronic kidney disease (CKD) stages was assessed by the Jonckheere–Terpstra trend test. Pairwise comparisons among the CKD stages were made by the Kruskal–Wallis test with Bonferroni adjustment. The discrimination abilities of several markers (i.e., serum CypA, uNGAL/Cr, serum CypA + uNGAL/Cr, and urine CypA/Cr) in diagnosing outcomes (including AKI, hemodialysis, and 90-day mortality) were assessed using the area under the receiver operating characteristic curve (AUROC). Subsequently, optimal cut-off points and the corresponding sensitivities/specificities were obtained according to the Youden index. The areas under the curve (AUCs) of different markers were compared by the DeLong test. All tests were two-tailed, and $p < 0.05$ was considered statistically significant. No adjustment for multiple testing (multiplicity) was made in this study. Data analyses were conducted using SPSS 22 (IBM SPSS Inc, Chicago, IL, USA).

3. Results

3.1. *Study Population Characteristics*

Overall, 186 adult patients (116 men and 70 women) with a mean age of 60 years were investigated. AKI was diagnosed in 92 (49.5%) patients. The patient characteristics, including age, sex, preoperative laboratory data, and surgical details, are listed in Table 1. Diabetes mellitus and congestive heart failure were recorded in 32.8% and 19.9% of the patients, respectively, during recruitment. The AKI patients exhibited significantly higher EuroSCORE II than the non-AKI patients ($p = 0.018$). Furthermore, the AKI patients exhibited lower platelet and albumin levels and higher Cr levels at baseline than the non-AKI patients ($p < 0.05$; Table 1). No significant differences were seen in other clinical and biochemical parameters between the AKI and non-AKI groups after the cardiac surgeries.

Table 1. Baseline characteristics of the patients with and without AKI after cardiac surgeries.

Characteristics	All Patients	AKI	Non-AKI	*p*
Patient number	186	92	94	-
Age, year	60.0 ± 14.6	60.7 ± 14.8	59.3 ± 14.5	0.504
Male gender, *n* (%)	116 (62.4)	55 (59.8)	61 (64.9)	0.545
Diabetes mellitus, *n* (%)	61 (32.8)	33 (35.9)	28 (29.8)	0.436
CHF NYHA III/IV, *n* (%)	37 (19.9)	22 (23.9)	15 (16.0)	0.201
Mean arterial pressure, mmHg	90.3 ± 14.4	89.5 ± 15.4	91.0 ± 13.3	0.475
LVEF, %	60.9 ± 15.5	59.9 ± 15.9	61.8 ± 15.3	0.394

Table 1. *Cont.*

Characteristics	All Patients	AKI	Non-AKI	*p*
Preoperative laboratory data				
Leukocyte count, 1000/mL	7.8 ± 3.4	7.7 ± 3.6	7.9 ± 3.2	0.730
Hemoglobin, g/dL	12.6 ± 2.4	12.3 ± 2.7	12.9 ± 2.0	0.083
Platelet count, 1000/mL	201 ± 75	189 ± 81	212 ± 66	0.038
ALT, u/L	30.2 ± 34.8	31.2 ± 43.3	29.1 ± 24.0	0.691
Serum creatinine, mg/dL	1.1 ± 1.0	1.3 ± 1.3	0.9 ± 0.4	0.013
Albumin, mg/dL	3.9 ± 0.5	3.9 ± 0.6	4.0 ± 0.4	0.044
EuroSCORE II	6.7 (6.1)	8.0 (7.2)	5.5 (4.5)	0.018
Surgical detail, *n* (%)				0.162
CABG	61 (32.8)	24 (26.1)	37 (39.4)	
Valve surgery	64 (34.4)	33 (35.9)	31 (33.0)	
CABG + valve surgery	17 (9.1)	12 (13.0)	5 (5.3)	
Aorta	34 (18.3)	19 (20.7)	15 (16.0)	
Others	10 (5.4)	4 (4.3)	6 (6.4)	

Continuous data are presented as means ± SDs or medians (interquartile range); AKI, acute kidney injury; CHF, congestive heart failure; NYHA, New York Heart Association; ALT, alanine aminotransferase; CABG, coronary artery bypass grafting.

Table 2 summarizes the postoperative biomarkers and clinical outcomes of the patients with and without AKI in this study. In the AKI and non-AKI groups, the median serum CypA levels were 5.8 ng/mL and 4.0 ng/mL ($p < 0.001$), respectively; the median uNGAL levels were 91 ng/mL and 31 ng/mL ($p < 0.001$), respectively; and the median urine CypA levels were 0.24 ng/mL and 0.17 ng/mL ($p = 0.035$), respectively. To compensate for perioperative variation in urine dilution, urine CypA and uNGAL were adjusted according to urine Cr. The median urine CypA/Cr levels in the AKI and non-AKI groups were 0.004 ng/mL and 0.002 ng/mL ($p = 0.003$), respectively, and the median uNGAL/Cr levels in the two groups were 1.73 ng/mL and 0.43 ng/mL ($p < 0.001$), respectively. Eventually, eleven (12%) of the AKI patients underwent hemodialysis. There were seven (7.6%) and five (5.4%) patients in the AKI group suffered from post-operative bleeding and sepsis respectively. Overall, 12 (6.5%) patients died within 90 days. Patients in the AKI group had a longer hospital stay and a higher incidence of postoperative bleeding and mortality than did those in the non-AKI group.

Table 2. Postoperative biomarkers and outcomes of the patients with and without AKI after cardiac surgeries.

Characteristics	All Patients	AKI	Non-AKI	*p*
Patient number	186	92	94	-
Postoperative biomarkers				
Urine NGAL, ng/mL	44 (104)	91 (141)	31 (39)	<0.001
Urine NGAL/urine creatinine	0.73 (1.9)	1.73 (6.51)	0.43 (0.65)	<0.001
CypA, ng/mL	5.2 (3.3)	5.8 (3.9)	4.0 (4.3)	<0.001
Urine CypA, ng/mL	0.19 (0.29)	0.24 (0.40)	0.17 (0.24)	0.035
Urine CypA/urine creatinine	0.003 (0.007)	0.004 (0.013)	0.002 (0.005)	0.003
Peak serum creatinine, mg/dL	1.6 ± 1.3	2.3 ± 1.8	1.0 ± 0.4	<0.001
Outcome				
AKI stage 1/2/3	-	48/23/21	-	-
Renal replacement therapy, *n* (%)	12 (6.5)	11 (12.0)	1 (1.1)	0.002
Postoperative bleeding, *n* (%)	8 (4.3)	7 (7.6)	1 (1.1)	0.034
Postoperative sepsis, *n* (%)	6 (3.2)	5 (5.4)	1 (1.1)	0.116
Stay of hospital, days	21.4 (15.0)	28.0 (18.5)	14.9 (11.0)	<0.001
Mortality in 90 days, *n* (%)	12 (6.5)	10 (10.9)	2 (2.1)	0.018

Continuous data are presented as means ± SDs or medians (interquartile range); AKI, acute kidney injury; NGAL, neutrophil gelatinase-associated lipocalin; CypA, cyclophilin A.

The patients in the AKI group exhibited significantly higher serum CypA and normalized uNGAL levels than those in the non-AKI group. The level of normalized uNGAL increased along with the more severe AKI stage, but there was no significant difference between the KDIGO 1 and KDIGO 2 stages (Figure 1A). The level of serum CypA was significantly different between the AKI and non-AKI groups, but there was no significant difference among the KDIGO stages 1–3 (Figure 1B).

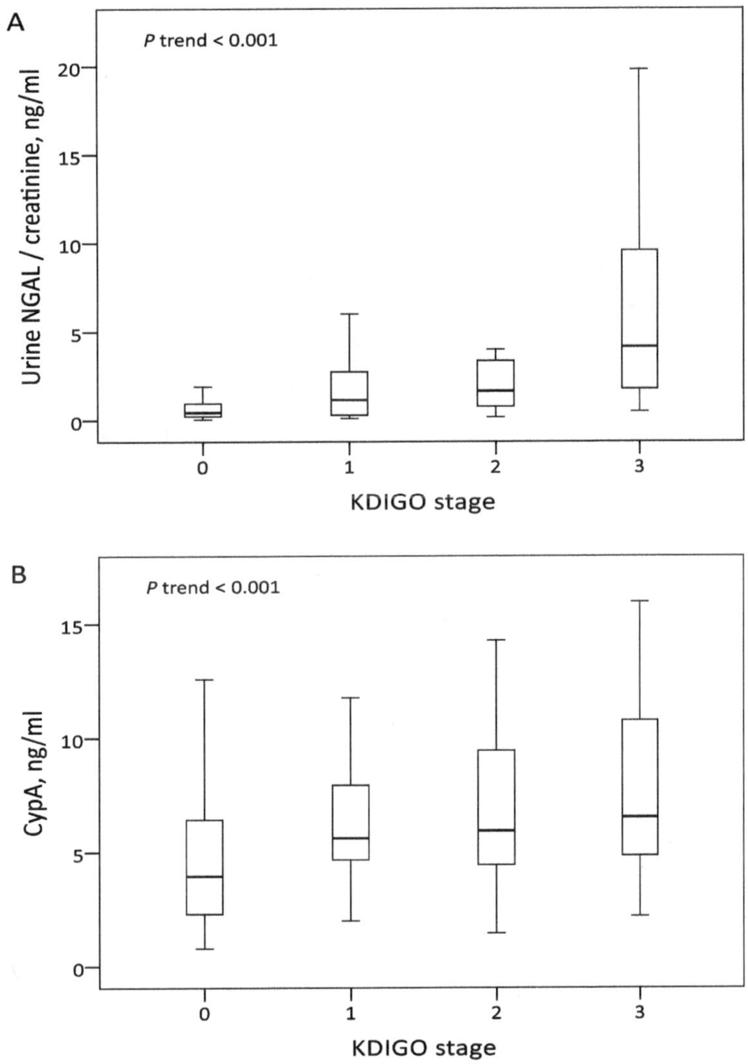

Figure 1. Levels of urine NGAL normalized by urine creatinine (**A**) and serum CypA (**B**) across KDIGO stages. Abbreviations: CypA, cyclophilin A; NGAL, neutrophil gelatinase-associated lipocalin; KDIGO, Kidney Disease Improving Global Outcomes.

3.2. Discrimination Abilities of Serum CypA and Normalized uNGAL in Detecting AKI, Dialysis-Requiring AKI, and 90-Day Mortality

The performances of serum CypA and normalized uNGAL in the detection of outcomes were assessed through AUROC analysis, as shown in Figure 2A–C. The ROC analysis of serum CypA and normalized uNGAL revealed AUROC values of 0.689 (95% confidence interval [CI], 0.618–0.755) and 0.752 (95% CI, 0.684–0.812), respectively, for predicting the future development of AKI. The combination of serum CypA and normalized uNGAL showed the highest AUC of 0.787 (95% CI, 0.721–0.843) in diagnosing AKI. In terms of using a single marker to predict dialysis-requiring AKI, serum CypA and normalized uNGAL had AUROCs of 0.738 (95% CI, 0.668–0.799) and 0.835 (95% CI, 0.773–0.885), respectively. Normalized urine CypA had an AUROC of 0.762 and exhibited a good specificity of 83.9%

for a cutoff value of 0.012. The combination of CypA and normalized uNGAL showed the highest AUC of 0.848 (95% CI, 0.788–0.896).

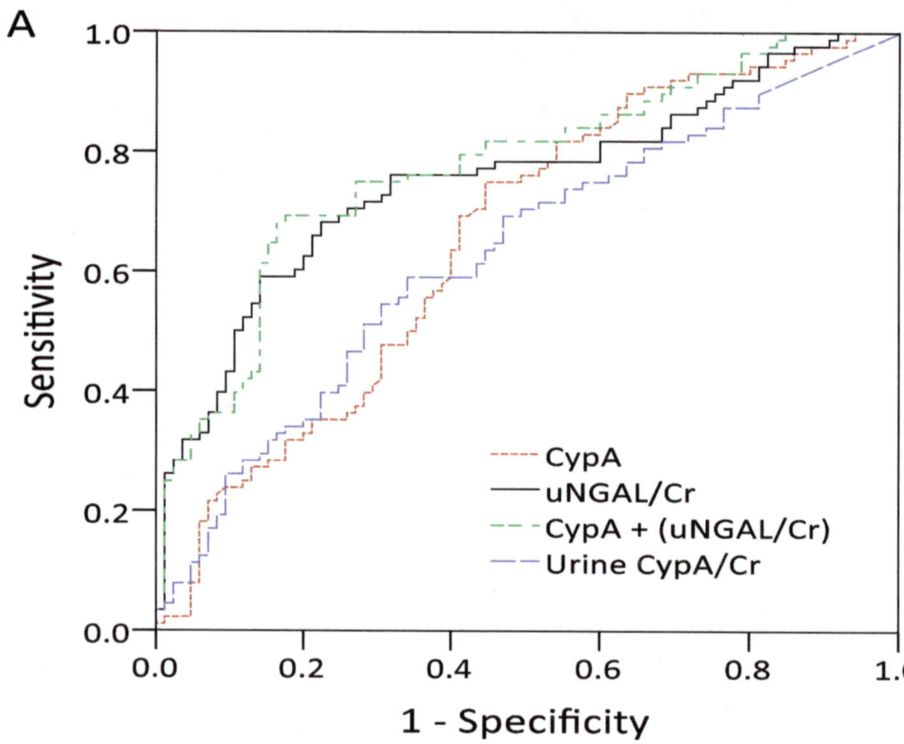

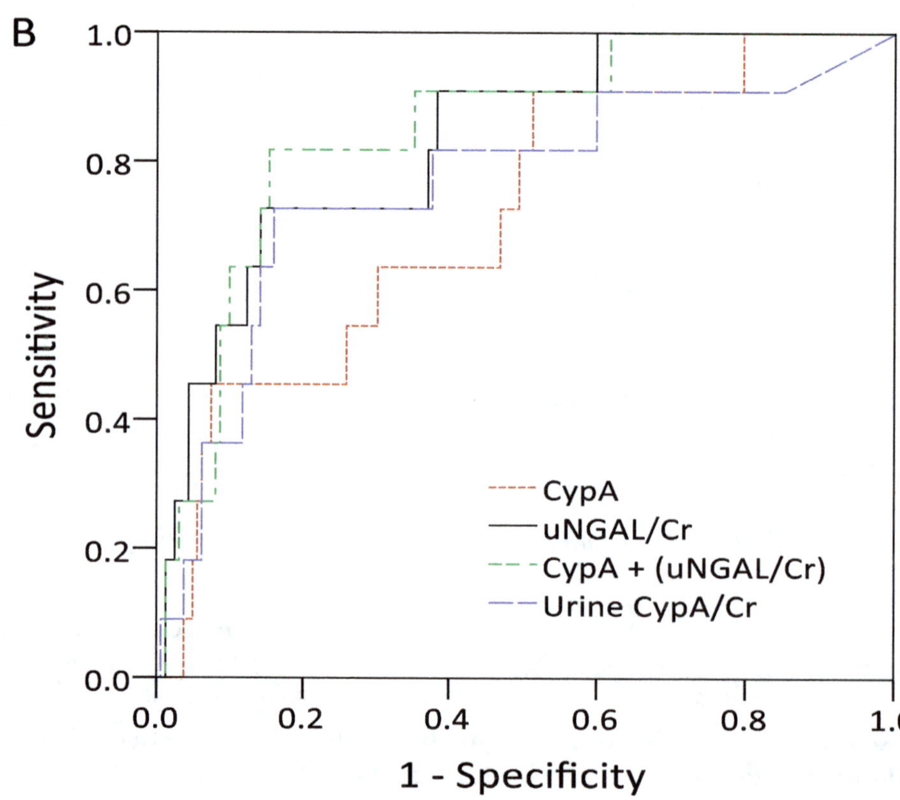

Figure 2. *Cont.*

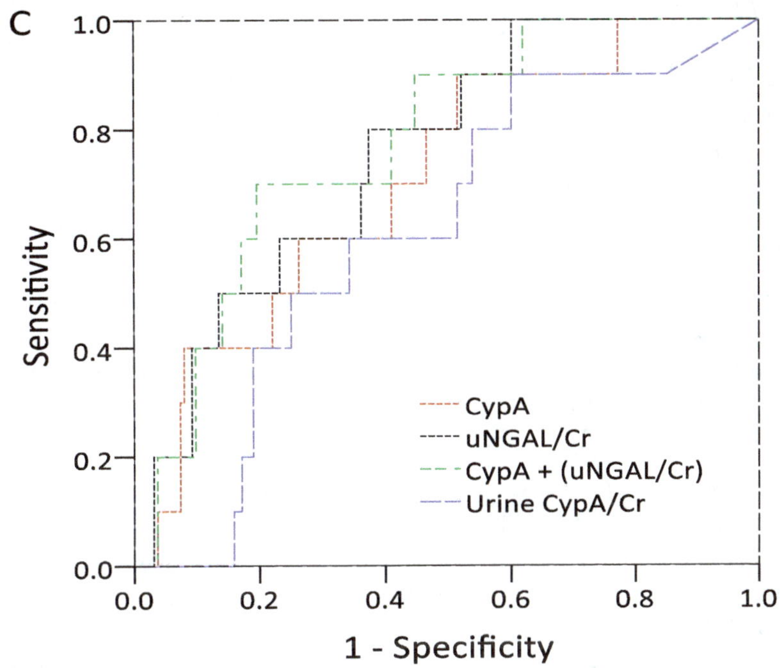

Figure 2. Area under the curves for serum CypA, urine NGAL normalized by urine Cr, serum CypA plus urine NGAL normalized by urine Cr, and urine CypA normalized by urine Cr in discriminating acute kidney injury (**A**), dialysis-requiring acute kidney injury (**B**), and 90-day mortality (**C**). Abbreviations: CypA, cyclophilin A; NGAL, neutrophil gelatinase-associated lipocalin; Cr, creatinine.

As for the detection of AKI, CypA exhibited a sensitivity of 76.1% and a specificity of 58.5% for a threshold value of 4.36 ng/mL, whereas normalized uNGAL exhibited a poor sensitivity of 68.5% and a specificity of 76.6% for a cut-off value of 0.85 (Table 3). However, there was no significant difference in the 90-day survival rates between the subgroups of high/low serum CypA and normalized uNGAL.

Table 3. Diagnostic property of markers in discriminating outcomes.

Outcome/Marker	AUC (95% CI)	Cut-Off #	Sensitivity (95% CI)	Specificity (95% CI)
Acute kidney injury				
CypA	68.9 (61.8–75.5)	>4.36	76.1 (66.1–84.4)	58.5 (47.9–68.6)
Urine NGAL/Cr	75.2 (68.4–81.2)	>0.85	68.5 (58.0–77.8)	76.6 (66.7–84.7)
CypA + (urine NGAL/Cr)	78.7 (72.1–84.3)	NA	NA	NA
Urine CypA/Cr	63.0 (55.3–70.2)	>0.003	59.1 (48.1–69.5)	65.9 (54.8–75.8)
Dialysis-requiring AKI				
CypA	73.8 (66.8–79.9)	>4.84	91.7 (61.5–99.8)	50.0 (42.3–57.7)
Urine NGAL/Cr	83.5 (77.3–88.5)	>3.09	75.0 (42.8–94.5)	85.1 (78.9–90.0)
CypA + (urine NGAL/Cr)	84.8 (78.8–89.6)	NA	NA	NA
Urine CypA/Cr	76.2 (69.2–82.3)	>0.012	72.7 (39.0–94.0)	83.9 (77.4–89.2)
90-day mortality				
CypA	67.0 (59.7–73.7)	>4.84	83.3 (51.6–97.9)	49.4 (41.8–57.1)
Urine NGAL/Cr	75.4 (68.5–81.4)	>1.12	83.3 (51.6–97.9)	62.6 (55.0–69.8)
CypA + (urine NGAL/Cr)	73.1 (66.2–79.4)	NA	NA	NA
Urine CypA/Cr	61.1 (53.4–68.4)	>0.0016	90.0 (55.5–99.7)	39.9 (32.3–47.8)

AUC, area under the curve; CI, confidence interval; CypA, cyclophilin A; NGAL, neutrophil gelatinase-associated lipocalin; Cr, creatinine; AKI, acute kidney injury; NA, not applicable; #, number by Youden index.

4. Discussion

The development of AKI is associated with unfavorable outcomes and high mortality in patients undergoing cardiac surgery. Because renal dysfunction is known as a well-established predictor of all-cause mortality in cardiac surgery, biomarkers for the early detection of AKI after cardiac surgery would be valuable for clinical practices, such as decision making, patient counseling, and optimization of post-operative care [21]. NGAL has been the most popular biomarker for the early identification of AKI following cardiac surgery. However, compared with the excellent discrimination reported in pediatric patients, studies of urinary NGAL in adult patients reported only moderate discrimination, with an AUROC of 0.72 (95% confidence interval, 0.66–0.79) [22]. Thus, new biomarkers with better performance are urgently needed. Strategies combining biomarkers with different types of pathophysiological relevance may also be beneficial in risk stratification. In this study, we found that both serum CypA and normalized urine CypA were elevated in the patients who developed AKI after sample collection. As we have shown, serum CypA is suitable for the early detection of AKI in patients undergoing cardiac surgery, with a good sensitivity and acceptable discriminative power comparable to those of normalized uNGAL. A combination of serum CypA and normalized uNGAL enhanced the overall performance for predicting the development of AKI and dialysis-requiring AKI, with AUROC values of 0.787 and 0.848, respectively.

Cyclophilins are a family of ubiquitous proteins that are evolutionarily well conserved and present in all prokaryotes and eukaryotes [23]. The most abundant member of this family is CypA, which accounts for about 0.1–0.6% of total cytosolic proteins [24]. Although CypA is present intracellularly and was originally identified as the primary cytosolic binding protein of the immunosuppressive drug cyclosporin A, it has been found to be secreted from cells in response to inflammatory stimuli, such as hypoxia, infection, and oxidative stress [25–28]. Secreted CypA has been demonstrated to be a damage-associated molecular pattern molecule that has a potent chemotactic effect on leukocytes, and, in turn, perpetuates the inflammatory response [15,27]. Moreover, high levels of extracellular CypA have also been detected in several different human inflammatory diseases, such as rheumatoid arthritis [29,30] and sepsis [17,31], and found to be correlated with the severity of those diseases. Our data are in accordance with these findings. The distinctive characteristics of cardiac surgery, including aortic clamping and cardiopulmonary bypass, which induce a systemic inflammatory response lead to the development of AKI [32]. Notably, our study also revealed that urine CypA is elevated in patients with AKI. Because CypA is an 18-kDa protein that theoretically can be freely filtered by renal glomeruli, higher levels of urine CypA in patients with AKI may just reflect an increase in serum CypA levels. An alternative explanation is that the actual source of urine CypA may be the injured renal tubular cells. Studies have demonstrated that CypA is highly expressed in the kidney, especially in the proximal tubular epithelial cells [33]. Tsai et al. also demonstrated that CypA is released by human proximal tubular cells in a dose-dependent manner after exposure to free radical treatment [18]. However, our study showed that normalized urine CypA only exhibited modest discrimination ability for predicting AKI, with an AUROC of 0.63. In addition, although normalized urine CypA exhibited a good specificity of 83.9% in predicting dialysis-requiring AKI for a cutoff value of 0.012, its overall performance was not better than that of the well-known marker normalized urine NGAL. Intriguingly, previous studies reported that not only urine soluble components, but human urine exosomes, contain CypA [15]. Whether the exosomal part of urine CypA can exhibit better discrimination power than soluble part of urine CypA alone in stratifying AKI risk needs further investigation.

Our study found that serum CypA levels were higher in the patients who subsequently developed AKI than in those who did not, but the levels were not significantly different among the AKI KDIGO stages 1–3. This might be explained by the notion that the AKI severity is more associated with changes in the serum CypA level over time than with the level at a single time. Indeed, some of the elevation in serum CypA levels in our patients might just reflect their underlying cardiac diseases. Extracellular CypA was previously found to contribute to cardiovascular diseases as a novel player not only through its proinflammatory actions but through its proatherogenic properties [10,11,34]. Yan et al. reported that serum CypA concentrations in patients with unstable angina and acute myocardial infarction were significantly higher than those in patients with stable angina and controls [12]. Serum CypA levels were also previously found to be associated with the clinical outcomes of coronary artery disease [35], ST-elevated myocardial infarction [36], and heart failure [37]. In addition to coronary artery disease, extracellular CypA was identified as a mediator in abdominal aortic aneurysm (AAA) progression. In human AAA lesions, CypA was highly expressed, especially in the area that expresses active metalloproteinase 2 (MMP-2) [14]. Using human AAA-derived vascular smooth muscle cells, angiotensin II induces the release of CypA and enhances vascular inflammation by activating MMP activity, which was significantly reduced by treatment with the CypA inhibitor. Based on these evidences, we hypothesized that increased serum CypA levels may partly be a consequence of underlying cardiovascular diseases, and that patients with more severe cardiovascular diseases might have hemodynamic instability, leading to higher baseline renal dysfunction. Further studies using preoperative serum CypA levels or serum CypA dynamics are needed to help clarify the relationship between CypA and the outcomes of cardiac surgery.

Our study showed that normalized uNGAL best predicted the development of AKI, and the level of normalized uNGAL increased along with the more severe AKI stage. This finding is consistent with previous reports that uNGAL is an early predictive biomarker of AKI following cardiac surgery [38,39]. NGAL was originally identified from neutrophils as a shuttle for iron transport, and its upregulation has been demonstrated in the proximal renal tubule after exposure to harmful insults, such as ischemia [40]. Consequently, increased level of NGAL is rapidly detectable in the urine before SCr is elevated, presumably resulting from acute tubular damage. Although the discrimination ability of CypA levels regarding the development of AKI was not superior to that of normalized uNGAL levels, our study found that normalized uNGAL had only modest sensitivity in predicting AKI and dialysis-requiring AKI. Meanwhile, we further found that the combination of these two biomarkers provides the most accurate predictive ability in these patients, suggesting that their combination is a reasonable strategy to improve the diagnostic performance of biomarkers. Our study also found a moderate discrimination ability of normalized urine CypA when predicting dialysis-requiring AKI, with comparable sensitivity and specificity ability when compared to the well-known marker normalized uNGAL. However, this study only considered AKI identified within a 7-day period; thus, studies focusing on longer-term outcomes, such as acute kidney disease [41], are warranted to clarify the potential pathogenic role of serum CypA or urine CypA in cardiac surgery-related kidney injury.

This study has several limitations. First, only one measurement of the CypA and NGAL levels was used in this cross-sectional study to predict the development of AKI. Repeated measurements to detect persistent or secondary kidney damage may improve the predictive ability. Second, the roles and expression of CypA in AKI require further investigation. Using animal models to evaluate the origin of CypA in urine may help determine the pathogenic role of urine CypA. Third, this research was conducted on a heterogeneous population with different cardiovascular diseases, and no subgroup analysis was conducted to explore the relationships between a specific disease type and the biomarkers. We also did not analyze the relationships between CypA levels and medications that may interfere with CypA levels. Finally, given the small sample size and observational design, additional prospective trials are warranted to explore the role of CypA in different etiologies of AKI.

In summary, both serum CypA and normalized uNGAL are suitable for the early detection of AKI in patients undergoing cardiac surgery, as both have acceptable discriminative power. Moreover, the combination of these two markers provides the highest AUROC and could serve as a new non-invasive test for use in clinical applications to differentiate AKI and RRT, potentially shortening the time to the initiation of appropriate therapy. Relatedly, the careful consideration of the appropriate medication, choice of therapy, and early intervention in patients exhibiting increased biomarker levels may improve AKI outcomes.

Author Contributions: C.-C.L. and C.-H.C. made substantial contribution to conception and design of the study. Y.-L.C., G.K. and S.-W.C. assisted in analysis and interpretation of the data. Y.-J.L. and Y.-T.C. assisted in laboratory analysis and interpretation of results. C.-C.L. and C.-H.C. wrote the manuscript and prepared the figures. C.-H.C., Y.-J.L. and Y.-C.T. supervised the study. All authors have read and agreed to the published version of the manuscript.

Acknowledgments: The authors thank all participants from the Kidney Research Center of Chang Gung Memorial Hospital, Linkou, Taiwan. The authors also thank Alfred Hsing-Fen Lin for his assistance in statistical analysis.

References

1. Hobson, C.E.; Yavas, S.; Segal, M.S.; Schold, J.D.; Tribble, C.G.; Layon, A.J.; Bihorac, A. Acute Kidney Injury Is Associated With Increased Long-Term Mortality After Cardiothoracic Surgery. *Circulation* **2009**, *119*, 2444–2453. [CrossRef] [PubMed]
2. Rydén, L.; Ahnve, S.; Bell, M.; Hammar, N.; Ivert, T.; Holzmann, M.J. Acute kidney injury following coronary artery bypass grafting: Early mortality and postoperative complications. *Scand. Cardiovasc. J.* **2012**, *46*, 114–120. [CrossRef] [PubMed]
3. Chertow, G.M.; Levy, E.M.; Hammermeister, K.E.; Grover, F.; Daley, J. Independent Association between Acute Renal Failure and Mortality following Cardiac Surgery. *Am. J. Med.* **1998**, *104*, 343–348. [CrossRef]
4. Zanardo, G.; Michielon, P.; Paccagnella, A.; Rosi, P.; Caló, M.; Salandin, V.; Da Ros, A.; Michieletto, F.; Simini, G. Acute renal failure in the patient undergoing cardiac operation. Prevalence, mortality rate, and main risk factors. *J. Thorac. Cardiovasc. Surg.* **1994**, *107*, 1489–1495. [CrossRef]
5. Mangano, C.M.; Diamondstone, L.S.; Ramsay, J.G.; Aggarwal, A.; Herskowitz, A.; Mangano, D.T. Renal dysfunction after myocardial revascularization: Risk factors, adverse outcomes, and hospital resource utilization. The Multicenter Study of Perioperative Ischemia Research Group. *Ann. Intern. Med.* **1998**, *128*, 194–203. [CrossRef] [PubMed]
6. Liotta, M.; Olsson, D.; Sartipy, U.; Holzmann, M.J. Minimal changes in postoperative creatinine values and early and late mortality and cardiovascular events after coronary artery bypass grafting. *Am. J. Cardiol.* **2014**, *113*, 70–75. [CrossRef]
7. Olsson, D.; Sartipy, U.; Braunschweig, F.; Holzmann, M.J. Acute Kidney Injury Following Coronary Artery Bypass Surgery and Long-term Risk of Heart Failure. *Circ. Heart Fail.* **2013**, *6*, 83–90. [CrossRef]
8. Rydén, L.; Ahnve, S.; Bell, M.; Hammar, N.; Ivert, T.; Sartipy, U.; Holzmann, M.J. Acute kidney injury after coronary artery bypass grafting and long-term risk of myocardial infarction and death. *Int. J. Cardiol.* **2014**, *172*, 190–195. [CrossRef]
9. Pickering, J.W.; James, M.T.; Palmer, S.C. Acute Kidney Injury and Prognosis After Cardiopulmonary Bypass: A Meta-analysis of Cohort Studies. *Am. J. Kidney Dis.* **2015**, *65*, 283–293. [CrossRef]
10. Nigro, P.; Satoh, K.; O'Dell, M.R.; Soe, N.N.; Cui, Z.; Mohan, A.; Abe, J.-I.; Alexis, J.D.; Sparks, J.D.; Berk, B.C. Cyclophilin A is an inflammatory mediator that promotes atherosclerosis in apolipoprotein E–deficient mice. *J. Exp. Med.* **2011**, *208*, 53–66. [CrossRef]
11. Rezzani, R.; Favero, G.; Stacchiotti, A.; Rodella, L.F. Endothelial and vascular smooth muscle cell dysfunction mediated by cyclophylin A and the atheroprotective effects of melatonin. *Life Sci.* **2013**, *92*, 875–882. [CrossRef] [PubMed]
12. Yan, J.; Zang, X.; Chen, R.; Yuan, W.; Gong, J.; Wang, C.; Li, Y. The clinical implications of increased cyclophilin A levels in patients with acute coronary syndromes. *Clin. Chim. Acta* **2012**, *413*, 691–695. [CrossRef] [PubMed]
13. Satoh, K.; Fukumoto, Y.; Sugimura, K.; Miura, Y.; Aoki, T.; Nochioka, K.; Tatebe, S.; Miyamichi-Yamamoto, S.; Shimizu, T.; Osaki, S.; et al. Plasma Cyclophilin A Is a Novel Biomarker for Coronary Artery Disease. *Circ. J.* **2013**, *77*, 447–455. [CrossRef] [PubMed]
14. Satoh, K.; Nigro, P.; Matoba, T.; O'Dell, M.R.; Cui, Z.; Shi, X.; Mohan, A.; Yan, C.; Abe, J.; Illig, K.A.; et al. Cyclophilin A enhances vascular oxidative stress and the development of angiotensin II-induced aortic aneurysms. *Nat. Med.* **2009**, *15*, 649–656. [CrossRef] [PubMed]
15. Dear, J.W.; Simpson, K.J.; Nicolai, M.P.; Catterson, J.H.; Street, J.; Huizinga, T.; Craig, D.G.; Dhaliwal, K.; Webb, S.; Bateman, D.N.; et al. Cyclophilin A is a damage-associated molecular pattern molecule that mediates acetaminophen-induced liver injury. *J. Immunol.* **2011**, *187*, 3347–3352. [CrossRef]
16. Seizer, P.; Geisler, T.; Bigalke, B.; Schneider, M.; Klingel, K.; Kandolf, R.; Stellos, K.; Schreieck, J.; Gawaz, M.; May, A.E. EMMPRIN and its ligand cyclophilin A as novel diagnostic markers in inflammatory cardiomyopathy. *Int. J. Cardiol.* **2013**, *163*, 299–304. [CrossRef]
17. Dear, J.W.; Leelahavanichkul, A.; Aponte, A.; Hu, X.; Constant, S.L.; Hewitt, S.M.; Yuen, P.S.; Star, R.A. Liver proteomics for therapeutic drug discovery: Inhibition of the cyclophilin receptor CD147 attenuates sepsis-induced acute renal failure. *Crit. Care Med.* **2007**, *35*, 2319–2328. [CrossRef]

18. Tsai, S.F.; Su, C.W.; Wu, M.J.; Chen, C.H.; Fu, C.P.; Liu, C.S.; Hsieh, M. Urinary Cyclophilin A as a New Marker for Diabetic Nephropathy: A Cross-Sectional Analysis of Diabetes Mellitus. *Medicine* **2015**, *94*, e1802. [CrossRef]
19. Palevsky, P.M.; Liu, K.D.; Brophy, P.D.; Chawla, L.S.; Parikh, C.R.; Thakar, C.V.; Tolwani, A.J.; Waikar, S.S.; Weisbord, S.D. KDOQI US Commentary on the 2012 KDIGO Clinical Practice Guideline for Acute Kidney Injury. *Am. J. Kidney Dis.* **2013**, *61*, 649–672. [CrossRef]
20. Nashef, S.A.M.; Roques, F.; Sharples, L.D.; Nilsson, J.; Smith, C.; Goldstone, A.R.; Lockowandt, U. EuroSCORE II. *Eur. J. Cardio-Thorac. Surg.* **2012**, *41*, 734–745. [CrossRef]
21. Lee, C.C.; Chang, C.H.; Chen, S.W.; Fan, P.C.; Chang, S.W.; Chen, Y.T.; Nan, Y.Y.; Lin, P.J.; Tsai, F.C. Preoperative risk assessment improves biomarker detection for predicting acute kidney injury after cardiac surgery. *PLoS ONE* **2018**, *13*, e0203447. [CrossRef] [PubMed]
22. Ho, J.; Tangri, N.; Komenda, P.; Kaushal, A.; Sood, M.; Brar, R.; Gill, K.; Walker, S.; MacDonald, K.; Hiebert, B.M.; et al. Urinary, Plasma, and Serum Biomarkers' Utility for Predicting Acute Kidney Injury Associated With Cardiac Surgery in Adults: A Meta-analysis. *Am. J. Kidney Dis.* **2015**, *66*, 993–1005. [CrossRef] [PubMed]
23. Wang, P.; Heitman, J. The cyclophilins. *Genome Biol.* **2005**, *6*. [CrossRef]
24. Dornan, J.; Taylor, P.; Walkinshaw, M.D. Structures of immunophilins and their ligand complexes. *Curr. Top. Med. Chem.* **2003**, *3*, 1392–1409. [CrossRef] [PubMed]
25. Handschumacher, R.E.; Harding, M.W.; Rice, J.; Drugge, R.J.; Speicher, D.W. Cyclophilin: A specific cytosolic binding protein for cyclosporin A. *Science* **1984**, *226*, 544–547. [CrossRef] [PubMed]
26. Jin, Z.-G.; Melaragno, M.G.; Liao, D.-F.; Yan, C.; Haendeler, J.; Suh, Y.-A.; Lambeth, J.D.; Berk, B.C. Cyclophilin A Is a Secreted Growth Factor Induced by Oxidative Stress. *Circ. Res.* **2000**, *87*, 789–796. [CrossRef]
27. Sherry, B.; Yarlett, N.; Strupp, A.; Cerami, A. Identification of cyclophilin as a proinflammatory secretory product of lipopolysaccharide-activated macrophages. 1992, 89, 3511–3515. *Proc. Natl. Acad. Sci. USA*.
28. Suzuki, J.; Jin, Z.-G.; Meoli, D.F.; Matoba, T.; Berk, B.C. Cyclophilin A Is Secreted by a Vesicular Pathway in Vascular Smooth Muscle Cells. *Circ. Res.* **2006**, *98*, 811–817. [CrossRef]
29. Billich, A.; Winkler, G.; Aschauer, H.; Rot, A.; Peichl, P. Presence of cyclophilin A in synovial fluids of patients with rheumatoid arthritis. *J. Exp. Med.* **1997**, *185*, 975–980. [CrossRef]
30. Wang, L.; Wang, C.H.; Jia, J.F.; Ma, X.K.; Li, Y.; Zhu, H.B.; Tang, H.; Chen, Z.N.; Zhu, P. Contribution of cyclophilin A to the regulation of inflammatory processes in rheumatoid arthritis. *J. Clin. Immunol.* **2010**, *30*, 24–33. [CrossRef]
31. Tegeder, I.; Schumacher, A.; John, S.; Geiger, H.; Geisslinger, G.; Bang, H.; Brune, K. Elevated serum cyclophilin levels in patients with severe sepsis. *J. Clin. Immunol.* **1997**, *17*, 380–386. [CrossRef] [PubMed]
32. O'Neal, J.B.; Shaw, A.D.; Billings, F.T. Acute kidney injury following cardiac surgery: Current understanding and future directions. *Crit. Care* **2016**, *20*, 187. [CrossRef] [PubMed]
33. Demeule, M.; Laplante, A.; Sepehr-Arae, A.; Murphy, G.M.; Wenger, R.M.; Beliveau, R. Association of cyclophilin A with renal brush border membranes: Redistribution by cyclosporine A. *Kidney Int.* **2000**, *57*, 1590–1598. [CrossRef] [PubMed]
34. Seizer, P.; Schönberger, T.; Schött, M.; Lang, M.R.; Langer, H.F.; Bigalke, B.; Krämer, B.F.; Borst, O.; Daub, K.; Heidenreich, O.; et al. EMMPRIN and its ligand cyclophilin A regulate MT1-MMP, MMP-9 and M-CSF during foam cell formation. *Atherosclerosis* **2010**, *209*, 51–57. [CrossRef] [PubMed]
35. Ohtsuki, T.; Satoh, K.; Omura, J.; Kikuchi, N.; Satoh, T.; Kurosawa, R.; Nogi, M.; Sunamura, S.; Yaoita, N.; Aoki, T.; et al. Prognostic Impacts of Plasma Levels of Cyclophilin A in Patients with Coronary Artery Disease. *Arter. Thromb. Vasc. Biol.* **2017**, *37*, 685–693. [CrossRef]
36. Huang, C.-H.; Chang, C.-C.; Kuo, C.-L.; Huang, C.-S.; Lin, C.-S.; Liu, C.-S. Decrease in Plasma Cyclophilin A Concentration at 1 Month after Myocardial Infarction Predicts Better Left Ventricular Performance and Synchronicity at 6 Months: A Pilot Study in Patients with ST Elevation Myocardial Infarction. *Int. J. Biol. Sci.* **2015**, *11*, 38–47. [CrossRef]
37. Zuern, C.S.; Müller, K.A.L.; Seizer, P.; Geisler, T.; Banya, W.; Klingel, K.; Kandolf, R.; Bauer, A.; Gawaz, M.; May, A.E. Cyclophilin A predicts clinical outcome in patients with congestive heart failure undergoing endomyocardial biopsy. *Eur. J. Heart Fail.* **2013**, *15*, 176–184. [CrossRef]
38. Bennett, M.; Dent, C.L.; Ma, Q.; Dastrala, S.; Grenier, F.; Workman, R.; Syed, H.; Ali, S.; Barasch, J.; Devarajan, P. Urine NGAL predicts severity of acute kidney injury after cardiac surgery: A prospective study. *Clin. J. Am. Soc. Nephrol.* **2008**, *3*, 665–673. [CrossRef]

39. Parikh, C.R.; Coca, S.G.; Thiessen-Philbrook, H.; Shlipak, M.G.; Koyner, J.L.; Wang, Z.; Edelstein, C.L.; Devarajan, P.; Patel, U.D.; Zappitelli, M.; et al. Postoperative biomarkers predict acute kidney injury and poor outcomes after adult cardiac surgery. *J. Am. Soc. Nephrol.* **2011**, *22*, 1748–1757. [CrossRef]
40. Paragas, N.; Qiu, A.; Zhang, Q.; Samstein, B.; Deng, S.X.; Schmidt-Ott, K.M.; Viltard, M.; Yu, W.; Forster, C.S.; Gong, G.; et al. The Ngal reporter mouse detects the response of the kidney to injury in real time. *Nat. Med.* **2011**, *17*, 216–222. [CrossRef]
41. Chawla, L.S.; Bellomo, R.; Bihorac, A.; Goldstein, S.L.; Siew, E.D.; Bagshaw, S.M.; Bittleman, D.; Cruz, D.; Endre, Z.; Fitzgerald, R.L.; et al. Acute kidney disease and renal recovery: Consensus report of the Acute Disease Quality Initiative (ADQI) 16 Workgroup. *Nat. Rev. Nephrol.* **2017**, *13*, 241–257. [CrossRef] [PubMed]

2

Mechanisms of Fasting-Mediated Protection against Renal Injury and Fibrosis Development after Ischemic Acute Kidney Injury

Pedro Rojas-Morales [1], Edilia Tapia [2], Juan Carlos León-Contreras [3], Susana González-Reyes [4], Angélica Saraí Jiménez-Osorio [5], Joyce Trujillo [6], Natalia Pavón [7], Jessica Granados-Pineda [1], Rogelio Hernández-Pando [3], Laura Gabriela Sánchez-Lozada [2], Horacio Osorio-Alonso [2] and José Pedraza-Chaverri [1,*]

1 Departamento de Biología, Facultad de Química, Universidad Nacional Autónoma de México, Ciudad de México 04510, Mexico
2 Departamento de Fisiopatología Cardio-Renal, Instituto Nacional de Cardiología Ignacio Chávez, Ciudad de México 14080, Mexico
3 Departamento de Patología, Instituto Nacional de Ciencias Médicas y Nutrición Salvador Zubirán, Ciudad de México 14080, Mexico
4 Laboratorio de Bioquímica, Facultad de Medicina y Psicología, Universidad Nacional Autónoma de Baja California, Tijuana 22390, Mexico
5 Laboratorio de Medicina Genómica, Hospital Regional Lic. Adolfo López Mateos, ISSSTE, Ciudad de México 01030, Mexico
6 Consejo Nacional de Ciencia y Tecnología-Consorcio de Investigación, Innovación y Desarrollo para las Zonas Áridas- Instituto Potosino de Investigación Científica y Tecnológica, San Luis Potosí 78216, Mexico
7 Departamento de Farmacología, Instituto Nacional de Cardiología Ignacio Chávez, Ciudad de México 14080, Mexico
* Correspondence: pedraza@unam.mx

Abstract: Ischemia-reperfusion injury of the kidney may lead to renal fibrosis through a combination of several mechanisms. We recently demonstrated that fasting protects the rat kidney against oxidative stress and mitochondrial dysfunction in early acute kidney injury, and also against fibrosis development. Here we show that preoperative fasting preserves redox status and mitochondrial homeostasis at the chronic phase of damage after severe ischemia. Also, the protective effect of fasting coincides with the suppression of inflammation and endoplasmic reticulum stress, as well as the down-regulation of the mechanistic target of rapamycin (mTOR) and extracellular signal-regulated kinase 1/2 (ERK1/2) signaling pathways in the fibrotic kidney. Our results demonstrate that fasting targets multiple pathophysiological mechanisms to prevent renal fibrosis and damage that results after renal ischemia-reperfusion injury.

Keywords: fasting; fibrosis; mitochondrial dysfunction; oxidative stress; inflammation; ER stress; ischemia-reperfusion injury

1. Introduction

Fibrosis is a hallmark and a driver of chronic kidney disease (CKD) [1]. It is a maladaptive repair process after severe acute kidney injury (AKI), leading to end-stage renal disease and increased mortality [2–4]. The molecular signature predisposing to fibrosis development after AKI is not fully understood. Multiple interrelated factors such as oxidative stress, mitochondrial dysfunction, endoplasmic reticulum (ER) stress, and an exacerbated inflammatory response contribute to extracellular matrix deposition, loss of kidney architecture, disruption of cellular homeostasis, and finally renal dysfunction [4–9]. Mechanistically, transforming growth factor β (TGF-β1) has been shown to play a direct role in fibrogenesis, as inhibition of TGF-β1 signaling by genetic or pharmacological means significantly abrogates fibrosis progression after severe kidney injury [10]. Emerging evidence also implicates extracellular signal-regulated kinase 1/2 (ERK1/2) and the mechanistic target of rapamycin (mTOR), which operate downstream of TGF-β1 signaling, in renal fibrosis development [11,12], thus expanding our understanding of CKD pathophysiology.

Mild food restriction has been known for many years to lead to multisystemic beneficial effects and activates cellular stress response pathways to protect cells and tissues from damage [13,14]. As such, dietary restriction regimens, namely calorie restriction, fasting, and intermittent fasting, confer protection against ischemic insults in organs like the liver, heart, brain, and the kidney [14,15]. By using a rat model of AKI induced by ischemia-reperfusion (IR), we recently demonstrated that preoperative fasting protects the kidney against redox and mitochondrial alterations seen early after IR, and also confers long-lasting protection against fibrosis development [16]. These findings led us to investigate the mechanisms that preoperative fasting regulates to protect against the chronic phase of damage induced by ischemia. To this end, we first tested the efficacy of fasting against fibrogenesis in a slightly different, yet more severe IR injury model than in our previous work. Then, oxidative stress, mitochondrial homeostasis, ER stress, inflammation, as well as the signal transducers mTOR and ERK1/2 were assessed two weeks later to understand the magnitude of the protective effect of fasting.

2. Materials and Methods

2.1. Reagents, Materials, and Antibodies

All chemicals used in this study were purchased from Sigma-Aldrich (St Louis, MO, USA). Commercial kits to measure blood urea nitrogen (BUN), creatinine, and glucose levels in plasma were obtained from SpinReact (Girona, Spain). The nitrocellulose membrane, the Chemiluminiscent Detection Kit, and the primary antibody for peroxisome proliferator-activated receptor gamma coactivator 1 alpha (PGC1α, #AB3242, 1:2,000) were from Merck Millipore (Burlington, MA, USA). The antibody against catalase (CAT, #219010, 1:2,500) was purchased from Calbiochem (San Diego, CA, USA). Antibodies against activating transcription factor 4 (ATF4, #GTX30070, 1:5,000), alpha smooth muscle actin (α-SMA, #GTX100034, 1:2,000), glutamate-cysteine ligase modifier subunit (GCLM, #GTX114075, 1:2,500), and glyceraldehyde-3-phosphate dehydrogenase (GAPDH, #GTX100118, 1:10,000) were purchased from GeneTex (Irvine, CA, USA). The antibody against nuclear factor kappa B p65 (NF-κB p65, #PA5-16545, 1:2,000) was purchased from Thermo Fisher Scientific (Waltham, MA, USA). The antibodies against NADH:Ubiquinone oxidoreductase subunit B8 (NDUFB8, #ab110242, 1:5,000), succinate dehydrogenase subunit B (SDHB, #ab14714, 1:5,000), cytochrome c oxidase subunit 1 (MTCO1, #ab14705, 1:2,000), ATP synthase F1 subunit α (ATP5A, #ab14748, 1:10,000), 8-hydroxy-2′-deoxyguanosine (8-OHdG, #ab62623, 1:200), and nucleotide-binding oligomerization domain (NOD)-like receptor protein 3 (NLRP3, #ab214185, 1:1,000) were from Abcam (Cambridge, MA, USA). Antibodies against mitofusin 2 (NFN2 #9482S, 1:2,000), phospho-ERK1/2 (p-ERK1/2, #4370, 1:2,000), ERK1/2 (#9102, 1:2,000), and phospho-S6 kinase (p-S6K, #9205, 1:2,000) were from Cell Signaling (Danvers, MA, USA). Antibodies against dynamin-related protein 1 (DRP1, #sc-32898, 1:1,000), interleukin 6 (IL-6, #sc-57315, 1:500), TGF-β1 (#sc-130348, 1:1,000), tumor necrosis factor alpha (TNFα, #sc-52746, 1:100) were from Santa Cruz Biotechnology (Dallas, TX, USA). Antibodies against collagen IV (Col IV, #SAB5200500, 1:4,000), glucose-regulated protein 94 (GRP94, #G4420, 1:2,000), and protein kinase RNA-like endoplasmic reticulum kinase (PERK, #P0074, 1:2,000) were from Sigma-Aldrich. Antibody against nicotinamide adenine dinucleotide phosphate oxidase 4 (NOX4, #NB110-58849, 1:1,000) was from Novus Biologicals (Centennial, CO, USA). Anti-rabbit (#7074S, 1:5,000) and anti-mouse (#7076S, 1:5,000) horseradish peroxidase (HRP)-conjugated secondary antibodies were purchased from Cell Signaling (Danvers). Goat polyclonal secondary antibody to mouse immunoglobulin G (Alexa Fluor 647, #ab150115, 1:1,000) was purchased from Abcam.

2.2. *Animals, Experimental Design, and Study Approval*

Eight nine-week-old male Wistar rats weighing 240–260 g were used in this study. Rats were maintained in standard laboratory conditions with normal rodent chow diet and water provided ad libitum until the beginning of experiments. After acclimatization for at least one week, rats were randomly assigned to either one of the following experimental groups ($n = 4$, each): sham control, IR only, and IR + Fasting. Rats enrolled in the IR + Fasting group were deprived of food (beginning at 10:00 am) for three days before surgery. Rats were subjected to unilateral renal ischemia for 45 min and then allowed to recover for two weeks (Figure 1). All animal experiments were approved by the Institutional Animal Care and Use Committee of Instituto Nacional de Cardiología Ignacio Chávez (#INC/CICUAL/005/2018).

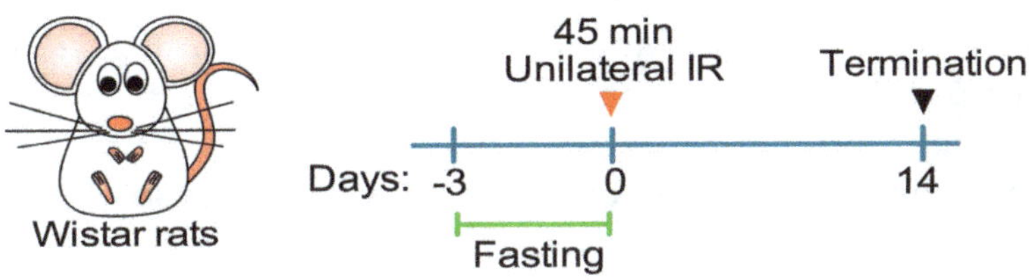

Figure 1. Schematic depiction of the experimental schedule. Fed or fasted rats were subjected to either sham surgery or 45 min of unilateral ischemia-reperfusion (IR). After surgery, all rats were fed and euthanized 14 days after IR.

2.3. *Unilateral Ischemia-Reperfusion Injury*

A unilateral IR injury model was used to induce severe tubular damage and fibrosis while avoiding unacceptable high mortality seen in bilateral IR injury models [17]. Fed or fasted rats were anesthetized with an intraperitoneal injection of sodium pentobarbital (60 mg/kg), and after exposing the left kidney through a midline abdominal incision, the left renal artery was occluded for 45 min using nontraumatic vascular clamps. Laparotomy without ischemia was performed in sham-operated rats, which served as control. After ischemia or sham operation, all rats were fed ad libitum and euthanized two weeks later to harvest blood and kidneys for histology, transmission electron microscopy, immunohistochemistry, and Western Blot analysis.

2.4. *Plasma Biochemistry*

The levels of blood urea nitrogen (BUN), creatinine, and glucose were measured in plasma samples using commercial kits according to the manufacturer's instructions.

2.5. *Histology and Transmission Electron Microscopy*

To assess kidney damage and fibrosis, kidneys were immersed in a 4% paraformaldehyde plus 1.5% glutaraldehyde solution, embedded in paraffin, sectioned at 4 μm, and stained with routine hematoxylin and eosin (H&E) or Masson trichrome. For automated morphometry, six random choice fields for each kidney were studied at 200× magnification (total area $3{,}1 \times 10^5$ μm^2), the total number of convoluted tubules and the percentage of atrophic or cystic tubules was determined using ImageJ (National Institute of Health, Bethesda, MD, USA), and the data were expressed as the percentage of atrophic tubules. For fibrosis determination, the same software program and the Masson trichrome stain were used, the total area at 200× magnification was measured in six random choice fields for each section and the percentage of interstitial fibrosis was determined from each rat.

For mitochondrial morphology visualization, paraformaldehyde/glutaraldehyde-fixed kidney fragments were post-fixed with 2% osmium tetroxide, embedded in epoxy resin, ultra-sectioned at 70–90 nm, and stained with uranyl acetate and lead citrate. Images were acquired with the Tecnai Spirit BioTWIN transmission electron microscope (Hillsboro, OR, USA).

2.6. *Immunohistochemistry and Immunofluorescence*

For immunodetection of DNA damage, paraffin-embedded kidney sections were dewaxed, rehydrated, and incubated for 2 h with the anti-8-OHdG (1:200) antibody. After several washes, tissue sections were incubated with an HRP-conjugated secondary antibody, revealed with 3,3′-diaminobenzidine and counterstained with hematoxylin. For immunofluorescence, kidney sections were incubated for 2 h with a primary antibody against TNFα (1:100) and then with the Alexa Fluor 647. Nuclei were stained with 1 μg/mL 4′,6-diamidino-2-fenilindol (DAPI). Images were acquired with an epifluorescence microscope.

2.7. *Subcellular Fractionation*

Mitochondria were isolated by differential centrifugation essentially as previously described [16]. Frozen kidney fragments were homogenized in ice-cold buffer containing 225 mM D-mannitol, 75 mM sucrose, 10 mM 4-(2-hydroxyethyl)-1-piperazineethanesulfonic acid (HEPES), 1 mM ethylenediamine tetraacetic acid (EDTA), and 0.5 mg/mL fatty acid-free bovine serum albumin (BSA), pH 7.4, using a Potter–Elvehjem tissue homogenizer, and then centrifuged at 800× *g* for 10 min. The obtained supernatant was separated into a new tube and centrifuged again at 10,000× *g* for another 10 min to obtain mitochondria (pellet) and cytosol (supernatant), which were prepared for western blot analysis.

2.8. *Western Blot*

Kidneys were homogenized in ice-cold lysis buffer containing 50 mM Tris pH 8.0, 150 mM NaCl, 5 m EDTA, 1 mM ethylene glycol-bis(2-aminoethylether)-N N N′N-tetraacetic acid (EGTA), sodium deoxycholate, 0.1% sodium dodecyl sulfate (SDS), 1% Nonidet P-40, and protease and phosphatase inhibitors, and then centrifuged at 15,000× *g* for 10 min at 4 °C. Twenty μg of total protein were subjected to polyacrylamide gel electrophoresis and subsequently transferred at 100 volts for 1.5 h to nitrocellulose membranes, which were then incubated for 2 h at room temperature with primary antibodies. After several washes, membranes were incubated at room temperature for 1 h with secondary antibodies, and specific proteins were detected by chemiluminescence, quantified using ImageJ (National Institute of Health, Bethesda, MD, USA), normalized to GAPDH, and finally expressed as fold-change vs. sham. For protein normalization, membranes were incubated at room temperature for 30 min with a stripping solution (100 mM glycine pH 2.5, 0.5% SDS), and then re-probed with anti-GAPDH.

2.9. *Enzyme-Linked Immunosorbent Assays*

Kidney homogenates were obtained, and the levels of interleukin 1 beta (IL-1β), IL-6, and TNFα were measured with an enzyme-linked immunosorbent assay (ELISA) (PeproTech, Rocky Hill, NJ, USA).

2.10. *Statistical Analysis*

Data are presented as mean ± standard error of the mean (SEM). Differences between groups were assessed by one-way analysis of variance (ANOVA) followed by the Tukey test using the GraphPad Prism 6 software (San Diego, CA, USA). The level of significance was set at $p < 0.05$.

3. Results

3.1. *Fasting Attenuates Tubular Injury and Fibrosis Induced by Ischemia-Reperfusion Injury*

Severe ischemic AKI results in chronic renal injury and interstitial fibrosis [2]. Rats studied two weeks after 45 min of unilateral renal ischemia presented no changes in BUN, creatinine, and plasma glucose (Figure 2A); however, they showed severe renal damage demonstrated by histological analysis of kidney sections H&E stained (Figure 2B). Kidney sections from the sham group exhibited normal morphology. In contrast, post-IR kidneys showed extensive tubular atrophy, manifested by cuboidal or flattened epithelium that was part of small or cystic tubules, many other tubules showed detachment of epithelial cells or hyaline casts; some glomeruli showed retracted capillary tuffs and were surrounded by fibrotic interstitium with chronic inflammatory infiltrate and numerous fibroblasts (Figure 2B). Masson Trichrome staining confirmed extensive tubule-interstitial fibrosis (Figure 2B), and automated morphometry showed significantly greater tubular damage and interstitial fibrosis in the kidneys of IR group. In addition, Western blot analysis showed increased protein expression of fibrosis markers such as TGF-β1, α-SMA, and Col IV (Figure 2C). In contrast, such increased damage and fibrotic index after IR were not observed in the kidneys of rats that were preoperatively fasted for three days (Figure 2B,C), indicating that fasting confers strong protection against tubular injury and fibrosis, which is consistent with our previous report [16].

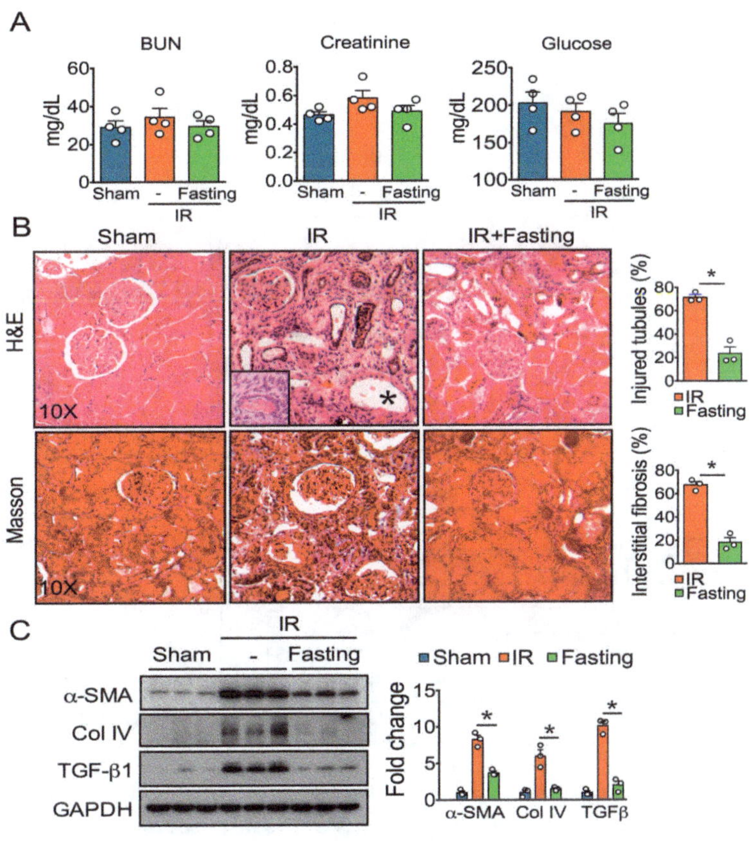

Figure 2. Effect of fasting on renal injury and development of fibrosis after two weeks of unilateral ischemia-reperfusion (IR) injury. (**A**) Plasma levels of blood urea nitrogen (BUN), creatinine, and glucose assessed 14 days post-IR or sham operation. (**B**) Representative hematoxylin & eosin (H&E)- and Masson trichrome-stained kidney sections (left) at 10× magnification from sham, IR, and IR + Fasting experimental groups at day 14 post-IR. Quantification (right) of injured tubules (H&E) and interstitial fibrosis (Masson) in IR and IR + Fasting experimental groups. In contrast to the normal kidney, histology showed by a rat from the sham group, kidney sections from the IR animal show extensive interstitial fibrosis with mild chronic inflammatory infiltrate, and numerous atrophic small tubules coated with cuboidal epithelial cells or with cystic appearance (asterisk). The inset shows a high-power micrograph of the interstitial fibrotic process, with numerous fusiform cells that correspond to fibroblasts around an atrophic tubule with the hyaline cast. Fasting decreased interstitial fibrosis and tubular atrophy. (**C**) Immunoblots (left) and quantification (right) of alpha-smooth muscle actin (α-SMA), collagen IV (Col IV), and transforming growth factor β1 (TGF-β1) in the kidney cortex of rats from sham, IR, and IR + Fasting experimental groups. GAPDH, glyceraldehyde-3-phosphate dehydrogenase. Data are expressed as mean ± standard error of the mean (SEM). $n = 3$ to 4 animals per group. * $p < 0.05$.

3.2. *Fasting Prevents Oxidative Stress Long after Ischemia-Reperfusion Injury*

Our previous study showed fasting protects against redox imbalance seen early (24 h) after ischemic AKI [16]. Increased oxidative deoxyribonucleic acid (DNA) damage, revealed by 8-OHdG immunostaining, was observed two weeks post-IR (Figure 3A), suggesting ischemia leads to persistent oxidative stress. Preoperative fasting reduced the oxidative damage induced by IR injury (Figure 3A), which was associated with increased protein levels of the hydrogen peroxide (H_2O_2)-degrading enzyme CAT and GCLM, the regulatory subunit of the glutamate-cysteine ligase enzyme involved in glutathione synthesis (Figure 3B). On the other hand, fasting reduced NOX4 protein expression, a major renal source of reactive oxygen species (ROS) [18] (Figure 3B). Thus, these data indicate fasting conferred long-lasting protection against IR-induced oxidative stress by activating antioxidant defenses and by down-regulating NOX4.

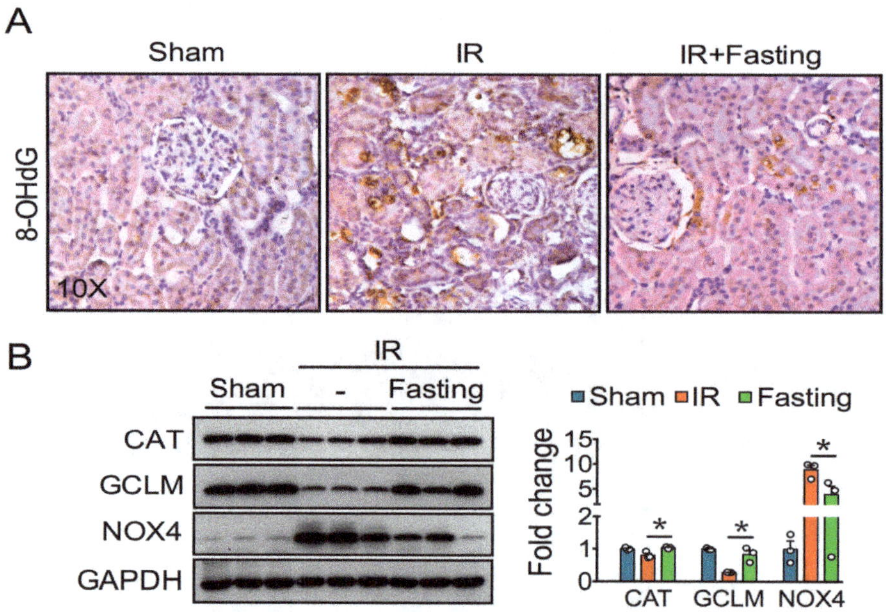

Figure 3. Fasting protects against oxidative stress resulting after two weeks of unilateral ischemia-reperfusion (IR) injury. (**A**) Representative kidney sections (10×) immunostained for 8-hydroxy-2′-deoxyguanosine (8-OHdG) in sham, IR, and IR + Fasting experimental groups at day 14 post-IR or sham surgery. (**B**) Immunoblots (left) and quantification (right) of catalase (CAT), glutamate-cysteine ligase modifier subunit (GCLM), and nicotinamide adenine dinucleotide phosphate oxidase 4 (NOX4) in the kidney cortex of rats from sham, IR, and IR + Fasting experimental groups. GAPDH, glyceraldehyde-3-phosphate dehydrogenase. Data are expressed as mean ± SEM. $n = 3$ animals per group. * $p < 0.05$.

3.3. *Fasting Protects Mitochondria Long After Ischemia-Reperfusion Injury*

Altered mitochondrial homeostasis has been observed long after severe ischemia [6]. Whereas IR reduced the levels of NDUFB8, SDHB, and MTCO1 oxidative phosphorylation (OXPHOS) proteins, fasting increased the levels of NDUFB8 and MTCO1, although not that of SDHB (Figure 4A). Consistent with these favorable changes, transmission electron microscopy showed that cristae effacement and fragmented mitochondria in proximal tubular epithelial cells from post-IR kidneys were also reduced by fasting (Figure 4B).

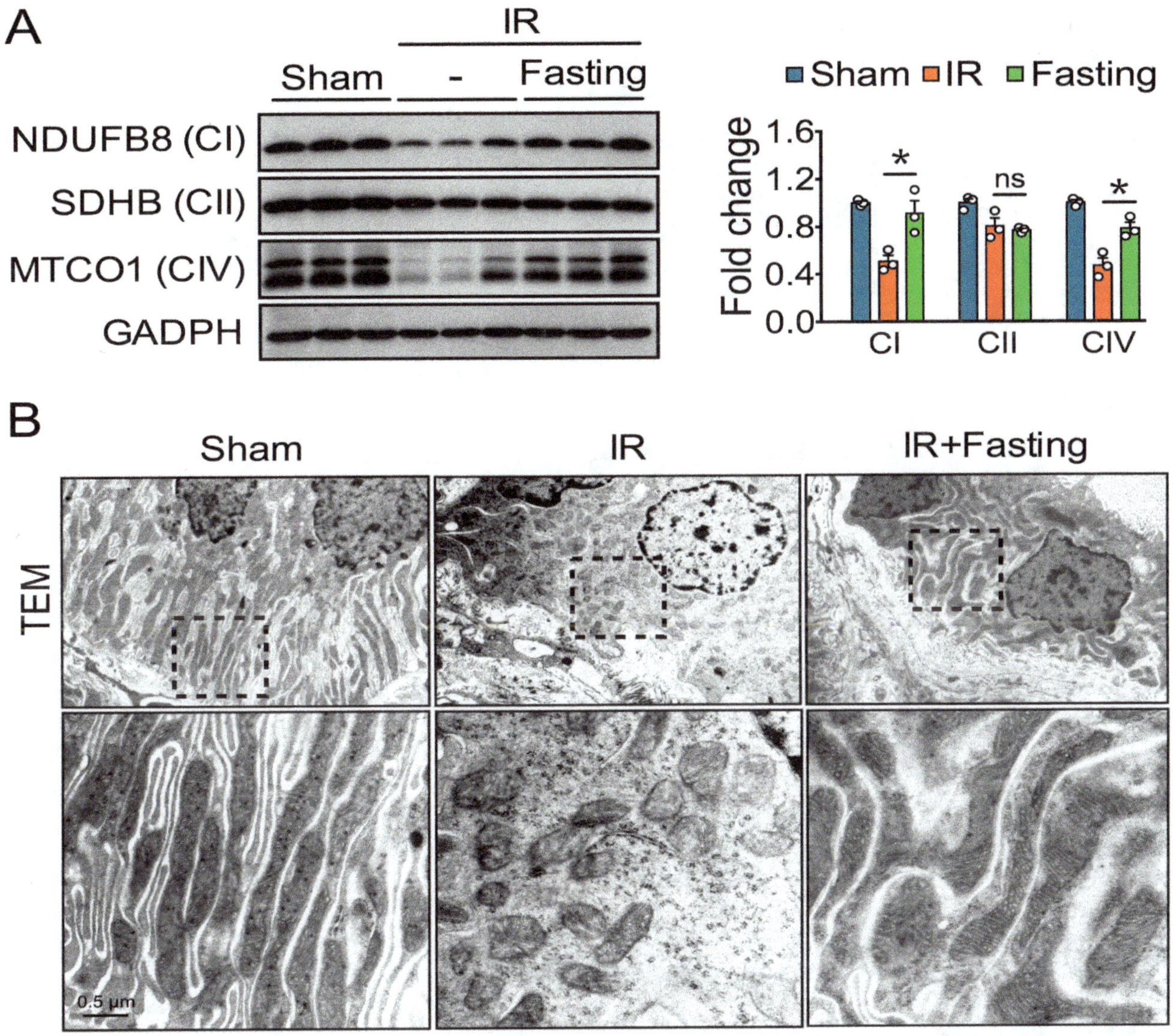

Figure 4. Fasting protects mitochondria long after ischemia-reperfusion (IR) injury. (**A**) Protein expression (left) and quantification (right) of respiratory-complex subunits in kidneys from fed or fasted rats two weeks after IR injury. NDUFB8, NADH:Ubiquinone oxidoreductase subunit B8; SDHB, succinate dehydrogenase subunit B; MTCO1, cytochrome c oxidase subunit 1; GAPDH, glyceraldehyde-3-phosphate dehydrogenase; ns, not significant. (**B**) Representative transmission electron microscopy (TEM) micrographs of mitochondria from proximal tubular epithelial cells two weeks after IR. Magnified areas (Insets) are taken from the black boxes with dash lines. Data are expressed as mean ± SEM. $n = 3$ animals per group. * $p < 0.05$.

Mitochondrial biogenesis and dynamics are required for maintaining a healthy mitochondrial pool and hence mitochondrial homeostasis [19]; therefore, we further assessed the levels of the mitochondrial fusion protein mitofusin 2 (MFN2), the mitochondrial fission protein dynamin-related protein 1 (DRP1), and PGC1α, a master transcriptional regulator of mitochondrial biogenesis [19]. While MFN2 remained mostly unaltered, DRP1 significantly increased in the IR group, and this increase was diminished by fasting. Also, we observed reduced levels of PGC1α in the IR group, but not in the fasted group (Figure 5A). To confirm the involvement of DRP1 in mitochondrial fragmentation after IR injury, we performed cellular fractionation and analyzed mitochondrial localization of DRP1. IR increased the levels of DRP1 at the mitochondria fraction, and this effect was prevented by fasting (Figure 5B). Again, we did not observe changes in MFN2. Thus, our results suggest that fasting partially protects mitochondria in renal fibrosis by regulating mitochondrial biogenesis and dynamics.

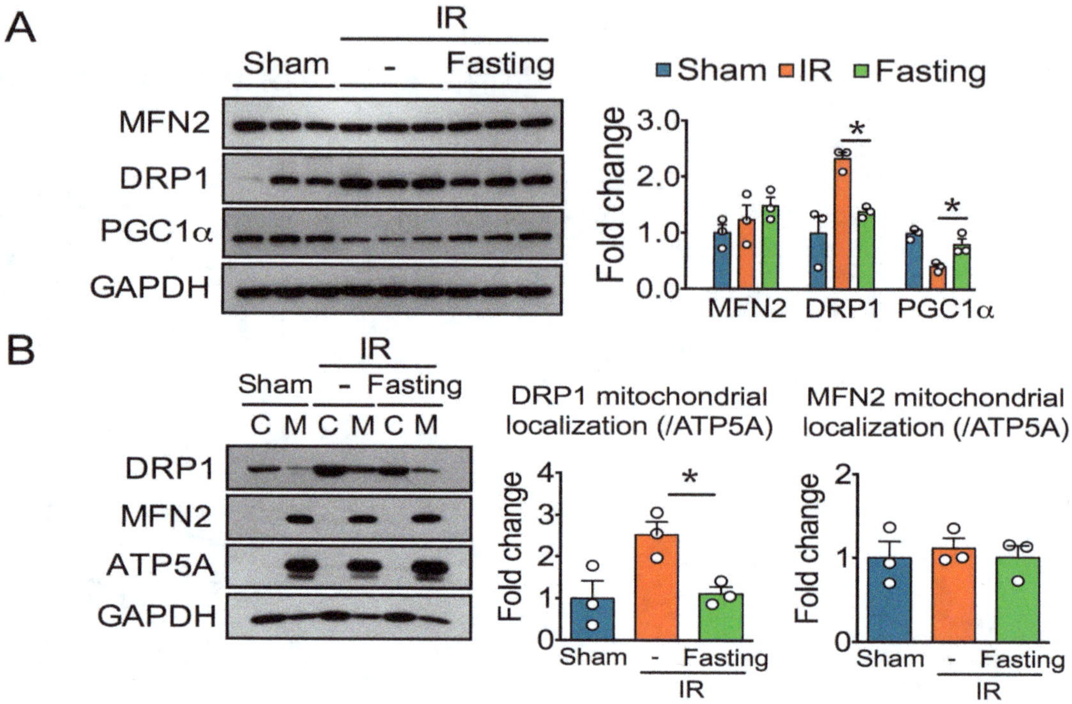

Figure 5. Fasting regulates disturbances in mitochondria dynamics and biogenesis induced by ischemia-reperfusion (IR) injury. (**A**) Immunoblots (left) and quantification (right) of mitofusin 2 (MFN2), dynamin-related protein 1 (DRP1), and peroxisome proliferator-activated receptor gamma coactivator 1 alpha (PGC1α) in total kidney homogenates of rats from sham, IR, and IR + Fasting experimental groups. (**B**) Representative immunoblots (left) and quantification (right) of DRP1 and MFN2 in isolated mitochondria from the experimental groups described. (**C**) cytoplasmic fraction; M, mitochondrial fraction; ATP5A, ATP synthase F1 subunit alpha; GAPDH, glyceraldehyde-3-phosphate dehydrogenase. Data are expressed as mean ± SEM. $n = 3$ animals per group. * $p < 0.05$.

3.4. Fasting Protects Against Ischemia-Reperfusion Induced Endoplasmatic Reticulum Stress

Emerging evidence indicates ER stress may contribute to fibrosis [7]. Perturbed ER homeostasis was observed in fibrotic kidneys. Unfolded protein response markers, such as GRP94, PERK, and ATF4, were increased in the IR group, compared to the non-fibrotic kidneys from the control sham-operated rats (Figure 6). Fasting, on the other hand, diminished ER stress proteins, thus suggesting that fasting maintains protein folding and quality control in post-ischemic kidneys.

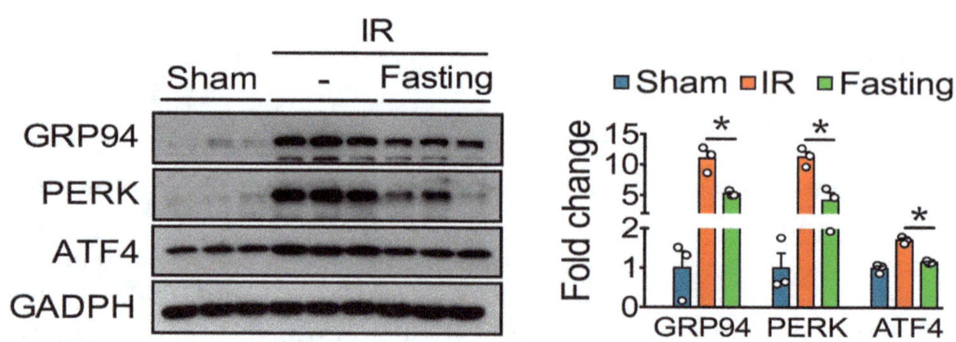

Figure 6. Fasting reduces endoplasmic reticulum (ER) stress induced by ischemia-reperfusion (IR) injury. Immunoblots (left) and quantification (right) of glucose-regulated protein 94 (GRP94), protein kinase RNA-like endoplasmic reticulum kinase (PERK), and activating transcription factor 4 (ATF4) in the kidney from the experimental groups described. GAPDH, glyceraldehyde-3-phosphate dehydrogenase. Data are expressed as mean ± SEM. $n = 3$ animals per group. * $p < 0.05$.

3.5. *Fasting Suppresses Inflammation Long After Ischemia-Reperfusion Injury*

Chronic inflammation is tightly associated with fibrosis development [20], so we evaluated the effect of IR and fasting on inflammatory markers. Our Western blot analysis showed that IR increased protein levels of the NLRP3 inflammasome, NF-κB, and IL-6 (Figure 7A), indicative of significant inflammation. Immunofluorescence microscopy revealed high levels of TNFα in renal tubular epithelial cells after IR injury (Figure 7B). In addition, IR increased the renal content of IL-1β, IL-6, and TNFα, revealed by ELISA assays (Figure 7C). On the other hand, preoperative fasting for three days diminished inflammatory markers, thus indicating that fasting exerts strong protection against chronic inflammation after IR.

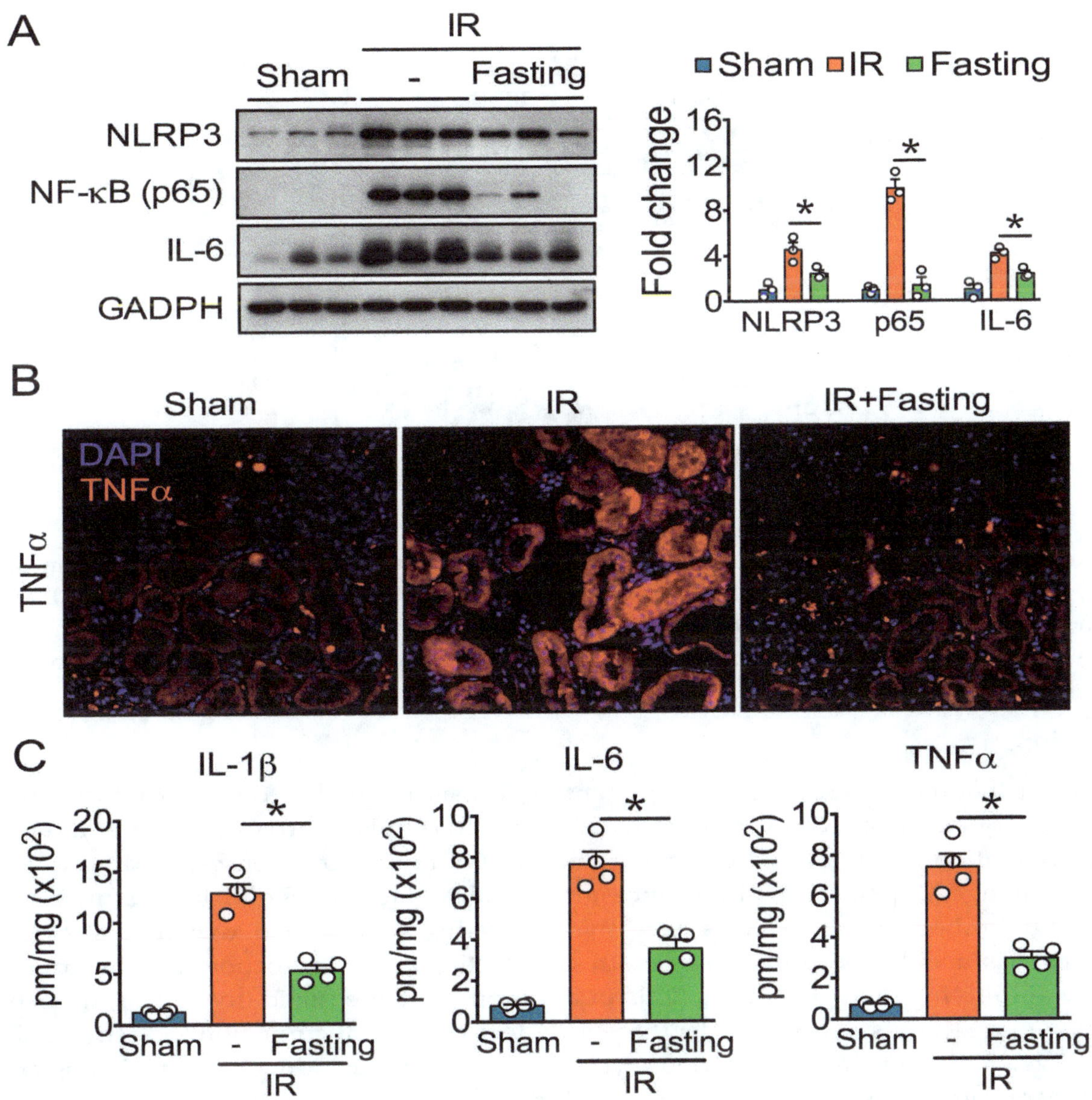

Figure 7. Fasting suppresses persistent inflammation induced by ischemia-reperfusion (IR) injury. (**A**) Immunoblots (left) and quantification (right) of nucleotide-binding oligomerization domain (NOD)-like receptor protein 3 (NLRP3) inflammasome, nuclear factor kappa B (NF-κB), and interleukin 6 (IL-6) in fed or fasted rats subjected to ischemia-reperfusion (IR). GAPDH, glyceraldehyde-3-phosphate dehydrogenase. (**B**) Representative kidney sections immunostained for tumor necrosis factor alpha (TNFα) and analyzed by fluorescence microscopy. (**C**) Renal content of interleukin 1 beta (IL-1β), IL-6, and TNFα. DAPI, 4′,6-diamidino-2-fenilindol. Data are expressed as mean ± SEM. n = 3 to 4 animals per group. * $p < 0.05$.

3.6. *Effect of Fasting on ERK and mTOR Signaling Pathway*

Several signaling pathways have been implicated in fibrosis development after ischemia, and various studies clearly indicate that both ERK1/2 and mTOR have multiple crosstalks with the pathophysiological mechanisms operating in CKD [11,12]. Although we observed that IR increased the levels of both phosphorylated and non-phosphorylated ERK1/2, densitometry analysis of the p-ERK1/2 to ERK1/2 ratio revealed no activation of these kinases after IR (Figure 8A). Also, although fasting diminished the levels of p-ERK1/2, it did not modify p-ERK1/2 to ERK1/2 ratio. On the other hand, we observed that the levels of the phosphorylated form of S6K, a downstream target and surrogated indicator of active mTOR, were significantly upregulated in fibrotic kidneys (Figure 8B). Fasting, on the other hand, diminished the levels of phospho-S6K.

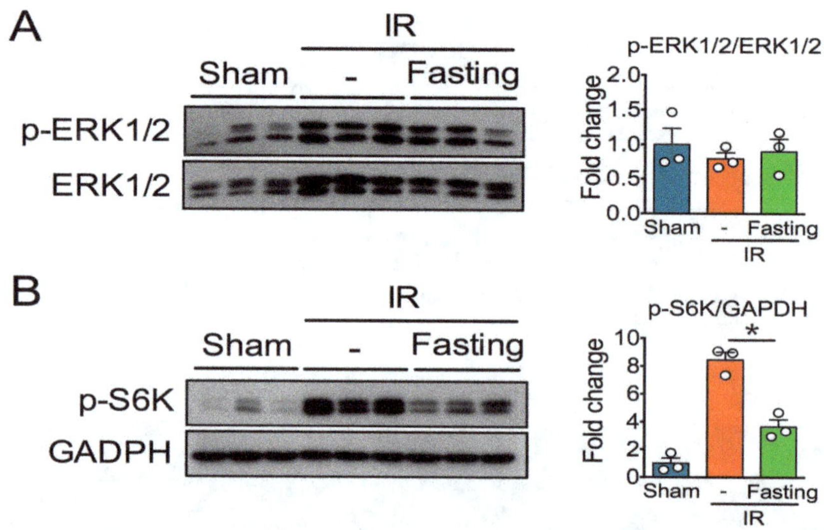

Figure 8. Effect of fasting on ischemia-reperfusion (IR)-associated signaling pathways. (**A**) Immunoblots (left) and quantification (right) of phospho-extracellular-regulated kinase 1/2 (p-ERK1/2) and ERK1/2 in the kidney cortex of rats from sham, IR, and IR + Fasting experimental groups. (**B**) Immunoblots (left) and quantification (right) of phospho-S6 kinase (p-S6K). GAPDH, glyceraldehyde-3-phosphate dehydrogenase. Data are expressed as mean ± SEM. $n = 3$ animals per group. * $p < 0.05$.

4. Discussion

It is clear that renal injury and development of fibrosis are mediated by an interplay of several mechanisms. For example, TGF-β1, a key regulator of extracellular matrix assembly and remodeling, promotes activation of NOX4 and down-regulation of antioxidant defenses, leading to oxidative stress and damage [21,22]. Redox imbalances, in turn, leads to mitochondrial dysfunction, and in turn, damaged mitochondria produce excessive free radicals [23]. Also, oxidative stress perturbs ER homeostasis and leads to proteotoxic stress, affecting again mitochondrial functioning and ultimately amplifying ROS generation [24]. In addition, sustained oxidative stress, mitochondrial dysfunction, and ER stress can independently contribute to chronic inflammation and activate fibrogenic signals [4,5,22,25,26], thus creating a vicious cycle that culminates in kidney malfunctioning and death.

Dietary restriction has been widely recognized as a strong non-genetic, non-pharmacological tool to increase multisystemic protection against stress and to postpone many aspects related to the onset, rate, and progression of age-related chronic diseases, mainly due to its antioxidant and anti-inflammatory properties [27]. However, we know very little about how dietary restriction protocols impact kidney physiology and disease. We and others have shown that fasting is renoprotective in early AKI, as this short-term dietary intervention diminishes tubular injury, cell death, inflammation, oxidative stress, and mitochondrial dysfunction seen 24 h after IR [16,28]. In the present work, we focused on the effect of preoperative fasting on tubular injury and renal fibrosis that develop long after AKI.

We used a unilateral renal IR without contralateral nephrectomy injury model that leads to tubular injury and interstitial fibrosis, to analyze the long-term protective effect of fasting. As expected, because in this model, rodents still have one intact kidney, no changes in plasma urea and creatinine were observed. However, at two weeks after 45 min of unilateral IR, fibrosis, oxidative stress, mitochondrial dysfunction, ER stress, and inflammation were prominent, and histology revealed severe tubular injury. Also, renal injury was accompanied by increased levels of phospho-ERK1/2 and phospho-S6K, which are engaged in fibrogenic processes. a recent study reported that pharmacological inhibition of ERK1/2 signaling significantly ameliorates collagen deposition and myofibroblast expansion during kidney fibrosis, a phenomenon that is explained by reduced mTOR, signal transducer and activator of transcription 3 (STAT3), small mothers against decapentaplegic 2/3 (Smad2/3), and NF-κB pathway activation [11].

We found that fasting primes the kidney to resist tubular injury and fibrosis development through various mechanisms (Figure 9). These include preservation of redox balance, maintenance of both mitochondria and ER homeostasis and suppression of inflammatory processes persisting long after the initial ischemic insult. Also, fasting abrogated ERK1/2 and mTOR signaling, both playing important roles in renal fibrosis development. Overall, our data provide further evidence into the long-term benefit of fasting preconditioning. Interestingly, others have shown that food restriction protects against polycystic kidney disease, a leading genetic cause of end-stage renal disease [29]. Also, protein restriction protects against renal IR injury [30] and ameliorates CKD in uremic rats [31]. Together, these findings illustrate how dietary approaches, other than pharmacological ones, may prove useful in improving the outcome of kidney diseases [32].

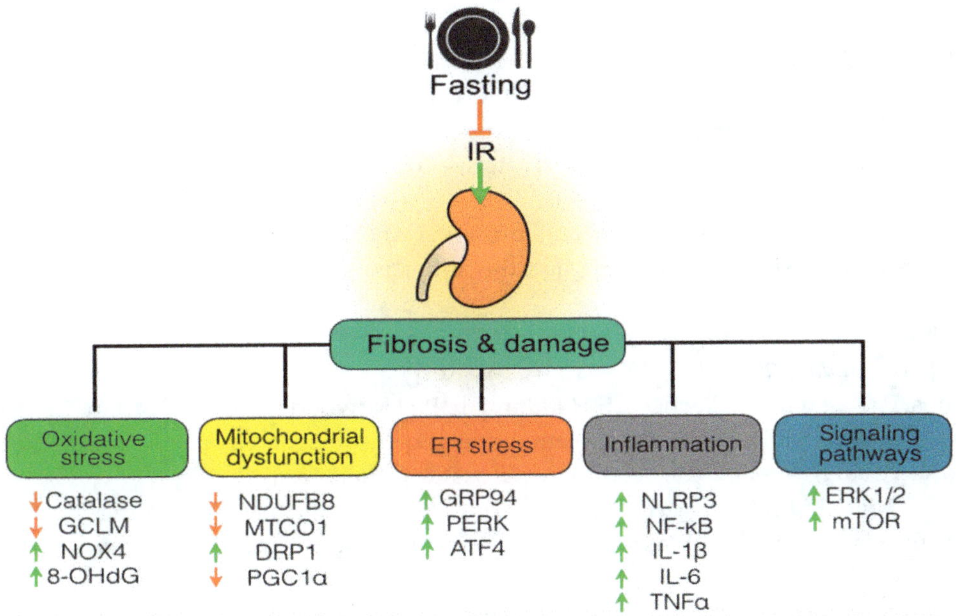

Figure 9. Protection against chronic damage and fibrosis development after ischemia-reperfusion (IR) injury by fasting. Preoperative fasting limits IR-induced fibrosis and renal damage by suppressing oxidative stress, mitochondrial dysfunction, endoplasmic reticulum (ER) stress, inflammation, and signaling pathways. GCLM, glutamate-cysteine ligase modifier subunit; NOX4, nicotinamide adenine dinucleotide phosphate oxidase 4; 8-OHdG, 8-hydroxy-2′-deoxyguanosine; NDUFB8, NADH:Ubiquinone oxidoreductase subunit B8; MTCO1, cytochrome c oxidase subunit 1; succinate dehydrogenase subunit B; DRP1, dynamin-related protein 1; PGC1α, peroxisome proliferator-activated receptor gamma coactivator 1 alpha; GRP94, glucose-regulated protein 94; PERK, protein kinase RNA-like endoplasmic reticulum kinase; ATF4, activating transcription factor 4; NLRP3, NOD-like receptor protein 3; NF-κB, nuclear factor kappa B; IL-1β, interleukin 1 beta; IL-6, interleukin 6; TNFα, tumor necrosis factor-alpha; ERK1/2, extracellular signal-regulated kinase 1/2; mTOR, mechanistic target of rapamycin.

5. Conclusions

Fasting is a strong nutritional intervention to abrogate multiple pathophysiological mechanisms implicated in tissue injury and fibrosis that develops after renal IR.

Author Contributions: Conceptualization—P.R.-M.; Methodology—P.R.-M., E.T., J.C.L.-C., N.P., J.G.-P.; Analysis and investigation—P.R.-M., S.G.-R., A.S.J.-O., J.T., and R.H.-P.; Original draft preparation—P.R.-M.; Review and editing—J.P.-C.; Resources—E.T., R.H.-P., L.G.S.-L., H.O.-A.; Supervision—J.P.-C.; Funding acquisition—E.T., and J.P.-C.

Acknowledgments: P.R.-M. is a doctoral student from Programa de Doctorado en Ciencias Bioquímicas, Universidad Nacional Autónoma de México (UNAM) and receives a scholarship from CONACyT.

References

1. Duffield, J.S. Cellular and molecular mechanisms in kidney fibrosis. *J. Clin. Investig.* **2014**, *124*, 2299–2306. [CrossRef] [PubMed]
2. Basile, D.P.; Bonventre, J.V.; Mehta, R.; Nangaku, M.; Unwin, R.; Rosner, M.H.; Kellum, J.A.; Ronco, C.; Group AXW. Progression after AKI: Understanding maladaptive repair processes to predict and identify therapeutic treatments. *J. Am. Soc. Nephrol.* **2016**, *27*, 687–697. [CrossRef] [PubMed]
3. Chawla, L.S.; Eggers, P.W.; Star, R.A.; Kimmel, P.L. Acute kidney injury and chronic kidney disease as interconnected syndromes. *N Engl. J. Med.* **2014**, *371*, 58–66. [CrossRef] [PubMed]
4. Humphreys, B.D. Mechanisms of renal fibrosis. *Annu. Rev. Physiol.* **2018**, *80*, 309–326. [CrossRef] [PubMed]
5. Lv, W.; Booz, G.W.; Fan, F.; Wang, Y.; Roman, R.J. Oxidative stress and renal fibrosis: Recent insights for the development of novel therapeutic strategies. *Front Physiol.* **2018**, *9*, 105. [CrossRef] [PubMed]
6. Galvan, D.L.; Green, N.H.; Danesh, F.R. The hallmarks of mitochondrial dysfunction in chronic kidney disease. *Kidney Int.* **2017**, *92*, 1051–1057. [CrossRef] [PubMed]
7. Cybulsky, A.V. Endoplasmic reticulum stress, the unfolded protein response and autophagy in kidney diseases. *Nat. Rev. Nephrol.* **2017**, *13*, 681–696. [CrossRef]
8. Eltzsching, H.K.; Eckle, T. Ischemia and reperfusion—From mechanisms to translation. *Nat. Medicine* **2011**, *17*, 1391–1401. [CrossRef]
9. He, L.; Wei, Q.; Liu, J.; Yi, M.; Liu, Y.; Liu, H.; Sun, L.; Peng, Y.; Liu, F.; Venkatachalam, M.A.; et al. AKI on CKD: Heightened injury, suppressed repair, and the underlying mechanisms. *Kidney Int.* **2017**, *92*, 1071–1083. [CrossRef]
10. Huynh, P.; Chai, Z. Transforming growth factor β (TGFβ) and related molecules in chronic kidney disease (CKD). *Clin. Sci. (London)* **2019**, *133*, 287–313. [CrossRef]
11. Andrikopoulos, P.; Kieswich, J.; Pacheco, S.; Nadarajah, L.; Harwood, S.M.; O'Riordan, C.E.; Thiemermann, C.; Yaqoob, M.M. The MEK inhibitor trametinib ameliorates kidney fibrosis by suppressing ERK1/2 and mTORC1 signaling. *J. Am. Soc. Nephrol.* **2019**, *30*, 33–49. [CrossRef] [PubMed]
12. Jiang, L.; Xu, L.; Mao, J.; Li, J.; Fang, L.; Zhou, Y.; Liu, W.; He, W.; Zhao, A.Z.; Yang, J.; et al. Rheb/mTORC1 signaling promotes kidney fibroblast activation and fibrosis. *J. Am. Soc. Nephrol.* **2013**, *24*, 1114–1126. [CrossRef]
13. Longo, V.D.; Mattson, M.P. Fasting: Molecular mechanisms and clinical applications. *Cell Metab.* **2014**, *19*, 181–192. [CrossRef] [PubMed]
14. Robertson, L.T.; Mitchell, J.R. Benefits of short-term dietary restriction in mammals. *Exp. Gerontol.* **2013**, *48*, 1043–1048. [CrossRef] [PubMed]
15. Brandhorst, S.; Harputlugil, E.; Mitchell, J.R.; Longo, V.D. Protective effects of short-term dietary restriction in surgical stress and chemotherapy. *Ageing Res. Rev.* **2017**, *39*, 68–77. [CrossRef] [PubMed]
16. Rojas-Morales, P.; León-Contreras, J.C.; Aparicio-Trejo, O.E.; Reyes-Ocampo, J.G.; Medina-Campos, O.N.; Jiménez-Osorio, A.S.; González-Reyes, S.; Marquina-Castillo, B.; Hernández-Pando, R.; Barrera-Oviedo, D.; et al. Fasting reduces oxidative stress, mitochondrial dysfunction and fibrosis induced by renal ischemia-reperfusion injury. *Free Radic. Biol. Med.* **2019**, *135*, 60–67. [CrossRef] [PubMed]
17. Fu, Y.; Tang, C.; Cai, J.; Chen, G.; Zhang, D.; Dong, Z. Rodent models of AKI-CKD transition. *Am. J. Physiol. Renal Physiol.* **2018**, *315*, F1098–F1106. [CrossRef] [PubMed]

18. Sedeek, M.; Nasrallah, R.; Touyz, R.M.; Hébert, R.L. NADPH oxidases, reactive oxygen species, and the kidney: Friend and foe. *J. Am. Soc. Nephrol.* **2013**, *24*, 1512–1518. [CrossRef] [PubMed]
19. Bhargava, P.; Schnellmann, R.G. Mitochondrial energetics in the kidney. *Nat. Rev. Nephrol.* **2017**, *13*, 629–646. [CrossRef] [PubMed]
20. Meng, X.M.; Nikolic-Paterson, D.J.; Lan, H.Y. Inflammatory processes in renal fibrosis. *Nat. Rev. Nephrol.* **2014**, *10*, 493–503. [CrossRef]
21. Jiang, F.; Liu, G.S.; Dusting, G.J.; Chan, E.C. NADPH oxidase-dependent redox signaling in TGF-β-mediated fibrotic responses. *Redox Biol.* **2014**, *2*, 267–272. [CrossRef] [PubMed]
22. Liu, R.M.; Desai, L.P. Reciprocal regulation of TGF-β and reactive oxygen species: a perverse cycle for fibrosis. *Redox Biol.* **2015**, *6*, 565–577. [CrossRef] [PubMed]
23. Cadenas, E.; Davies, K.J. Mitochondrial free radical generation, oxidative stress, and aging. *Free Radic. Biol. Med.* **2000**, *29*, 222–230. [CrossRef]
24. Malhotra, J.D.; Kaufman, R.J. Endoplasmic reticulum stress and oxidative stress: a vicious cycle or a double-edged sword? *Antioxid. Redox Signal.* **2007**, *9*, 2277–2293. [CrossRef] [PubMed]
25. Mittal, M.; Siddiqui, M.R.; Tran, K.; Reddy, S.P.; Malik, A.B. Reactive oxygen species in inflammation and tissue injury. *Antioxid. Redox Signal.* **2014**, *20*, 1126–1167. [CrossRef] [PubMed]
26. Zhang, K.; Kaufman, R.J. From endoplasmic-reticulum stress to the inflammatory response. *Nature* **2008**, *454*, 455–462. [CrossRef] [PubMed]
27. Fontana, L.; Partridge, L. Promoting health and longevity through diet: From model organisms to humans. *Cell* **2015**, *161*, 106–118. [CrossRef] [PubMed]
28. Mitchell, J.R.; Verweij, M.; Brand, K.; van de Ven, M.; Goemaere, N.; van den Engel, S.; Chu, T.; Forrer, F.; Müller, C.; de Jong, M.; et al. Short-term dietary restriction and fasting precondition against ischemia reperfusion injury in mice. *Aging Cell* **2010**, *9*, 40–53. [CrossRef]
29. Warner, G.; Hein, K.Z.; Nin, V.; Edwards, M.; Chini, C.C.; Hopp, K.; Harris, P.C.; Torres, V.E.; Chini, E.N. Food restriction ameliorates the development of polycystic kidney disease. *J. Am. Soc. Nephrol.* **2016**, *27*, 1437–1447. [CrossRef]
30. Jongbloed, F.; Saat, T.C.; Verweij, M.; Payan-Gomez, C.; Hoeijmakers, J.H.; van den Engel, S.; van Oostrom, C.T.; Ambagtsheer, G.; Imholz, S.; Pennings, J.L.; et al. a signature of renal stress resistance induced by short-term dietary restriction, fasting, and protein restriction. *Sci. Rep.* **2017**, *7*, 40901. [CrossRef]
31. Hostetter, T.H.; Meyer, T.W.; Rennke, H.G.; Brenner, B.M. Chronic effects of dietary protein in the rat with intact and reduced renal mass. *Kidney Int.* **1986**, *30*, 509–517. [CrossRef] [PubMed]
32. Wang, S.Y.; Cai, G.Y.; Chen, X.M. Energy restriction in renal protection. *Br. J. Nutr.* **2018**, *120*, 1149–1158. [CrossRef] [PubMed]

3

Acute Kidney Injury in Pediatric Patients on Extracorporeal Membrane Oxygenation

Panupong Hansrivijit [1], Ploypin Lertjitbanjong [2], Charat Thongprayoon [3,*], Wisit Cheungpasitporn [4,*], Narothama Reddy Aeddula [5], Sohail Abdul Salim [4], Api Chewcharat [3], Kanramon Watthanasuntorn [2], Narat Srivali [6], Michael A. Mao [7], Patompong Ungprasert [8], Karn Wijarnpreecha [7], Wisit Kaewput [9] and Tarun Bathini [10]

1 Department of Internal Medicine, University of Pittsburgh Medical Center Pinnacle, Harrisburg, PA 17105, USA; hansrivijitp@upmc.edu

2 Department of Internal Medicine, Bassett Medical Center, Cooperstown, NY 13326, USA; ploypinlert@gmail.com (P.L.); kanramon@gmail.com (K.W.)

3 Division of Nephrology and Hypertension, Mayo Clinic, Rochester, MN 55905, USA; api.che@hotmail.com

4 Division of Nephrology, University of Mississippi Medical Center, Jackson, MS 39216, USA; sohail3553@gmail.com

5 Department of Internal Medicine, Deaconess Health System, Evansville, IN 47747, USA; dr.anreddy@gmail.com

6 Division of Pulmonary and Critical Care Medicine, St. Agnes Hospital, Baltimore, MD 21229, USA; nsrivali@gmail.com

7 Department of Medicine, Mayo Clinic, Jacksonville, FL 32224, USA; mao.michael@mayo.edu (M.A.M.); dr.karn.wi@gmail.com (K.W.)

8 Department of Rheumatic and Immunologic Diseases, Cleveland Clinic, Cleveland Clinic Lerner College of Medicine of Case Western Reserve University, Cleveland, OH 44106, USA; p.ungprasert@gmail.com

9 Department of Military and Community Medicine, Phramongkutklao College of Medicine, Bangkok 10400, Thailand; wisitnephro@gmail.com

10 Department of Internal Medicine, University of Arizona, Tucson, AZ 85721, USA; tarunjacobb@gmail.com

* Correspondence: charat.thongprayoon@gmail.com (C.T.); wcheungpasitporn@gmail.com (W.C.)

Abstract: Background: Acute kidney injury (AKI) is a well-established complication of extra-corporal membrane oxygenation (ECMO) in the adult population. The data in the pediatric and neonatal population is still limited. Moreover, the mortality risk of AKI among pediatric patients requiring ECMO remains unclear. Thus, this meta-analysis aims to assess the incidence of AKI, AKI requiring renal replacement therapy and AKI associated mortality in pediatric/neonatal patients requiring ECMO. **Methods:** A literature search was performed utilizing MEDLINE, EMBASE, and the Cochrane Database from inception through June 2019. We included studies that evaluated the incidence of AKI, severe AKI requiring renal replacement therapy (RRT) and the risk of mortality among pediatric patients on ECMO with AKI. Random-effects meta-analysis was used to calculate the pooled incidence of AKI and the odds ratios (OR) for mortality. **Results:** 13 studies with 3523 pediatric patients on ECMO were identified. Pooled incidence of AKI and AKI requiring RRT were 61.9% (95% confidence interval (CI): 39.0–80.4%) and 40.9% (95%CI: 31.2–51.4%), respectively. A meta-analysis limited to studies with standard AKI definitions showed a pooled estimated AKI incidence of 69.2% (95%CI: 59.7–77.3%). Compared with patients without AKI, those with AKI and AKI requiring RRT while on ECMO were associated with increased hospital mortality ORs of 1.70 (95% CI, 1.38–2.10) and 3.64 (95% CI: 2.02–6.55), respectively. **Conclusions:** The estimated incidence of AKI and severe AKI requiring RRT in pediatric patients receiving ECMO are high at 61.9% and 40.9%, respectively. AKI among pediatric patients on ECMO is significantly associated with reduced patient survival.

Keywords: AKI; ECMO; extracorporeal membrane oxygenation; incidence; mortality

---

1. Introduction

For the past 20 years, extra-corporal membrane oxygenation (ECMO) use has remarkably increased, as it has become an essential rescue therapy for severe refractory cardiac and pulmonary dysfunction in both adults and children [1]. In general, ECMO provides temporary support for patients who have a predicted mortality rate of 80% and above [2]. Indications for ECMO can be categorized into: (1) Respiratory Support and (2) Cardiac Support. Based on the indication for ECMO, the modality of ECMO is adapted for the patient. Veno-venous (VV) ECMO provides only respiratory support, and requires patients to have stable hemodynamics, whereas veno-arterial (VA) ECMO provides dual cardiac and respiratory support [1–7]. In VA ECMO, the blood bypasses both the heart and lungs. Generally, there is minimal vascular pulsatility in VA ECMO, while there is considerable pulsatility in VV ECMO. Pulsatility has been suggested to be essential in maintaining optimal perfusion to the vital organs, including the brain, heart and kidneys [8]. For instance, Pappalardo et al. [9] has shown that the incidence of acute ischemic stroke in VV ECMO is 1.4% compared to 3.8% in VA ECMO [10].

A recent meta-analysis has demonstrated that the pooled incidence of AKI and severe AKI requiring renal replacement therapy (RRT) among adult patients on ECMO was 63% and 45%, respectively. Furthermore, adult ECMO patients with AKI requiring RRT have a significantly increased mortality with a pooled odds ratio (OR) of 3.73 [11]. Although the incidence and associated mortality of AKI in adults on ECMO are widely reported, comparable data in the pediatric population are limited. While one study has reported a mortality rate of 27.4 and 41.6%, respectively, for neonatal and pediatric patients who received ECMO support for non-cardiac indications [12], the impact of AKI and its severity on outcomes is less clear. Furthermore, the need for RRT during ECMO is considered an independent risk factor for the failure to wean from ECMO [13]. Therefore, we performed this meta-analysis to assess the incidence rate of AKI and its associated mortality in pediatric patients receiving ECMO for various indications. The results of our study will help define the burden of AKI and its clinical impact on pediatric patients receiving ECMO, and allow comparisons to the adult counterpart.

2. Method

2.1. Literature Review and Search Strategy

We conducted a systematic literature review of Ovid MEDLINE, EMBASE and the Cochrane Database of Systematic Reviews until June 2019 to assess the incidence and mortality risk of AKI in pediatric patients on ECMO. Independent reviewers (C.T. and P.L.) conducted a systematic literature search using a search strategy that incorporated the search terms "extracorporeal membrane oxygenation" OR "ECMO" AND "acute kidney injury" OR "acute renal failure", as shown in Supplementary Data S1. A manual search for potentially relevant studies utilizing the references of the initial included articles was subsequently performed. There was no language limitation. This systematic review was conducted following the PRISMA (Preferred Reporting Items for Systematic Reviews and Meta-Analysis) [14].

2.2. Selection Criteria

Inclusion criteria consisted of observational studies or clinical trials that evaluated both the incidence of acute kidney injury (AKI) and/or severe AKI requiring RRT and mortality risk of AKI in pediatric patients (aged younger than 18 years old) on ECMO. Retrieved articles were individually assessed for study eligibility by the two investigators previously noted. Any discrepancies were resolved by mutual consensus.

2.3. Data Abstraction

A data collecting form was utilized to derive the following information from the individual studies: Title, study year, publication year, name of authors, country where the study was performed, ECMO type, definition of AKI, incidence rate of AKI, incidence rate of AKI requiring RRT and risk of mortality in pediatric patients on ECMO with AKI.

2.4. Statistical Analysis

Analyses were performed using the Comprehensive Meta-Analysis 3.3 software (version 3; Biostat Inc, Englewood, NJ, USA). Pooled AKI incidence and mortality risk of included studies were incorporated by the generic inverse variance method of DerSimonian-Laird, which indicated the weight of each study depending on its variance [15]. Because of the likelihood of inter-observation variance, we utilized a random-effects model for meta-analyses of the incidence and mortality risk of AKI among pediatric patients receiving ECMO. Statistical heterogeneity of studies was evaluated by the Cochran's Q test (statistically significant as $p < 0.05$) and the I^2 statistic (≤25% represents insignificant heterogeneity, 26% to 50% represents low heterogeneity, 51% to 75% represents moderate heterogeneity, and ≥75% represents high heterogeneity) [16]. Publication bias was evaluated via the Egger test [17].

3. Results

Our search strategy produced a total of 1741 potentially eligible articles. 887 articles were excluded because they were duplicated. and 684 articles because they were case reports, correspondences, review articles, in vitro studies, or animal studies. 170 articles remained for full-length review. Forty one articles were subsequently excluded because the study cohort was an adult patient population, and 116 studies were excluded due to a lack of data on the outcomes of interest. Consequently, 13 cohort studies [12,18–29] comprised of 3523 pediatric patients on ECMO were identified in this systematic review. The systematic review process is presented in Figure 1. The characteristics of the included studies are demonstrated in Table 1. The kappa coefficient (0.87) indicated that agreement between the authors was acceptable.

Table 1. Included studies in this systematic review of acute kidney injury (AKI) incidence and mortality in pediatric patients requiring ECMO.

Study	Year	Country	Patient Population	Number	Definition of AKI	Incidence of AKI	Mortality
Kolovos et al. [18]	2003	USA	Patients on ECMO within seven days after cardiac surgery	74	RRT	RRT 26/74 (35%)	Hospital mortality RRT 20/26 (77%)
Hoover et al. [19]	2008	USA	Patients aged 1 month to 18 years with respiratory failure requiring ECMO	86	CRRT	CRRT 26/86 (30%)	Hospital mortality RRT 7/26 (27%)
Gbadegesin et al. [20]	2009	USA	Patients aged < 3 years requiring ECMO after cardiac surgery	104	CRRT	CRRT 42/104 (40%)	Hospital mortality RRT 35/42 (83%)
Gadepalli et al. [21]	2010	USA	Congenital diaphragmatic hernia patients requiring ECMO	68	AKI: RIFLE	AKI 48/68 (71%) RIFLE—failure AKI 33/68 (49%) CRRT 11/68 = 16%	Mortality RIFLE—failure AKI 24/33 (73%)
Goto et al. [22]	2011	USA	Patients aged 19 days to 20 years with respiratory failure and/or heart failure requiring ECMO	14	RRT	RRT 7/14 (50%)	Hospital mortality RRT 2/7 (29%)
Askenazi et al. [12]	2011	USA	All non-cardiac patients requiring ECMO	9903 Neonates -7941 Children -1962	SCr > 1.5 mg/dL or ICD-9 for acute renal failure	Neonates AKI—638/7941 (8%) RRT—1786/7941 (22%) Children AKI—402/1962 (20%) RRT—840/1962 (43%)	Neonates Hospital mortality AKI—413/638 (65%) RRT—863/1786 (48%) Children Hospital mortality AKI—264/402 (66%) RRT—487/840 (58%)
Ricci et al. [23]	2012	Italy	Patients aged 13 days to 13 years on VA ECMO after cardiac surgery	10	CRRT	CRRT 3/10 (30%)	Hospital mortality RRT 2/3 (66%)
Hoffman et al. [24]	2013	USA	Patients with persistent hypoxia or cardiovascular instability requiring ECMO	10	AKI; (1) urine output < 1 ml/kg/h with SCr > 1 mg/dL for 24 hours, (2) SCr of > 1.5 mg/dL, (3) failure to improve creatinine clearance by > 50%	AKI 5/10 (50%)	N/A
Zwiers et al. [25]	2013	Netherlands	Neonates aged < 28 days requiring ECMO	242	AKI: RIFLE	AKI 153/242 (63%)	Hospital mortality AKI 43/153 (28%)

Table 1. *Cont.*

Study	Year	Country	Patient Population	Number	Definition of AKI	Incidence of AKI	Mortality
Fleming et al. [26]	2016	USA	Pediatric patients aged < 18 requiring ECMO	832	AKI: KDIGO	AKI by SCr—502/832 (60%) AKI by SCr + renal support therapy—615/832 (74%)	N/A
Yang et al. [27]	2016	China	Patients aged 1 to 13 years with refractory cardiopulmonary failure requiring ECMO	12	CRRT	CRRT 1/12 (8%)	Hospital mortality RRT 0/1 (0%)
Elella et al. [28]	2017	Saudi Arabia	Pediatric patients requiring VA-ECMO after cardiac surgery	59	AKI pRIFLE	AKI 53/59 (90%) RRT 29/59 (49%)	Hospital mortality AKI 33/53 (62%)
Borasino et al. [29]	2018	USA	Pediatric cardiac patient on ECMO in CICU	50	AKI: increase in SCr of 200% from baseline	AKI 35/50 (70%) RRT 26/50 (52%)	Hospital mortality RRT 16/26 (61%)

Abbreviations: AKIN, Acute Kidney Injury Network; COPD, chronic obstructive pulmonary disease; CRRT, continuous renal replacement therapy; KDIGO, Kidney Disease Improving Global Outcomes; pRIFLE, Pediatric Risk, Injury, Failure, Loss of kidney function; RIFLE, Risk, Injury, Failure, Loss of kidney function, and End-stage kidney disease; RRT, renal replacement therapy; SCr, serum creatinine; ECMO, extra-corporal membrane oxygenation.

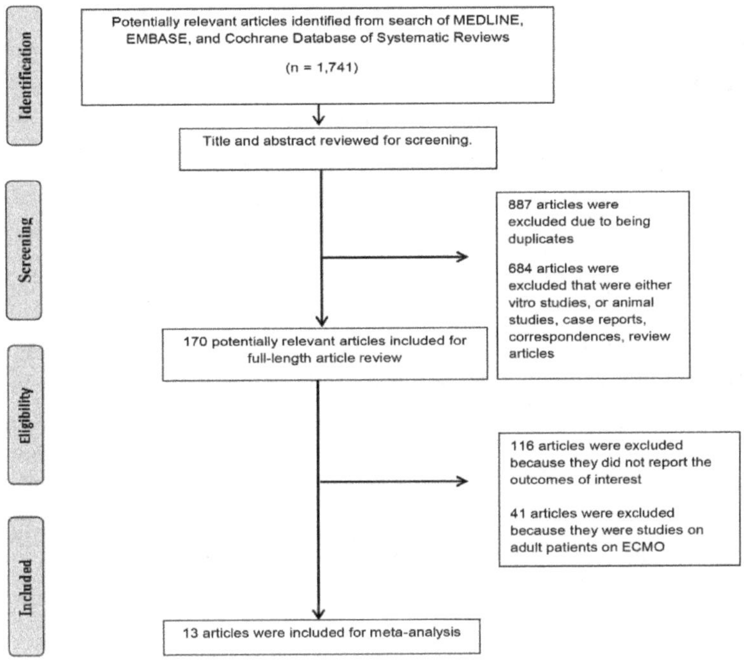

Figure 1. Flow diagram of our search strategy.

3.1. Incidence of AKI among Pediatric Patients on ECMO

Pooled estimated incidence of AKI and severe AKI requiring RRT were 61.9% (95%CI: 39.0–80.4%, $I^2 = 98\%$, Figure 2A) and 40.9% (95%CI: 31.2–51.4%, $I^2 = 86\%$, Figure 2B), respectively. We additionally performed a meta-analysis limited to studies using standard AKI definitions; this showed a pooled estimated AKI incidence of 69.2% (95%CI: 59.7–77.3%, $I^2 = 83\%$, Figure S1).

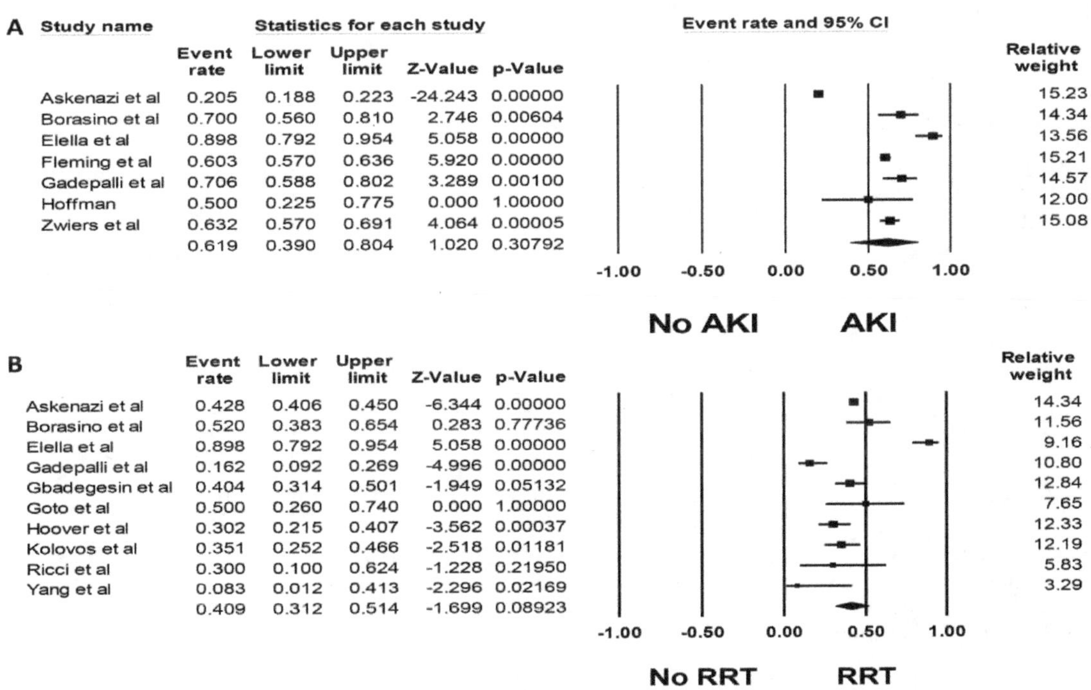

Figure 2. Forest plots of included studies on pediatric patients requiring extra-corporal membrane oxygenation (ECMO) that evaluated (**A**) incidence of AKI and (**B**) incidence of AKI requiring renal replacement therapy (RRT).

Subgroup analysis based on patient population (cardiac surgery vs. non-cardiac surgery) was performed. Pooled incidence of AKI was 81.4% (95%CI: 54.4–94.2%, I^2 = 84%, Figure S2) among patients after cardiac surgery and 52.3% (95%CI: 27.3–76.2%, I^2 = 99%, Figure S2) among non-cardiac surgery patients. Pooled incidence of AKI requiring RRT was 52.2% (95%CI: 32.5–71.2%, I^2 = 88%, Figure S3) among patients after cardiac surgery and 30.2% (95%CI: 18.7–44.9%, I^2 = 84%, Figure S3) among non-cardiac surgery patients.

3.2. Mortality in Pediatric ECMO Patients with AKI

Tables 1 and 2 demonstrate the AKI-associated mortality rate and risk in pediatric patients on ECMO, respectively. Pooled estimated hospital or 90-day mortality rates of pediatric ECMO patients with AKI and AKI requiring RRT were 51.7% (95%CI: 26.5–76.0%, I^2 = 96%, Figure S4) and 61.8% (95%CI: 48.8–73.4%, I^2 = 74%, Figure S5), respectively.

Table 2. Mortality Risk of AKI among pediatric patients requiring ECMO.

Study	Mortality Rate	OR for Mortality
Kolovos et al. [18]	Hospital mortality RRT 20/26 (77%)	Hospital mortality RRT: OR 5.6 (1.8–17.9)
Hoover et al. [19]	Hospital mortality RRT 7/26 (27%)	Hospital mortality CRRT: 1.55 (0.42–5.70)
Gbadegesin et al. [20]	Hospital mortality RRT 35/42 (83%)	Hospital mortality CRRT: 9.8 (3.7–25.7)
Gadepalli et al. [21]	Mortality RIFLE—failure AKI 24/33 (73%)	Hospital mortality RIFLE—Failure AKI: 10.67 (3.45–32.96)
Goto et al. [22]	Hospital mortality RRT 2/7 (29%)	Hospital mortality RRT: 0.53 (0.06–4.91)
Askenazi et al. [12]	Neonates Hospital mortality AKI—413/638 (65%) RRT—863/1786 (48%) Children Hospital mortality AKI—264/402 (66%) RRT—487/840 (58%)	Hospital mortality Neonates AKI: 3.2 (2.6–4.0) RRT: 1.9 (1.6–2.2) Children AKI: 1.7 (1.3–2.3) RRT: 2.5 (1.9–3.2)
Ricci et al. [23]	Hospital mortality RRT 2/3 (66%)	Hospital mortality CRRT: 2.67 (0.16–45.14)
Zwiers et al. [25]	Hospital mortality AKI 43/153 (28%)	Hospital mortality AKI: 1.35 (0.73–2.48)
Fleming et al. [26]	N/A	Hospital mortality AKI-SCr: 1.77 (1.22–2.55) AKI-SCr+RST: 2.50 (1.61–3.90)
Yang et al. [27]	Hospital mortality RRT 0/1 (0%)	Hospital mortality CRRT: 0/1 vs. 4/11
Elella et al. [28]	Hospital mortality AKI 33/53 (62%)	Hospital mortality AKI: 8.25 (0.90–75.79)
Borasino et al. [29]	Hospital mortality RRT 16/26 (61%)	Hospital morality RRT: 2.67 (0.85–8.37)

Abbreviations: AKIN, Acute Kidney Injury Network; COPD, chronic obstructive pulmonary disease; CRRT, continuous renal replacement therapy; KDIGO, Kidney Disease Improving Global Outcomes; pRIFLE, Pediatric Risk, Injury, Failure, Loss of kidney function; RIFLE, Risk, Injury, Failure, Loss of kidney function, and End-stage kidney disease; RRT, renal replacement therapy; RST, renal support therapy; SCr, serum creatinine.

The hospital mortality pooled OR in pediatric ECMO patients with AKI and severe AKI requiring RRT were 1.70 (95% CI: 1.38–2.10, I^2 = 0%, Figure 3A) and 3.64 (95% CI, 2.02–6.55, I^2 = 58%, Figure 3B), respectively. Meta-regression analysis was additionally performed, and it demonstrated that year of study was not correlated with either mortality risk associated with AKI ($p = 0.65$) or AKI requiring RRT ($p = 0.46$).

A

Study name	Odds ratio	Lower limit	Upper limit	Z-Value	p-Value	Relative weight
Askenazi et al	1.700	1.273	2.270	3.597	0.00032	53.87
Elella et al	8.250	0.924	73.688	1.889	0.05891	0.94
Fleming et al	1.770	1.224	2.559	3.036	0.00240	33.14
Zwiers et al	1.350	0.732	2.488	0.962	0.33609	12.04
	1.701	1.376	2.103	4.905	0.00000	

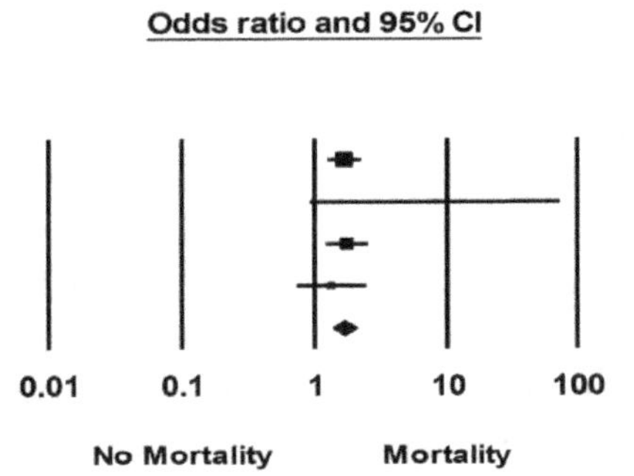

B

Study name	Odds ratio	Lower limit	Upper limit	Z-Value	p-Value	Relative weight
Askenazi et al	2.500	1.931	3.236	6.960	0.00000	24.73
Borasino et al	2.670	0.851	8.378	1.683	0.09234	13.08
Gadepalli et al	10.670	3.452	32.980	4.112	0.00004	13.26
Gbadegesin et al	9.800	3.718	25.828	4.616	0.00000	15.21
Goto et al	0.530	0.059	4.794	-0.565	0.57207	5.58
Hoover et al	1.550	0.421	5.710	0.659	0.51007	11.39
Kolovos et al	5.600	1.776	17.659	2.940	0.00328	13.03
Ricci et al	2.670	0.159	44.847	0.682	0.49506	3.71
	3.639	2.022	6.546	4.311	0.00002	

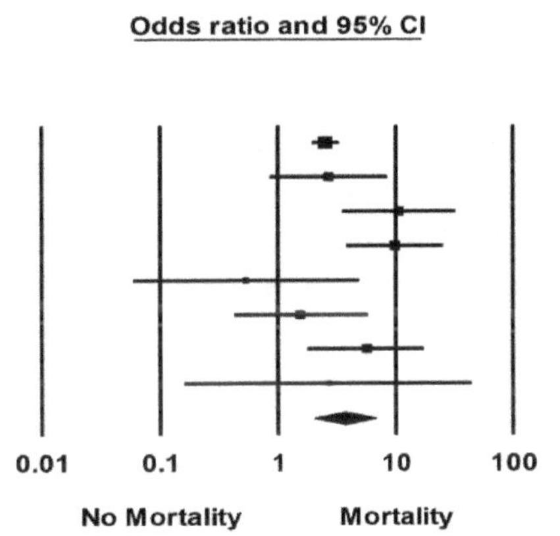

Figure 3. Forest plots of included studies on pediatric patients requiring ECMO that evaluated (**A**) hospital mortality with AKI and (**B**) hospital mortality with AKI necessitating RRT.

3.3. Assessment for Publication Bias

Funnel plots (Figures S6 and S7) and Egger's regression asymmetry tests were used to evaluate for publication bias. We found no significant publication bias for the incidence of AKI and severe AKI requiring RRT ($p = 0.16$ and $p = 0.74$, respectively).

4. Discussion

In this study, we have shown that the incidence of AKI and severe AKI in the pediatric population requiring ECMO is high (62% and 41%, respectively), especially in cardiac surgery patients requiring ECMO. AKI is associated with high mortality (OR 3.64) and AKI-associated mortality did not change over time. Similar to the adult population, our study in pediatric patients concurs that ECMO is associated with a higher risk of AKI and hospital mortality [11].

The mechanism by which ECMO support predisposes patients to AKI is not well established. Certainly, patients requiring ECMO often possess many known comorbidities and risk factors for AKI, such as low cardiac output, septic shock, anemia, diabetes, exposure to nephrotoxic drugs, etc. [30,31]. In general, there are fewer comorbidities among pediatric patients. Conversely, their renal reserve may not have fully developed [12].

However, it is proposed that ECMO itself is capable of inducing AKI via detrimental (1) hemodynamic alterations; (2) hormonal imbalances; and (3) systemic inflammatory cytokines [11,30,31]. Hemodynamic alterations may include the potential loss of pulsatility with VA ECMO versus the maintenance of pulsatility with VV ECMO. Evidence is supportive of the vital impact of pulsatility on maintaining renal cortical perfusion, thus helping to prevent acute tubular necrosis [8]. Slight hemodynamic changes could potentiate a significant reduction in renal perfusion. Current data on ECMO-associated hormonal changes show conflicting evidence. Saito et al. hypothesized that upregulation of plasma renin activity may be an adaptive response to the loss of pulsatile renal perfusion [32]. However, Semmekrot et al. observed a reduction of atrial natriuretic peptide (ANP) level, plasma renin activity (PRA) and angiotensin II levels in neonates requiring VA ECMO [33]. Further clinical investigation is needed to better understand the impact and interaction of different hormones on renal perfusion. Finally, studies have demonstrated that the continuous exposure of blood to the non-endothelialized/non-biological ECMO interface results in an activation of proinflammatory cytokines, such as tumor necrosis factor-alpha (TNF-α), IL (interleukin)-1β, IL-6, IL-8 [34,35].

Our study shows that the incidence of AKI, severe AKI requiring RRT and AKI-associated hospital mortality between adults and pediatric patients are similar [11]. This further supports ECMO as a potential independent predictor for AKI. However, we found a significant higher incidence of AKI and RRT in pediatric patients that the indication for ECMO was after cardiac surgery, than those who required ECMO for non-cardiac surgery related conditions. Despite improved knowledge of the indications for ECMO, patient comorbidities, and associated risk factors that may contribute to ECMO-associated AKI, ECMO as an independent risk factor for AKI cannot be determined from this meta-analysis alone. A pooled meta-analysis of both adult and pediatric patients assessing the incidence of AKI and mortality following ECMO support would be useful. Furthermore, a subgroup analysis comparing adult and pediatric patients would further elaborate whether ECMO is associated with AKI and increased mortality.

There were a few limitations in this study. Most of the included studies defined AKI based on serum creatinine levels, while studies utilizing the more sensitive urine output criteria or use of novel AKI biomarkers were limited [36]. Moreover, our meta-analysis is primarily based on observational studies, making it impossible to establish a causal relationship. Future data from population-based studies or prospective clinical trials focusing on AKI prevention in ECMO patients would be beneficial.

5. Conclusions

Our study demonstrates that AKI is common following ECMO in pediatric patients with an incidence of 68%. Approximately 40% of pediatric patients on ECMO develop severe AKI requiring RRT. We have also shown that presence of AKI is associated with a higher risk of hospital mortality. There is no difference in mortality between recent and remote studies. Clinical trials focusing on preventive measures for AKI with ECMO therapy is also encouraged.

Supplementary Materials: Data S1: Search terms for systematic review, Figure S1: Forest plots of the included studies assessing incidence of AKI limited to studies with standard AKI definitions was performed and demonstrated the pooled estimated incidence of AKI, Figure S2: Forest plots of the included studies assessing incidence of AKI based on cardiac surgery status, Figure S3: Forest plots of the included studies assessing incidence of severe AKI requiring RRT based on cardiac surgery status, Figure S4: Forest plots of the included studies assessing hospital and/or 90-day mortality rates of pediatric patients on ECMO with AKI, Figure S5: Forest plots of the included studies assessing hospital and/or 90-day mortality rates of pediatric patients on ECMO with severe AKI requiring RRT, Figure S6: Funnel plot evaluating for publication bias evaluating incidence of AKI while on ECMO, Figure S7: Funnel plot evaluating for publication bias evaluating incidence of severe AKI requiring RRT while on ECMO.

Author Contributions: Conceptualization, P.H., C.T., W.C., S.A.S., A.C., N.S., M.A.M., P.U., K.W. (Karn Wijarnpreecha), W.K. and T.B.; Data curation, C.T.; Formal analysis, T.B.; Funding acquisition, T.B.; Investigation, P.H., P.L., C.T. and T.B.; Methodology, P.H., P.L., C.T., W.C., W.K. and T.B.; Project administration, P.H., W.K. and T.B.; Resources, P.L., K.W. (Kanramon Watthanasuntorn) and T.B.; Software, K.W. (Kanramon Watthanasuntorn) and T.B.; Supervision, W.C., N.R.A., S.A.S., A.C., N.S., M.A.M., P.U., K.W. (Karn Wijarnpreecha), W.K. and T.B.; Validation, P.L., C.T., W.C. and T.B.; Visualization, P.L., S.A.S., A.C. and N.S.; Writing—original draft, P.H.; Writing—review & editing, P.H., P.L., C.T., W.C., N.R.A., S.A.S., A.C., K.W. (Kanramon Watthanasuntorn), N.S., M.A.M., P.U., K.W. (Karn Wijarnpreecha), W.K. and T.B.

References

1. Makdisi, G.; Wang, I.W. Extra Corporeal Membrane Oxygenation (ECMO) review of a lifesaving technology. *J. Thorac. Dis.* **2015**, *7*, 166–176.
2. Askenazi, D.J.; Selewski, D.T.; Paden, M.L.; Cooper, D.S.; Bridges, B.C.; Zappitelli, M. Renal replacement therapy in critically ill patients receiving extracorporeal membrane oxygenation. *Clin. J. Am. Soc. Nephrol.* **2012**, *7*, 1328–1336. [CrossRef] [PubMed]
3. De Jesus-Brugman, N.; Hobson, M.J.; Herrmann, J.L.; Friedman, M.L.; Cordes, T.; Mastropietro, C.W. Improved outcomes in neonates who require venoarterial extracorporeal membrane oxygenation after the Norwood procedure. *Int. J. Artif. Organs* **2019**. [CrossRef] [PubMed]
4. Constantinescu, A.R.; Adler, J.L.; Watkins, E.; Negroni-Balasquide, X.L.; Laufenberg, D.; Scholl, F.G.; Lavandosky, G.J. Aquapheresis (AQ) in Tandem with Extracorporeal Membrane Oxygenation (ECMO) in Pediatric Patients. *J. Extra Corpor. Technol.* **2019**, *51*, 163–168.
5. Lopez-Herce, J.; Casado, E.; Diez, M.; Sanchez, A.; Fernandez, S.N.; Bellon, J.M.; Santiago, M.J. Renal function in children assisted with extracorporeal membrane oxygenation. *Int. J. Artif. Organs* **2019**. [CrossRef]
6. Mallory, P.P.; Selewski, D.T.; Askenazi, D.J.; Cooper, D.S.; Fleming, G.M.; Paden, M.L.; Murphy, L.; Sahay, R.; King, E.; Zappitelli, M.; et al. Acute Kidney Injury, Fluid Overload, and Outcomes in Children Supported With Extracorporeal Membrane Oxygenation for a Respiratory Indication. *ASAIO J.* **2019**. [CrossRef]
7. Chen, S.W.; Lu, Y.A.; Lee, C.C.; Chou, A.H.; Wu, V.C.; Chang, S.W.; Fan, P.C.; Tian, Y.C.; Tsai, F.C.; Chang, C.H. Long-term outcomes after extracorporeal membrane oxygenation in patients with dialysis-requiring acute kidney injury: A cohort study. *PLoS ONE* **2019**, *14*, 0212352. [CrossRef]
8. Nemoto, M. Experimental evaluation of the influence of complete artificial circulation on renal circulation and tissue metabolism -comparative study of pulsatile vs nonpulsatile circulation. *Ann. Thorac. Cardiovasc. Surg.* **2003**, *9*, 355–364.
9. Pappalardo, F.; Montisci, A. Neurologic complications during V-V extracorporeal membrane oxygenation: Still counting. *J. Thorac. Dis.* **2017**, *9*, 2774–2776. [CrossRef]
10. Thiagarajan, R.R.; Barbaro, R.P.; Rycus, P.T.; McMullan, D.M.; Conrad, S.A.; Fortenberry, J.D.; Paden, M.L. Extracorporeal Life Support Organization Registry International Report 2016. *Asaio J.* **2017**, *63*, 60–67. [CrossRef]
11. Thongprayoon, C.; Cheungpasitporn, W.; Lertjitbanjong, P.; Aeddula, N.R.; Bathini, T.; Watthanasuntorn, K.; Srivali, N.; Mao, M.A.; Kashani, K. Incidence and Impact of Acute Kidney Injury in Patients Receiving Extracorporeal Membrane Oxygenation: A Meta-Analysis. *J. Clin. Med.* **2019**, *8*, 981. [CrossRef] [PubMed]
12. Askenazi, D.J.; Ambalavanan, N.; Hamilton, K.; Cutter, G.; Laney, D.; Kaslow, R.; Keith, G.; Douglas, C.B.; Reed, A.D. Acute kidney injury and renal replacement therapy independently predict mortality in neonatal and pediatric noncardiac patients on extracorporeal membrane oxygenation. *Pediatr. Crit. Care Med.* **2011**, *12*, 1–6. [CrossRef] [PubMed]
13. Wu, M.Y.; Lin, P.J.; Tsai, F.C.; Haung, Y.K.; Liu, K.S.; Tsai, F.C. Impact of preexisting organ dysfunction on extracorporeal life support for non-postcardiotomy cardiopulmonary failure. *Resuscitation* **2008**, *79*, 54–60. [CrossRef] [PubMed]
14. Moher, D.; Liberati, A.; Tetzlaff, J.; Altman, D.G. Preferred reporting items for systematic reviews and meta-analyses: The PRISMA statement. *PLoS ONE Med.* **2009**, *6*, 1000097.
15. DerSimonian, R.; Laird, N. Meta-analysis in clinical trials. *Control. Clin. Trials* **1986**, *7*, 177–188. [CrossRef]
16. Higgins, J.P.; Thompson, S.G.; Deeks, J.J.; Altman, D.G. Measuring inconsistency in meta-analyses. *BMJ* **2003**, *327*, 557–560. [CrossRef]
17. Easterbrook, P.J.; Berlin, J.A.; Gopalan, R.; Matthews, D.R. Publication bias in clinical research. *Lancet* **1991**, *337*, 867–872. [CrossRef]
18. Kolovos, N.S.; Bratton, S.L.; Moler, F.W.; Bove, E.L.; Ohye, R.G.; Bartlett, R.H.; Kulik, T.J. Outcome of pediatric patients treated with extracorporeal life support after cardiac surgery. *Ann. Thorac. Surg.* **2003**, *76*, 1435–1441. [CrossRef]
19. Hoover, N.G.; Heard, M.; Reid, C.; Wagoner, S.; Rogers, K.; Foland, J.; Paden, M.L.; Fortenberry, J.D. Enhanced fluid management with continuous venovenous hemofiltration in pediatric respiratory failure patients receiving extracorporeal membrane oxygenation support. *Intensive Care Med.* **2008**, *34*, 2241–2247. [CrossRef] [PubMed]

20. Gbadegesin, R.; Zhao, S.; Charpie, J.; Brophy, P.D.; Smoyer, W.E.; Lin, J.J. Significance of hemolysis on extracorporeal life support after cardiac surgery in children. *Pediatr. Nephrol.* **2009**, *24*, 589–595. [CrossRef]
21. Gadepalli, S.K.; Selewski, D.T.; Drongowski, R.A.; Mychaliska, G.B. Acute kidney injury in congenital diaphragmatic hernia requiring extracorporeal life support: An insidious problem. *J. Pediatr. Surg.* **2011**, *46*, 630–635. [CrossRef] [PubMed]
22. Goto, T.; Suzuki, Y.; Suzuki, Y.; Osanai, A.; Aoki, K.; Yamazaki, A.; Daitoku, K.; Fukuda, I. The impact of extracorporeal membrane oxygenation on survival in pediatric patients with respiratory and heart failure: Review of our experience. *Artif. Organs* **2011**, *35*, 1002–1009. [CrossRef] [PubMed]
23. Ricci, Z.; Morelli, S.; Favia, I.; Garisto, C.; Brancaccio, G.; Picardo, S. Neutrophil gelatinase-associated lipocalin levels during extracorporeal membrane oxygenation in critically ill children with congenital heart disease: Preliminary experience. *Pediatr. Crit. Care Med.* **2012**, *13*, 51–54. [CrossRef] [PubMed]
24. Hoffman, S.B.; Massaro, A.N.; Soler-Garcia, A.A.; Perazzo, S.; Ray, P.E. A novel urinary biomarker profile to identify acute kidney injury (AKI) in critically ill neonates: A pilot study. *Pediatr. Nephrol.* **2013**, *28*, 2179–2188. [CrossRef]
25. Zwiers, A.J.; de Wildt, S.N.; Hop, W.C.; Dorresteijn, E.M.; Gischler, S.J.; Tibboel, D.; Cransberg, K. Acute kidney injury is a frequent complication in critically ill neonates receiving extracorporeal membrane oxygenation: A 14-year cohort study. *Crit. Care* **2013**, *17*, R151. [CrossRef]
26. Fleming, G.M.; Sahay, R.; Zappitelli, M.; King, E.; Askenazi, D.J.; Bridges, B.C.; Paden, M.L.; Selewski, D.T.; Cooper, D.S. The Incidence of Acute Kidney Injury and Its Effect on Neonatal and Pediatric Extracorporeal Membrane Oxygenation Outcomes: A Multicenter Report From the Kidney Intervention During Extracorporeal Membrane Oxygenation Study Group. *Pediatr. Crit. Care Med.* **2016**, *17*, 1157–1169. [CrossRef]
27. Yang, Z.H.; Ning, B.T.; Zhang, C.M.; Lin, R.; Ye, S.; Liu, T. Clinical application of extracorporeal membrane oxygenation in children with refractory cardiopulmonary failure. *World J. Pediatr.* **2016**, *12*, 364–367. [CrossRef]
28. Elella, R.A.; Habib, E.; Mokrusova, P.; Joseph, P.; Aldalaty, H.; Ahmadi, M.A.; Al Halees, Z. Incidence and outcome of acute kidney injury by the pRIFLE criteria for children receiving extracorporeal membrane oxygenation after heart surgery. *Ann. Saudi Med.* **2017**, *37*, 201–206. [CrossRef]
29. Borasino, S.; Kalra, Y.; Elam, A.R.; Carlisle O'Meara, L.; Timpa, J.G.; Goldberg, K.G.; Leslie Collins Gaddis, J.; Alten, J.A. Impact of Hemolysis on Acute Kidney Injury and Mortality in Children Supported with Cardiac Extracorporeal Membrane Oxygenation. *J. Extra Corpor. Technol.* **2018**, *50*, 217–224.
30. Lin, C.Y.; Chen, Y.C.; Tsai, F.C.; Tian, Y.C.; Jenq, C.C.; Fang, J.T.; Yang, C.W. RIFLE classification is predictive of short-term prognosis in critically ill patients with acute renal failure supported by extracorporeal membrane oxygenation. *Nephrol. Dial. Transplant.* **2006**, *21*, 2867–2873. [CrossRef]
31. Bhatia, I.; Ho, K.C.; Rocha, B.A.; Yam, N.; Lun, K.S.; Yung, T.C.; Au, W.K.T. Pediatric ventricular assist device therapy for advanced heart failure-Hong Kong experience. *J. Artif. Organs* **2019**, 1–7. [CrossRef] [PubMed]
32. Saito, S.; Westaby, S.; Piggot, D.; Dudnikov, S.; Robson, D.; Catarino, P.A.; Clelland, C.; Nojiri, C. End-organ function during chronic nonpulsatile circulation. *Ann. Thorac. Surg.* **2002**, *74*, 1080–1085. [CrossRef]
33. Semmekrot, B.A.; Pesman, G.J.; Span, P.N.; Sweep, C.G.; van Heijst, A.F.; Monnens, L.A.; van de Bor, M.; Tanke, R.B.; van der Staak, F.H.J.M. Serial plasma concentrations of atrial natriuretic peptide, plasma renin activity, aldosterone, and antidiuretic hormone in neonates on extracorporeal membrane oxygenation. *Asaio J.* **2002**, *48*, 26–33. [CrossRef] [PubMed]
34. Hu, Y.; Yu, W.; Shi, J.; Chen, Q.; Shen, J.; Lin, Z.; He, C.; Li, N.; Li, J. Effects of continuous renal replacement therapy on renal inflammatory cytokines during extracorporeal membrane oxygenation in a porcine model. *J. Cardiothorac. Surg.* **2013**, *8*, 113.
35. McI, R.B.; Timpa, J.G.; Kurundkar, A.R.; Holt, D.W.; Kelly, D.R.; Hartman, Y.E.; Neel, M.L.; Karnatak, R.K.; Schelonka, R.L.; Anantharamaiah, G.M.; et al. Plasma concentrations of inflammatory cytokines rise rapidly during ECMO-related SIRS due to the release of preformed stores in the intestine. *Lab. Investig.* **2010**, *90*, 128–139.
36. Kashani, K.; Cheungpasitporn, W.; Ronco, C. Biomarkers of acute kidney injury: The pathway from discovery to clinical adoption. *Clin. Chem. Lab. Med.* **2017**, *55*, 1074–1089. [CrossRef]

4

Novel Variants of Angiotensin Converting Enzyme-2 of Shorter Molecular Size to Target the Kidney Renin Angiotensin System

Jan Wysocki [1], Arndt Schulze [1,2] and Daniel Batlle [1,*]

1 Department of Medicine, Division of Nephrology and Hypertension, Feinberg School of Medicine, Northwestern University, Chicago, IL 60611-3008, USA; j-wysocki@northwestern.edu (J.W.); arndt.schulze@northwestern.edu (A.S.)

2 Department of Medicine, Charité-Universitätsmedizin, D-10117 Berlin, Germany

* Correspondence: d-batlle@northwestern.edu.

Abstract: ACE2 is a monocarboxypeptidase which generates Angiotensin (1–7) from Angiotensin II (1–8). Attempts to target the kidney Renin Angiotensin System using native ACE2 to treat kidney disease are hampered by its large molecular size, 100 kDa, which precludes its glomerular filtration and subsequent tubular uptake. Here, we show that both urine and kidney lysates are capable of digesting native ACE2 into shorter proteins of ~60–75 kDa and then demonstrate that they are enzymatically very active. We then truncated the native ACE2 by design from the C-terminus to generate two short recombinant (r)ACE2 variants (1-605 and 1-619AA). These two truncates have a molecular size of ~70 kDa, as expected from the amino acid sequence and as shown by Western blot. ACE2 enzyme activity, measured using a specific substrate, was higher than that of the native rACE2 (1-740 AA). When infused to mice with genetic ACE2 deficiency, a single i.v. injection of 1-619 resulted in detectable ACE2 activity in urine, whereas infusion of the native ACE2 did not. Moreover, ACE2 activity was recovered in harvested kidneys from ACE2-deficient mice infused with 1-619, but not in controls (23.1 ± 4.3 RFU/µg creatinine/h and 1.96 ± 0.73 RFU/µg protein/hr, respectively). In addition, the kidneys of ACE2-null mice infused with 1-619 studied ex vivo formed more Ang (1–7) from exogenous Ang II than those infused with vehicle (AUC 8555 ± 1933 vs. 3439 ± 753 ng/mL, respectively, $p < 0.05$) further demonstrating the functional effect of increasing kidney ACE2 activity after the infusion of our short ACE2 1-619 variant. We conclude that our novel short recombinant ACE2 variants undergo glomerular filtration, which is associated with kidney uptake of enzymatically active proteins that can enhance the formation of Ang (1–7) from Ang II. These small ACE2 variants may offer a potentially useful approach to target kidney RAS overactivity to combat kidney injury.

Keywords: ACE2; Renin Angiotensin System; Acute Kidney Injury; Angiotensin II; Angiotensin (1-7)

---

1. Introduction

Angiotensin Converting Enzyme-2 (ACE2) is a monocarboxypeptidase that degrades several substrates, of which Ang II is most relevant because of the extensive biologic effects of this peptide and the attendant formation of Ang (1–7), which has actions generally opposite to those of Ang II [1–9]. ACE2 protein in its full-length form is an 805 amino-acid (AA) type-I transmembrane protein (110–120 kDa) that contains an extracellular domain (AA 1–740), a transmembrane region (AA 741–768), and an intracellular tail (769–805) [10,11]. The extracellular part of ACE2 (1-740 AA), here referred as "native" ACE2, contains the catalytic domain and is fully catalytically active. In our previous studies, the administration of native rACE2 (1-740 AA) resulted in a marked increase in circulating ACE2 activity, but neither kidney nor urinary ACE2 activity increased [6,12,13].

The lack of increase in urinary ACE2 activity after injection of native rACE2 was attributed to the lack of glomerular filtration of native rACE2, consistent with its large molecular size of 100–110 kDa [12,13]. While markedly increased circulatory levels of ACE2 activity after native rACE2 administration are capable of effectively lowering blood pressure in models of Ang II-induced hypertension [6,7,14] or renin overexpression in the circulation [15], their use is not suitable for treatment of other forms of kidney disease. For instance, in a diabetic model with local kidney but not systemic RAS over-activity [13], long-term augmentation of circulating ACE2 activity was not sufficient to alter glomerular pathology, GFR or albuminuria [13]. These observations provide the rationale for the development of shorter forms of ACE2 with a molecular size that render them filtrable by the kidney and, therefore, potentially useful therapeutically to amplify ACE2 activity in forms of kidney disease with an overactive local RAS in the kidney [13,16].

ACE2 is a tissue enzyme with low levels of activity in plasma [13,17]. In urine, enzymatic ACE2 activity is substantial [12,18,19]. Two distinctive ACE2-specific bands have been reported in mice and human urine [18–21]. One ACE2-immunoreactive band, at about 100–110 kD, corresponds to the expected molecular weight of native ACE2 at 110 kD [12]. This 100–110 kD ACE2-immunoreactive band is likely the result of shedding from the kidney apical tubular membrane, where ACE2 protein is abundantly expressed [22–24]. The other ACE2-imunoractive band detectable in mouse urine is of a lower size (~75 kD) and its origin and whether or not it is active remains unclear [12]. Based on these observations, we hypothesized that ACE2 variants of a shorter molecular size could be generated and still retain enzymatic activity. Accordingly, we sought to develop short ACE2 variants small enough, so that they could be filtered and subsequently re-absorbed by the kidney tubules. The kidney uptake of these small ACE2 variants, in turn, would foster Ang (1–7) formation from Ang II, thereby providing a novel and direct approach to target the kidney RAS, which is overactive in some forms of kidney disease, including acute kidney injury.

2. Methods

2.1. *Degradation of Native rACE2 in Urine and Kidney Lysates from ACE2KO Mice*

Kidney cortex total protein fractions were extracted as previously described [23,24]. Urines (500 µL; each containing 1–5 mg total protein) and kidney cortex lysates (each containing 1–2.5 mg total protein) from ACE2-deficient mice (C57BL/6 genetic background) were mixed with 50 mM HEPES, pH 7.4, NaCl (150 mM), Triton X-100 (0.5%), $ZnCl_2$ (12.5uM end-concentration) and incubated with 1 µg of native mouse mrACE2 (10 nM) at 37 °C constantly shaking at 800 rpm for up to 48 h. At specified time points of incubation, a 50 µL aliquot was taken and mixed with an equal volume of PBS buffer containing EDTA-free inhibitor cocktail (Roche, Basel, Switzerland) and immediately frozen. Each of the aliquots was then used for measuring ACE2 activity using Mca-APK-Dnp substrate and to detect ACE2 protein on Western blot. For Western blot, proteins were separated by SDS-PAGE, and transferred to nitrocellulose membranes. The membranes were blocked in non-fat dry milk (5–7% wt/vol) solubilized in Tris-buffered saline solution containing 0.1% Tween 20. The nitrocellulose membranes were incubated with primary anti-ACE2 antibody [AF3437 (R&D Systems, Minneapolis, MN, USA) or Ab38888 (Abcam, Cambridge, MA, USA)] and horseradish peroxidase-conjugated secondary antibody (Santa Cruz Biotechnology). The specificity of the ACE2 antibodies was confirmed by the absence of any bands in Western blot using ACE2KO samples, as previously reported [12]. Bands were visualized using chemiluminescence system (Super Signal Pico, Pierce, Rockford, IL, USA).

2.2. *Design of Short ACE2 Variants*

To generate short ACE2 fragments that exhibit ACE2 activity, a series of *ace2* DNA constructs of varying lengths were generated through truncation from the C terminus (Supplementary Materials Figure S1). The cDNA of short *ace2* was generated by PCR amplification using as a template the cDNA of the intact soluble mouse *ace2* (coding amino acids 1-740). To gradually shorten ACE2, we used specific primers that determine the length of the shorter ACE2 cDNA to be amplified and have compatibility with the expression vector restriction sites (pcDNA, Invitrogen, Carlsbad, CA, USA). The absence of mutations in the amplified cDNA was verified by sequencing. The plasmids with the inserted cDNAs of the short ACE2 variants were then expressed by transient transfection in HEK293 cells. ACE2 activity was measured in the conditioned culture medium using the fluorometric substrate Mca-APK-Dnp [7] (Supplementary Materials Figure S1). The native rACE2 that contained the full extracellular domain (1-740 AA) was used as a positive control. As a negative control, conditioned media from mock-transfected cells was used. In addition, Western blot using a polyclonal antibody raised against the entire extracellular domain of ACE2 (R&D Systems, AF3437) was used to detect the transgenes and confirm the molecular size of the over-expressed small ACE2 variants.

2.3. *Production and Purification of Selected Short ACE2 Variants*

Two short and enzymatically active ACE2 variants were selected for large scale production and purification. From stably transfected HEK cells, single clones were selected and expanded to 220 mL flasks. Conditioned serum-free medium from a clone of stably transfected HEK 293 cells that overexpressed the two short ACE2 variants was subjected to anion exchange Q-column on AKTA chromatography system in 25 mM Tris-HCl, pH 8.0 and eluted by applying increasing concentration of NaCl. Eluted fractions were screened for ACE2 activity was using Mca-APK-Dnp substrate. Fractions containing ACE2 activity were applied to SDS-PAGE, transferred to PVDF membrane and stained with Brilliant Blue to assess protein purity (Supplementary Materials Figure S2, showing ACE2-1-619 as an example).

2.4. *Enzyme Activity*

To compare the enzymatic activities of highly purified, enzymatically active short ACE2 proteins, we tested their ability to cleave its main natural substrate, Ang II (1–8), to form Ang (1–7). This was measured by an assay measuring the release of the C-terminal amino acid, phenylalanine, which is formed as a byproduct in the cleavage of Ang II (1-8) to Ang (1-7) [25]. The relative enzymatic potency of the short rACE2 fragments was determined by comparison with equivalent molar amounts of the intact rACE2 (740 AA long), which was used as a benchmark. For assessment of activity levels, the Michaelis–Menten model was used to derive the parameters of catalytic kinetics such as Km and Kcat [15].

2.5. *Acute Blood Pressure Response Ising Ang II-Induced Hypertension Mouse Model*

To study the effect of small rACE2 variants on Ang II-induced hypertension, we injected 10–20 week old male C57bl/6 mice i.p. with either vehicle (PBS), mouse rACE2 1-619 or mouse rACE2 1-605 (both 1 μg/g of body weight). After 1 h, mice were anesthetized with an i.p. injection of ketamine (150 mg/kg of body weight). Mice were then placed on a temperature-controlled platform for 10 min immediately after anesthesia was induced. Systolic BP was monitored noninvasively every 30 s for a period of 20 min, as previously described [6,7]. After five minutes of baseline SBP recording, acute hypertension in anesthetized mice was induced with an i.p. bolus injection of Ang II (0.2 mg/kg of body weight), and the SBP was monitored in a consecutive mode, at the same 30 s intervals throughout the remaining 15 min time period.

2.6. *Recovery of Urinary ACE2 after Recombinant ACE2 Infusion to ACE2-Deficient mice and the Effect of Blocking Tubular Reabsorption with L-lysine*

Immediately after the ACE2-deficient mice [26,27] voided urine (baseline urine collection), purified mouse recombinant ACE2 proteins were administered as a single i.v. bolus injection at a dose of 1.0 μg/g body weight. In order to determine the impact of ACE2 protein reabsorption in the proximal tubule, lysine, a blocker of proximal tubular reabsorption [28,29] was also administered (0.4 mg/g body weight) as a single i.p. injection. The timeline of the experiment was as follows: mice were weighted, followed by collection of baseline urine levels, and, within 5–10 min after voiding urine, mice were administered mrACE2 proteins in a single i.v. injection (0.2 mL/mouse, 1 µg/g BW). Then, immediately after i.v. injection, to collect urine, mice were placed for 2 h in urine collection cages with access to water and food. Afterwards, L-lysine was injected i.p. Urine was collected again within 2 h after the subsequent i.p. injection of the tubular reabsorption blocker, L-lysine (0.4 mg/g body weight).

2.7. *Pharmacokinetics Analysis*

The pharmacokinetic profiles of mouse rACE2 1-619 and 1-605 were assessed in Balb/c mice as compared to those of native mouse rACE2 1-740. The mice received a single i.v. or i.p. injection of each purified small rACE2 variant at a dose of 1 µg/g body weight. Blood samples were collected by tail bleeding either before or at a number of indicated time points after injection. Blood samples collected in heparinized capillaries were left undisturbed on ice, and plasma was isolated by centrifugation at 1850 g for 10 min at 4 °C. Mca-APK(Dnp) substrate (Bachem, Bubendorf, BL, Switzerland), PA) was used to measure ACE2 enzyme activity in plasma. The half-life ($t_{1/2}$), area under the plasma activity time curve and mean residence time of rACE2 species were calculated [15] using Prism 8 software (GraphPad, La Jolla, CA, USA).

2.8. *Statistical Analyses*

For comparison of two independent groups, a two-tailed t-test was used if data was normally distributed. The normality of the distribution was assessed using Shapiro-Wilk test. For not normally distributed data, a Mann–Whitney test was used. For comparison of more than two independent groups, one-way ANOVA was employed, followed by Tukey's multiple comparisons test. For comparisons of Ang (1–7) formation and SBP over time, 2-way Anova was used. A p-value < 0.05 was considered statistically significant. Results are presented as mean ± SE.

3. Results

3.1. *Degradation of Native rACE2 to Shorter Enzymatically Active ACE2 Truncates*

In mouse urine, two ACE2-immunoreactive bands are present [12]. In fresh kidney lysates, however, only a 100–110 kD ACE2 band was found to be consistent with the molecular size of native mouse ACE2 [12]. It was unclear whether the lower 75 kD band was a product of native ACE2 degradation or a distinct protein. We therefore decided to examine the possibility that the 75 kD band could be a proteolytic digestion product of the 110 kD ACE2 band. To study the hypothesis of ACE2 proteolysis, urines and kidneys from ACE2-deficient mice were spiked with native mrACE2 that we had generated, over-expressed and purified. This native recombinant mouse (mr)ACE2 has a molecular size of 100–110 kD (740 amino acid long) and contains a poly-His tag on its C-terminus [7]. Samples from ACE2 knockout mice were used to eliminate any interference arising from endogenous ACE2.

After spiking with the native 100–110 kD, mrACE2, ACE2KO urines and kidneys were incubated for up to 48 h at 37 °C to enable proteolysis of the native mrACE2 by urinary and kidney proteases, respectively. Small samples of the reaction mixture were taken for analysis at different time points within the 48 h incubation time. In ACE2KO [23,27] kidney lysates, the extended incubation resulted not only in the formation of a 75 kD band, but also a shorter ~60–70 kD ACE2 immunoreactive band that had significant ACE2 activity (Figure 1). The spiking of native mrACE2 into urine from ACE2 KO resulted similarly in the appearance of a 75 kD band and a gradual fading of the native 100–110 kD mrACE2. In kidney lysate, at 24 and 48 h of incubation, there was a band and no activity, which was not seen in the ACE2KO urine.

To confirm the consistency of the time course degradation studies just described, three different ACE2KO urines and three different kidney lysates were then incubated with the native 100–110 kD mrACE2 at 37 °C. The six hour timepoint was chosen for the robustness of the bands found in urine and kidney lysates. Consistent with data shown in Figure 1, the 100–110 kD native mrACE2 protein was converted in ACE2KO urines and kidney lysates into a band of an apparent molecular size of 75 kD (Figure 2). This 75 kD ACE2 immunoreactive band appeared to exhibit high specific enzyme activity, similar to that of the original 100–110 kD rACE2 band that has been used for spiking (Figure 2). This suggests that kidney and urine contain proteases capable of digesting native ACE2 into an enzymatically active truncate of ~75 kD.

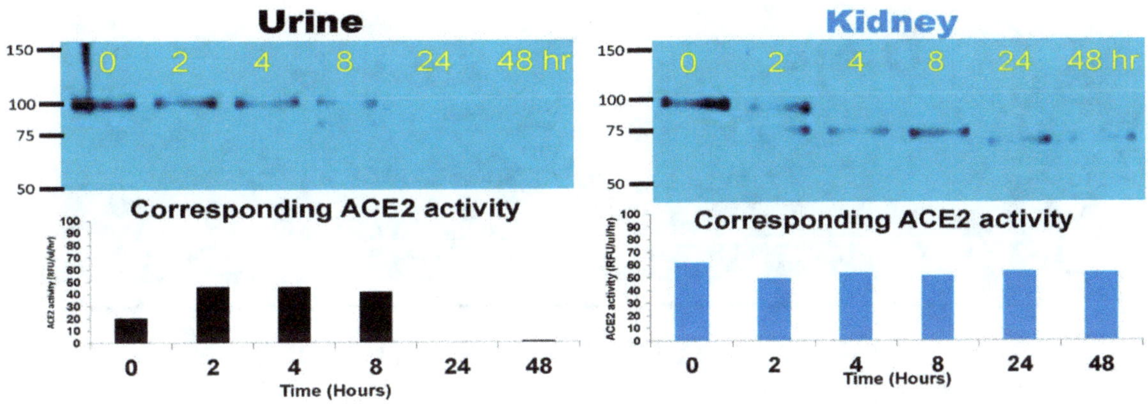

Figure 1. Native mouse recombinant (mr)ACE2 (100–110 kD) was spiked into ACEKO urine (**Left**) or kidney cortex lysate (10 nM mrACE2/~1 mg total protein of the lysate) from one ACE2KO mouse (**Right**) and incubated at 37 °C for 48 h. Spiked native mrACE2 samples at 0, 2, 4, 8, 24 and 48 h of incubation were subsequently probed in Western blot. **Left Panel.** Western blot image of ACE2KO urine spiked with native mrACE2 shows gradual weakening of the 100–110 kD native mrACE2 band and the appearance of smaller 75 kD ACE2 immunoreactive band for up to 8 h. At 24 and 48 h, no ACE2 immunoreactive bands and no ACE2 activity are detectable anymore. **Right Panel.** Western blot image shows the disappearance of the 100–110 kD mrACE2 band and, first the appearance of a smaller 75 kD ACE2 immunoreactive band, and then a ~60–70 kD band in kidney lysates from ACE2KO mice. In the lower panel, ACE2 activity is depicted showing similar enzyme activities of the 75 and ~60 kD bands versus the original 110 kD mrACE2 band throughout the incubation period; a single time-course experiment for kidney and for urine is shown.

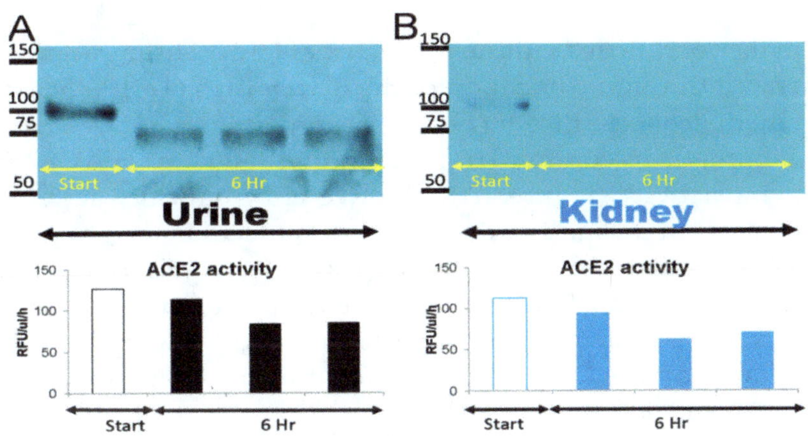

Figure 2. Native mouse recombinant (mr)ACE2 1-740 AA (100–110kD) was spiked into urine (10 nM mrACE2/~0.5 mL urine) (**A**) and kidney cortex lysates (10 nM mrACE2/~1 mg total protein of the lysate) from three ACE2KO mice (**B**) and incubated at 37 °C for 6 h. Spiked mrACE2 samples at 0 h (Start) and at 6 h of incubation were subsequently probed in Western blot using an anti-ACE2 antibody. Western blot image shows the disappearance of the 100–110 kD mrACE2 band and the appearance of a smaller 75 kD ACE2 immunoreactive band at 6 h in urine and kidney lysates from ACE2KO mice. In the lower panel, ACE2 activity is depicted showing the enzyme activity of the 75 kD band and the spiked original 100–110 kD native mrACE2 band; urines and kidney lysates from three independent degradation experiments.

The native mrACE2 that was used for spiking contains a C-terminal 10-His tag. Re-probing of the membranes with anti-His antibody revealed a band of the size of the original native mrACE2 at 100–110 kDa but failed to detect the lower band at ~75 kD (Figure 3). While N-terminal cleavage of native ACE2 cannot be disproved, this finding clearly shows that proteolysis by mouse urine and kidneys takes place at the C-terminal site.

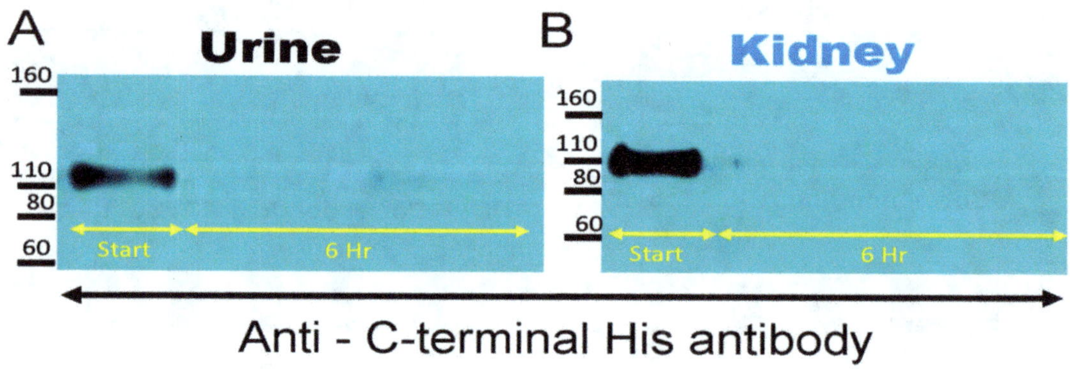

Figure 3. The native mrACE2 spiked into urine (**A**) and kidney (**B**) samples from ACE2KO mice had a c-terminal 10-His tag. The Western blot membrane shown in Figure 2 was re-probed using an anti-His antibody. Western blot image shows disappearance of the 100–110 kD mrACE2 band and no appearance of a smaller 75 kD ACE2 immunoreactive band in urine and kidney lysates from ACE2KO mice, suggesting the proteolysis of native mrACE2 from its c-terminal end; urines and kidney lysates from three independent degradation experiments.

3.2. Design of Small ACE2 Variants and Demonstration of Their Enzyme Activity and Molecular Size

Based on the above findings, we then generated C-terminally truncated recombinant mouse ACE2 proteins 1-522, 1-605 and 1-619 (see Methods and Supplementary Materials Figure S1). The molecular size and sequences of three short ACE2 variants, 1-522, 1-605 and 1-619, are provided in the supplement (Supplementary Figure S3). The enzyme activity of those variants was evaluated in conditioned medium and compared to the over-expressed native rACE2 1-740, which was used as a benchmark.

Enzyme activity in the conditioned culture media, from HEK cells transiently transfected with the ACE2 constructs generated through truncation of the C terminus (1-619 AA and 1-605 AA), was at least as high as in the media collected from cells overexpressing the native rACE2 1-740, as judged by the kinetic slope (Figure 4). In contrast, transfection with a shorter ACE2 fragment (1-522 AA) did not show any enzyme activity (Figure 4A). The two enzymatically active short ACE2 variants (619 and 605) appeared as a single band at the apparent molecular weight of ~70 kDa, as expected from the amino acid sequence deducted using the Expasy Informatics tool (Figure 4B and Figure S3). The enzymatically inactive variant 1-522 appeared, in addition to the expected size of ~50–60 kD, in oligomerized forms of 2–3 bands of higher molecular weight (Figure 4B). This suggests that the minimal length requirement on the C-terminal end for murine ACE2 to be enzymatically active is contained between AA 522 and 605.

3.3. Enzyme Activities and Kinetic Constants of Purified Short Recombinant ACE2 Variants Using Angiotensin II as a Substrate

Clonal HEK293 cell lines stably expressing the two ACE2 variants (1-605 and 1-619) were established, and the recombinant proteins were purified from the culture medium by strong anion-exchange chromatography, as shown in Supplementary Figure S1A [see details in Methods]. Purified native rACE2 1-740 [7] was used as a control to compare the enzymatic activities of the two short ACE2 variants. The catalytic efficiency of the two short ACE2 variants (Kcat/Km) to cleave the synthetic fluorogenic ACE2 substrate, Mca-APK-(Dnp) [7], was higher as compared to native rACE2.

In fact, for the rACE2 1-619, it was four-fold and for rACE2 1-605 three-fold higher as compared to enzymatic activity of the native rACE2 1-740 (Figure 5A). Using Ang II, the natural substrate of ACE2, catalytic efficiencies [K_{cat}/K_m (M^{-1} s^{-1})] were found to be not different for native rACE2 1-740 (1.97×10^6) and for the two shorter proteins rACE2 1-619 (1.02×10^6) and rACE2 1-605 (1.22×10^6) (Figure 5B) (n = 3–4 experiments for each protein).

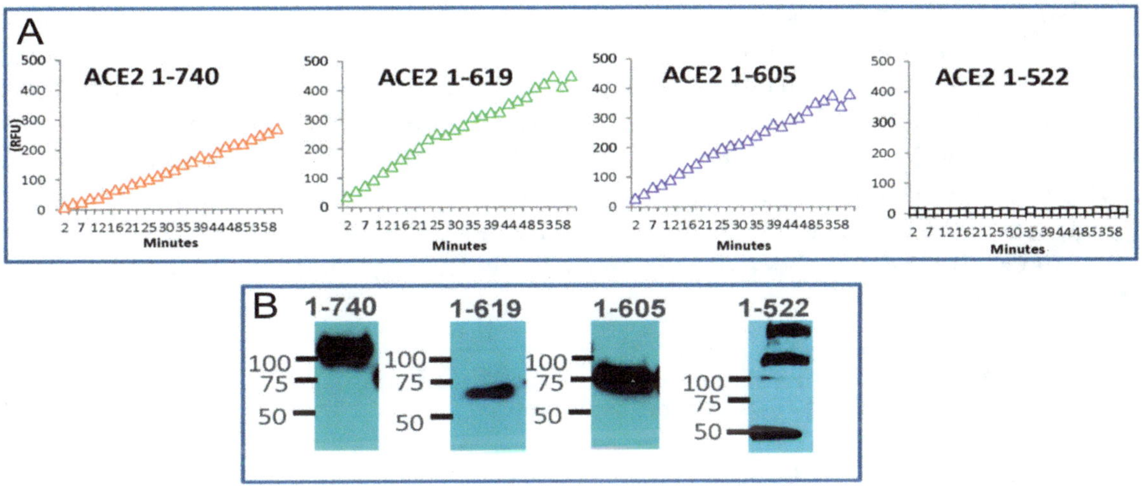

Figure 4. Enzyme activity and molecular size of shorter recombinant ACE2 protein variants. Relative activity of mouse small recombinant ACE2variants and ACE2 protein detection in conditioned media collected 40–60 h after transfection. (**A**) The cleavage rate of the synthetic fluorogenic substrate Mca-AKP(Dnp) over one hour (shown in relative fluorescence units—RFU) for native rACE2 and small ACE2 variants. Similar to native soluble mrACE2 1-740, mrACE2 variants, 1-619- and 1-605- showed enzymatic activity, respectively, while 1-522 did not exhibit any ACE2 activity. (**B**) Presence and estimated molecule size were confirmed by Western Blot with antibody against ACE2 ectodomain.

A

rACE2	Km (um)	Vmax (min^{-1})	K_{cat}/K_m
1-740	7.06	1195	169
1-619	7.67	7139	931
1-605	6.63	4289	647

B

rACE2	K_m (um)	K_{cat} (s^{-1})	K_{cat}/K_m ($M^{-1}s^{-1}$)
1-740	21.19	41.71	1.97×10^6
1-619	50.45	51.50	1.02×10^6
1-605	32.93	40.03	1.22×10^6

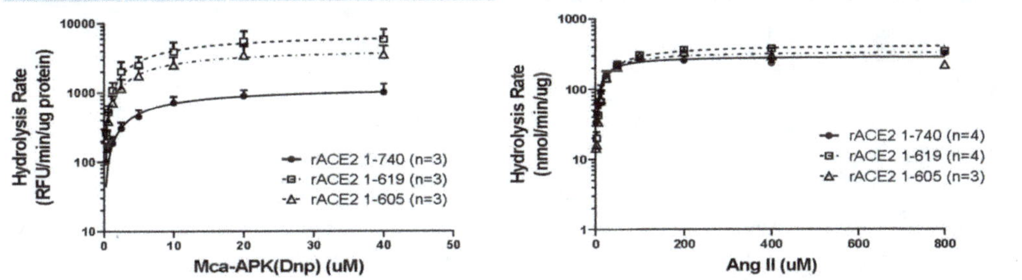

Figure 5. Summary of ACE2-activity assessment of highly purified mouse recombinant ACE2 1-619 and ACE2 1-605 compared to native rACE2 1-740 with a synthetic fluorogenic substrate Mca-APK(Dnp) (**A**) and with the natural substrate, angiotensin II (**B**). A higher catalytic activity (Kcat/Km) was found by cleavage of Mca-APK(Dnp) for rACE2 1-619 and rACE2 1-605 than for native rACE2 1-740 (**Panel A**). The catalytic efficiency to convert Angiotensin II to Angiotensin (1–7) (Kcat/Km) was similar for native rACE2 1-740 and for the small rACE2 variants 1-619 and 1-605 (**Panel B**). For assessment of activity levels, a Michaelis–Menten model was used to derive the parameters of catalytic kinetics such as Km and Kcat. The values were calculated from three to four independent experiments.

3.4. Pharmacokinetics

Pharmacokinetic profiles were determined in mice for rACE2 (1-619) and rACE2 (1-605) as compared to rACE2 (1-740) using the Mca-APK(Dnp) assay to measure ACE2 activity in serum collected in a time series. Following a single i.v. injection of each the rACE2 forms (1 μg/g BW) (see Methods), each had a relatively short distribution phase in the blood, followed by a longer elimination phase (Figure 6, Table 1). The distribution phase half-life of the 1-605 (58 ± 24 min) was not different from that of 1-619 (19 ± 5 min) and of native rACE2 (13 ± 2 min). Both 1-605 and 1-619 had a three times longer elimination phase half-life of 4.0 ± 0.5 ($p = 0.054$) and 4.2 ± 1.07 h ($p = 0.029$), respectively, compared to 1.35 ± 0.21 h for 1-740 (Table 1). The calculated area under the curve, which reflects the overall in vivo pharmacological efficacy, was also higher (around 4–5 times) for the two small rACE2 variants ($p < 0.05$ for both) as compared to native rACE2 1-740 (Table 1). In addition, the maximum serum activity of the two short ACE2 proteins was much higher than that of native rACE2 (Figure 6). The mean residence time was also higher for the rACE2 1-605 than for native rACE2 ($p = 0.038$), while for rACE2 1-619 variant the difference did not reach statistical significance (Table 1).

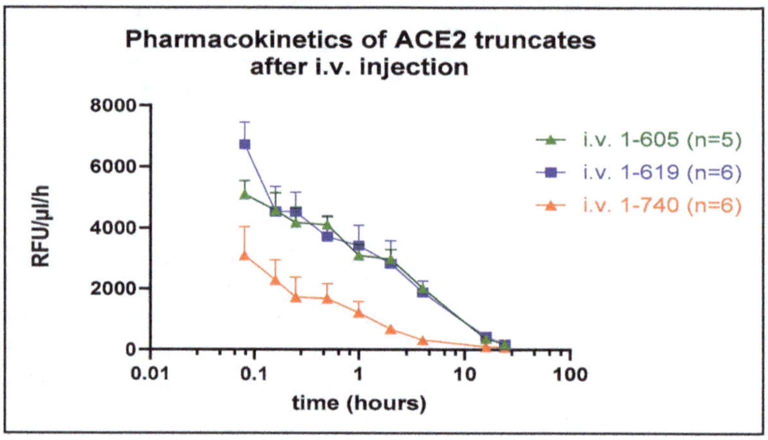

(A)

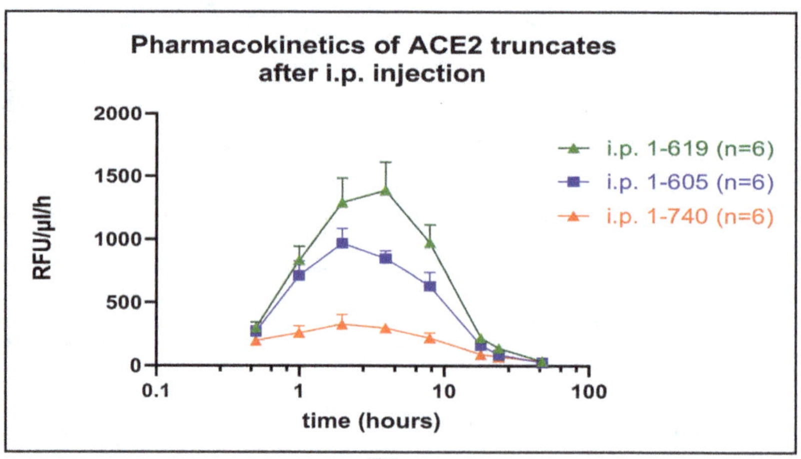

(B)

Figure 6. Pharmacokinetics of small ACE2 variants in vivo after i.v. (**A**) or i.p. injection (**B**). Wild-type mice (n = 5–6 per experiment) were injected with 1 μg/g BW of native murine rACE2 1-740 (reference protein) or mouse small rACE2 variants 1-619 and 1-605. Venous blood was collected at defined time points after bolus rACE2 injection and ACE2 activity measured using Mca-APK-Dnp fluorogenic substrate; RFU—relative fluorescence unit.

Table 1. Mean ± SE pharmacokinetic parameters of native rACE2 1-740 and the small ACE2 variants 1-619 and 1-605 in blood circulation in mice after **i.v.** administration.

	ACE2 1-740 (n = 6)	ACE2 1-619 (n = 6)	ACE2 1-605 (n = 5)
Distribution Phase ($t_{1/2\alpha}$) (min)	13 ± 2	19 ± 5	58 ± 24
Elimination Phase ($t_{1/2\beta}$) (h)	1.35 ± 0.21	4.2 ± 1.07 *	4.0 ± 0.5
AUC	6437 ± 1639	27,636 ± 6297 *	28,257 ± 1901 *
MRT (h)	0.86 ± 0.12	2.20 ± 0.8	3.30 ± 0.72 *

* denotes $p < 0.05$ or $p < 0.01$ vs. ACE2 1-740.

Following i.p. infusion, a method of delivery used in previous studies [6,7,15], as expected, there was a delay in achieving peak blood activity levels for both short rACE2s (1-619 and 1-605) and for rACE2-1-740 (Figure 6, Table 2) compared to levels obtained using i.v. administration (Table 1). Similar to the i.v. injections, after i.p. administration the maximum serum activity and the calculated AUC of native rACE2 1-740 was lower than that of the two shorter ACE2 variants (Figure 6). The elimination phase half-life and the mean residence time, however, were not lower compared to the two shorter ACE2 proteins (Table 2).

Table 2. Mean ± SE pharmacokinetic parameters of native rACE2 1-740 and ACE2 1-619 and 1-605 truncates in blood circulation in mice after **i.p.** administration.

	ACE2 1-740 (n = 6)	ACE2 1-619 (n = 6)	ACE2 1-605 (n = 6)
Distribution Phase ($t_{1/2\alpha}$) (min)	123 ± 47	70 ± 8	62 ± 9
Elimination Phase ($t_{1/2\beta}$) (h)	8.68 ± 0.79	5.62 ± 0.32 *	6.77 ± 0.67
AUC	5145 ± 683	17,792 ± 2288 *	11,753 ± 1250 *
MRT (h)	15.0 ± 1.71	14.9 ± 1.16	12.9 ± 0.95

* denotes $p < 0.05$, $p < 0.01$ or $p < 0.01$ vs. ACE2 1-740.

Overall, the small ACE2 variants 1-605 and 1-619 exhibited a higher serum activity than native rACE2 1-740 both after i.v and i.p. administration, and the 1-605 variants had the longest circulatory residence time after i.v injection (Tables 1 and 2).

3.5. *Demonstration of In Vivo Activity as Reflected by Blood Pressure-Lowering Effect of Short rACE2 Variants during Acute Ang II Infusion in Mice*

The effect of short rACE2 on acute hypertension was examined in a model of angiotensin II-induced hypertension as previously described by us [6,7,15]. Mice were pretreated with either vehicle (PBS), rACE2 1-605 or rACE2 1-619, by a single i.p. injection at 1 h before receiving a bolus injection of Ang II (Figure 7). Blood pressure in mice was monitored continuously under light anesthesia in a time series at 30 s intervals that started five minutes before Ang II injection (see Methods). The injection of Ang II resulted in a rapid increase in systolic blood pressure (peak of 204 ± 5 and 169 ± 8 mm Hg) from a baseline (124 ± 9 and 114 ± 9 mm Hg) in the control groups that had received PBS as pre-injection vehicle (Figure 7A,B, respectively). This increase in SBP was efficiently mitigated to a similar extent in the both rACE2 treatment groups (Figure 7A,B).

3.6. *Recovery of Urinary ACE2 Activity after Administration of Short rACE2 Variants to ACE2-Deficient Mice*

Since normally ACE2 is present in the urine, to better assess whether there is any increase in urinary ACE2 activity after administration of short ACE2 variants, we injected them to ACE2 deficient (ACE2-/-) mice [26,27]. Urinary ACE2 activity was measured using the Mca–APK–Dnp fluorogenic substrate.

As expected, no enzymatic ACE2 activity was detectable in baseline urines collected before infusion to ACE2-deficient mice ((−0.1 ± 0.2 RFU/μg creat/h, n = 5). The i.v. infusion of 1-619 and

1-605 resulted in increased ACE2 activity in mice ($n = 5$) to about the same extent (4.5 ± 1.8 and 5.1 ± 1.9, respectively). Urine was collected 1–2 h after the injection. Western blots, moreover, showed an ACE2-immunoreactive band after the rACE2 1-619 i.v. infusion (Figure 8).

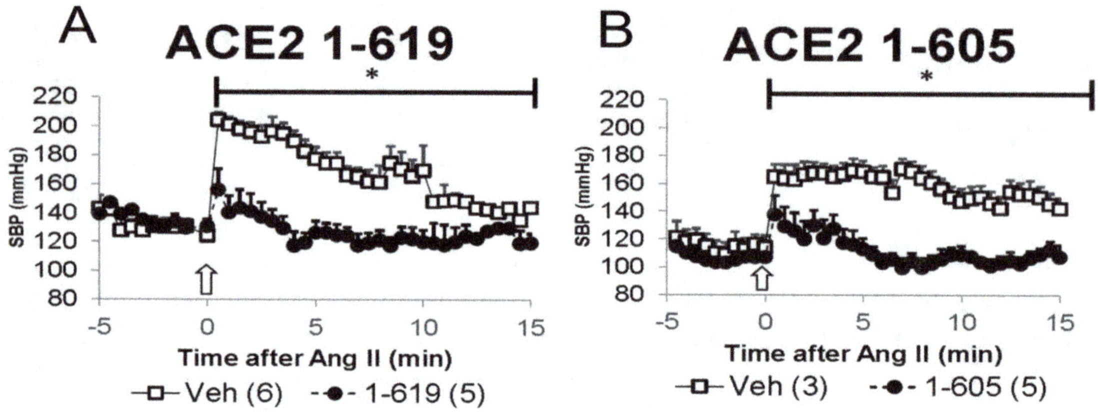

Figure 7. Pre-infusion of 1-619 (**A**) or 1-605 (**B**) rACE2 variants (filled circles) cause a faster recovery from acute Ang II-induced hypertension as compared to respective mice pre-infused with PBS as a vehicle (Veh; empty squares). *Y*-axis is SBP and *X*-axis indicates time (min) from Ang II bolus (arrow; 0.2 µg/g BW). Two-way ANOVA over time was used for comparisons of the experimental groups; * denotes $p < 0.01$.

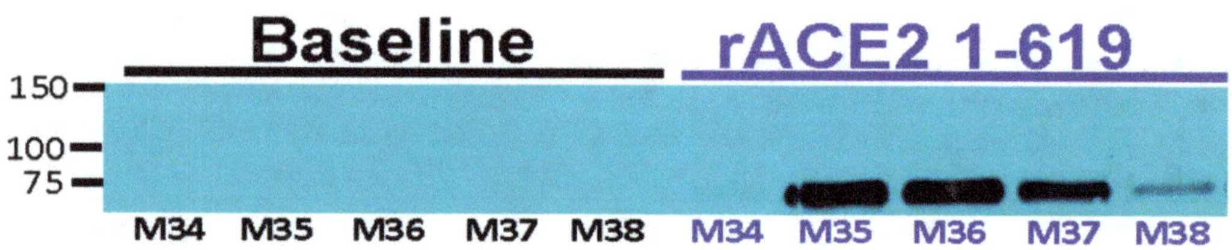

Figure 8. Western blot of urines collected before (Baseline) and after i.v. bolus of ACE2 1-619 variant (0–2 h) from five ACE2-deficient mice, showing an ACE2-immunoreactive band at the expected size of ~70 kD, consistent with the molecular size of the short rACE2 1-619 variant after, but not before, the injection. M34-M38 are ID numbers of the individual ACE2 deficient mice ($n = 5$) from which urines were obtained at baseline and within 2 h after mrACE2 1-619 infusion. Equal volumes (36 µL) of urines with similar creatinine concentrations (~10–20 mg/dL) were loaded per well.

3.7. Glomerular Filtration and Kidney Uptake of Small rACE2 Variants in ACE2-Deficient Mice

To examine whether, after glomerular filtration, a tubular uptake of filtered rACE2s takes place, ACE2-deficient mice were infused with either rACE2-1-605, 1-619 or the native rACE2 1-740 as negative control. Subsequently, L-lysine (a blocker of proximal tubular protein reabsorption) was injected i.p. (Figure 9).

Before injection and after native rACE2 injection, urinary ACE2 activity was not detectable, consistent with the lack of glomerular filtration of the large native rACE2. The tubular reabsorption blocker, L-lysine, moreover, did not result in an appreciable gain in urinary ACE2 activity (Figure 9).

In contrast, both small recombinant variants (1-619 and 1-605) when infused to ACE2-deficient mice, resulted in a clear gain in urinary ACE2 activity. Blocking with L-lysine further increased urinary ACE2 activity, demonstrating that the two truncates are both filtered and reabsorbed by the tubules (Figure 9). In the aggregate, these data show that rACE2-605 and rACE2-619 must undergo glomerular filtration and subsequent proximal tubular reabsorption.

To examine whether kidneys from ACE2-deficient mice infused with ACE2 1-619 gain substantial ACE2 activity, the ACE2 619 truncate was injected and kidneys harvested after infusion (Figure 10). In isolated kidney cortices from ACE2-deficient mice, ACE2 activity was not detectable in either in PBS- or rACE2 1-740-infused mice. In contrast, kidney cortex ACE2 activity after rACE2 1-619 was clearly detectable (2.7 ± 0.7 RFU/μg prot./h) and significantly higher than in PBS (0.2 ± 0.1 RFU/μg prot./h, $p < 0.05$) and rACE2 1-740 groups (−0.2 ± 0.8 RFU/μg prot./h, $p < 0.01$) (Figure 10A). In ex vivo experiments, kidneys from 1-619-infused mice, when spiked with Ang II, also exhibited significantly higher Ang 1–7 formation than kidneys from PBS-mice ($p < 0.001$) or native rACE2- 1-740-infused mice ($p < 0.01$) by 2-way Anova (Figure 10B). This shows that kidney uptake translates into increased kidney ACE2 activity and capability of Ang II to Ang 1–7 conversion.

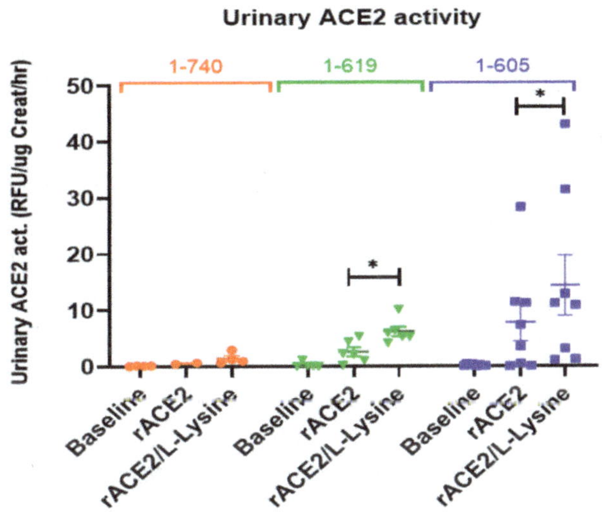

Figure 9. Glomerular filtration and tubular uptake of 1-605- (blue, $n = 8$) and 1-619-mACE2 (green, $n = 6$) as compared to native 1-740 rACE2 (red, $n = 4$) in ACE2-deficient mice. Immediately after voiding (baseline urine collection), ACE2-deficient mice were injected i.v. with 1 μg/g BW rACE2. Urine was collected again within the first 2 h after ACE2-injection ("rACE2"). L-Lysine was injected i.p. two hours after rACE2-injection and urine was collected within the next 2 h. ("rACE2/L-Lysine"). Recovery of ACE2-activity in the urine normalized to creatinine excretion is depicted. Repeated measures one-way ANOVA was used for comparisons within the experimental groups, followed by post-hoc analysis; * denotes $p < 0.05$ or $p < 0.01$.

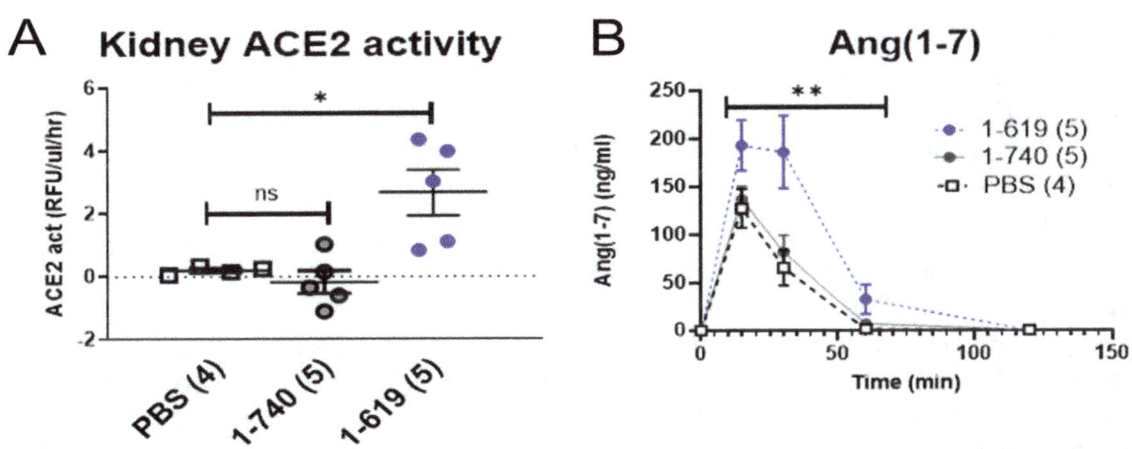

Figure 10. ACE2-deficient mice were infused i.v. with a bolus of PBS, native mouse rACE2 (1-740) or mouse rACE2 1-619 (1 μg/g BW). After 2 h, mice were perfused with saline and the kidneys removed. (**A**) A gain in kidney ACE2 activity was only appreciated in 1-619-infused mice. (**B**) In an ex vivo setting, kidney lysates (2 mg) were incubated with Ang II (10^{-5}M) to assess Ang 1–7 formation over time by 2-way Anova. Higher Ang 1–7 formation was seen in 1-619 mice as compared to the two other groups; ** denotes $p < 0.01$ against 1-740 and $p < 0.001$ against PBS.

4. Discussion

In this study, we describe the design and testing of novel recombinant mouse ACE2 proteins of a molecular size (~69–71 kD) much shorter than the native ACE2. The two short ACE2 variants are very active systemically, but of a molecular size short enough to render them filterable through the kidney glomerular filtration barrier. These short variants, moreover, are re-absorbable by the kidney tubules and thus capable of amplifying kidney ACE2 activity and fostering the formation of Ang 1–7 from Ang II. This feature should make them attractive to combat a vast array of kidney diseases where the RAS is over-active, such as acute kidney injury.

We and others have previously identified two main ACE2-immunoreactive bands in mouse urine [12,18–21]. One band at about 110 kD corresponded to the molecular weight of native ACE2 and was likely a product of shedding, likely mediated by the metalloprotease ADAM17 [20,30,31] from the kidney apical tubular membrane, where ACE2 is abundantly expressed [12,31]. These observations prompted us to investigate if these shorter forms of about 75 kD are enzymatically active and, if so, to design shorter ones and test them for potential activity in vitro and in vivo. Here, we demonstrate that the natural ACE2 of 100–110 kDa can be degraded in the urine and kidney to shorter ACE2 fragments which retain ACE2 enzyme activity. That the 75 kD ACE2 band is a result of a proteolytic cleavage of the 110 kDa ACE2 was determined by demonstrating that a recombinantly generated native recombinant, ACE2 110 kDa, can be digested by kidney and urine proteases to a shorter band of similar size to the 75 kDa ACE2 fragment that was naturally observed in the urine (Figures 1 and 2). In these experiments, we were also able to ascertain that the C-terminal end is the site, which is removed from native rACE2 without a loss in enzyme activity (Figure 3). This finding is consistent with crystallographic and homology studies for human ACE2 that indicated that on the C-terminal end there is a fairly large structural portion that has non-enzymatic function [11,32].

We next proceeded to demonstrate that longer exposure of the 110 kDa native rACE2 to proteases from kidneys resulted in the formation of even a shorter ~60–70 kDa band and showed that it still had very high ACE2 enzymatic activity (Figure 1). By contrast, in the urine, extended incubation of native rACE2 ultimately led to the disappearance of the 75 kDa ACE2 band and a loss of ACE2 activity. This suggests that, unlike the kidney, in which ACE2 truncates can prevail for an extended period of time, the urine is equipped with a repertoire of proteases that inactivate ACE2 by digesting it to small inactive fragments. We did not investigate, however, the specific proteases responsible for the cleavage of ACE2 or the cleavage site. Such studies should be done in the future.

Based on the findings of the ex vivo proteolysis of native rACE2, we then generated short ACE2 variants of varying lengths which were gradually truncated from the C-terminal end of ACE2. The shortest active variant was 605 AA long (~69 kDa) and all other longer variants exhibited enzymatic activity as well. In contrast, the short variant of 522 AA was enzymatically inactive (Figure 4). From this, our preliminary conclusion is that the minimum length requirement for ACE2 to be active has to be somewhere between 522 and 605 AA.

The two active short proteins 1-619 and 1-605 were then purified and their in vivo effects were compared with the native rACE2 and the half-lives of the injected recombinant proteins were evaluated (Figure 6; Tables 1 and 2). Compared to the native rACE2's blood half-life of 1.4 h after i.v. administration, ACE2 1-619 and 1-605 had a substantially extended half-life of around 4 h. In addition, the area under the curve for the short ACE2 proteins was about 4–5-fold higher than that of the native rACE2 after i.v. injection (Table 1) and 2–3-fold higher after i.p. administration (Table 2). It is also noteworthy that, with the same dose, the peak plasma ACE2 activity after the infusion of both short variants was substantially higher than that of native rACE2 (Figure 6), further suggesting a better pharmacological profile, as compared to the native rACE2 form. It should be noted, however, that this pharmacokinetic profile was based on ACE2 activity assessed against an artificial substrate. The catalytic efficiency towards the artificial substrate, likewise, was much higher than that of the native ACE2 (Figure 5A). In contrast, when the catalytic efficiency was assessed using the natural substrate,

Ang II, then there were no significant differences between the short ACE2 variants and the native ACE2 (Figure 5B).

To test the systemic effect of the short ACE2 variants 1-605 and 1-619 in vivo, we used an established protocol for acute Ang II-induced hypertension [6,7]. Using this protocol previously, we have demonstrated that lowering plasma Ang II using native rACE2 effectively mitigated an increase in blood pressure caused by Ang II administration [7]. Similar to native ACE2 [6,7], both small ACE2 variants blunted the peak increase in blood pressure after Ang II infusion which normalized faster within five minutes or less. This shows that both small ACE2 variants efficiently degrade the excess of systemic circulating Ang II, thereby enhancing blood pressure recovery. Having demonstrated the systemic effect on blood pressure, we further studied whether both small ACE2 variants have any added effect to their systemic action at the local urinary and kidney level. ACE2 is normally present in the urine, and to better assess whether there is any increase in urinary ACE2 activity after administration of the short ACE2 variants, ACE2-deficient mice were used. In contrast to native rACE2 injection, both small recombinant variants resulted in a gain in urinary ACE2 activity. L-lysine, a tubular reabsorption blocker [28,29], further increased urinary ACE2 activity, suggesting that the two short ACE2 variants are both filtered and reabsorbed by the tubules. That the short ACE2 protein variant that is taken up by the kidney is indeed enzymatically active was shown by the presence of ACE2 activity in kidneys from ACE2 deficient mice that had been injected with ACE2 1-619. In addition, kidney cortex lysates from ACE2 1-619-injected mice were able to form significantly more Ang (1–7) from Ang II than kidney lysates from PBS- or native rACE2-injected mice. In the aggregate, these data show that mouse short ACE2 variants are active, and sufficiently small to be filtered by the kidney and, moreover, capable of increasing kidney ACE2 activity to the extent that Ang 1–7 formation from Ang II is increased (Figure 10). As a limitation of this study, we acknowledge that our studies were not performed in a blinded fashion and that a potential bias in the measurements of activity of ACE2 in the urine and at the kidney level were not prevented by stratified randomization of the treated animals. In this regard, the ACE2 knockout allowed us to demonstrate urine and kidney activity after injection of our short ACE2 variants relatively easily and show that this was not the case after the infusion of native ACE2. The use of native rACE2 as a control enhances the results obtained with the novel short ACE2 variants and is a strength of our design. Even though the pharmacokinetic data show the clear superiority of short rACE2 variants as compared to the native rACE2, we caution to emphasize that this effect may be dependent on the artificial substrate used to measure ACE2 activity.

Knowing that the kidney ACE2 activity can be increased by the administration of short ACE2 variants, the natural question is under what clinical conditions such kidney amplification could be useful. We speculate that disease conditions where the local kidney RAS is over-active would be the natural target. Several studies using diabetic models show activation of the RAS locally within the kidney by glucose, including an increase in Ang II production [33–36]. Additional evidence comes from findings of increased RAS components in the kidney and urines from rodent models of diabetic kidney disease (DKD) and in patients with DKD [16,37] and non-diabetic CKD [38,39]. There is a need for new approaches to counteract RAS overactivity that expand and improve on the existing ones which are based on blockade of Ang II formation or action. We have chosen ACE2 as a therapeutic target because this enzyme cleaves Ang II to form Ang (1–7) with the highest efficiency [6,26,40].

There are several potential indications of our small ACE2 variants for the treatment of kidney disease. In particular, we think that Acute Kidney Injury (AKI) may benefit from the administration of our small ACE2 variants as a way to calm down the kidney RAS, which is overactive in this clinical syndrome. The pathogenesis of AKI is complex, often involving hemodynamic and non-hemodynamic mechanisms [41–44]. Alterations in the RAS have been shown to contribute to the development of AKI and are associated with adverse outcomes both in experimental and clinical studies [45–50]. Several components of the kidney RAS, such as urine Angiotensinogen and Ang II, the main active peptide, are increased in experimental AKI caused by ischemia-reperfusion AKI [45–47,51–56] ACE inhibitors (ACEi) and angiotensin receptor antagonists (ARBs) may attenuate renal inflammation, injury and improve renal function in the ischemia-reperfusion model of AKI [57–60]. Intrarenal Ang II is reportedly elevated in AKI, which may worsen kidney tissue injury independently of its hemodynamic effect that helps maintain renal circulation [61–63]. Based on these considerations, we are currently studying the effect of ACE2 1-619 in a mouse model of AKI.

In summary, we have developed short ACE2 variants with improved pharmacokinetic properties, as compared to the native rACE2. The short ACE2 protein variants, unlike the intact ACE2 protein, undergo glomerular filtration and tubular uptake. The kidney uptake of enzymatically active short ACE2 variants can enhance the local formation of Ang (1–7) from Ang II. The administration of active small ACE2 variants offers therapeutic potential in the prevention and treatment of acute kidney injury by directly reducing kidney RAS overactivity while retaining their systemic effect on ACE2 activity amplification.

Author Contributions: J.W. and D.B. conceived and designed the research J.W. and A.S. performed experiments; J.W., A.S., and D.B. analyzed data; J.W., A.S. and D.B. interpreted results of experiments; J.W., A.S. and D.B. edited and revised manuscript; J.W. and A.S. prepared figures; D.B. and J.W. wrote the manuscript; J.W., A.S. and D.B. approved final version of manuscript.

Acknowledgments: We would like to thank Minghao Ye for his support and oversight of our lab activities, Pan Liu and Jing Jin for their advice and help in purifying proteins and the George M. O'Brien Kidney Research Core Center (NU GoKidney) supported by the award P30 DK114857 of the National Institute of Diabetes and Digestive and Kidney Diseases).

References

1. Batlle, D.; Wysocki, J.; Soler, M.J.; Ranganath, K. Angiotensin-converting enzyme 2: Enhancing the degradation of angiotensin II as a potential therapy for diabetic nephropathy. *Kidney Int.* **2012**, *81*, 520–528. [CrossRef] [PubMed]
2. Ortiz-Melo, D.I.; Gurley, S.B. Angiotensin converting enzyme 2 and the kidney. *Curr. Opin. Nephrol. Hypertens.* **2016**, *25*, 59–66. [CrossRef] [PubMed]
3. Santos, R.A.; Simoes e Silva, A.C.; Maric, C.; Silva, D.M.; Machado, R.P.; de Buhr, I.; Heringer-Walther, S.; Pinheiro, S.V.; Lopes, M.T.; Bader, M.; et al. Angiotensin-(1-7) is an endogenous ligand for the G protein-coupled receptor Mas. *Proc. Natl. Acad. Sci. USA* **2003**, *100*, 8258–8263. [CrossRef] [PubMed]
4. Zimmerman, D.; Burns, K.D. Angiotensin-(1-7) in kidney disease: A review of the controversies. *Clin. Sci.* **2012**, *123*, 333–346. [CrossRef] [PubMed]
5. Ferrario, C.M.; Jessup, J.; Gallagher, P.E.; Averill, D.B.; Brosnihan, K.B.; Ann Tallant, E.; Smith, R.D.; Chappell, M.C. Effects of renin-angiotensin system blockade on renal angiotensin-(1-7) forming enzymes and receptors. *Kidney Int.* **2005**, *68*, 2189–2196. [CrossRef] [PubMed]
6. Wysocki, J.; Ye, M.; Rodriguez, E.; Gonzalez-Pacheco, F.R.; Barrios, C.; Evora, K.; Schuster, M.; Loibner, H.; Brosnihan, K.B.; Ferrario, C.M.; et al. Targeting the degradation of angiotensin II with recombinant angiotensin-converting enzyme 2: Prevention of angiotensin II-dependent hypertension. *Hypertension* **2010**, *55*, 90–98. [CrossRef] [PubMed]
7. Ye, M.; Wysocki, J.; Gonzalez-Pacheco, F.R.; Salem, M.; Evora, K.; Garcia-Halpin, L.; Poglitsch, M.; Schuster, M.; Batlle, D. Murine recombinant angiotensin-converting enzyme 2: Effect on angiotensin II-dependent hypertension and distinctive angiotensin-converting enzyme 2 inhibitor characteristics on rodent and human angiotensin-converting enzyme 2. *Hypertension* **2012**, *60*, 730–740. [CrossRef]
8. Li, N.; Zimpelmann, J.; Cheng, K.; Wilkins, J.A.; Burns, K.D. The role of angiotensin converting enzyme 2 in the generation of angiotensin 1-7 by rat proximal tubules. *Am. J. Physiol. Ren. Physiol.* **2005**, *288*, F353–F362. [CrossRef] [PubMed]

9. Ross, M.J.; Nangaku, M. ACE2 as therapy for glomerular disease: The devil is in the detail. *Kidney Int.* **2017**, *91*, 1269–1271. [CrossRef] [PubMed]
10. Jiang, F.; Yang, J.; Zhang, Y.; Dong, M.; Wang, S.; Zhang, Q.; Liu, F.F.; Zhang, K.; Zhang, C. Angiotensin-converting enzyme 2 and angiotensin 1-7: Novel therapeutic targets. *Nat. Rev. Cardiol.* **2014**, *11*, 413–426. [CrossRef]
11. Towler, P.; Staker, B.; Prasad, S.G.; Menon, S.; Tang, J.; Parsons, T.; Ryan, D.; Fisher, M.; Williams, D.; Dales, N.A.; et al. ACE2 X-ray structures reveal a large hinge-bending motion important for inhibitor binding and catalysis. *J. Biol. Chem.* **2004**, *279*, 17996–18007. [CrossRef] [PubMed]
12. Wysocki, J.; Garcia-Halpin, L.; Ye, M.; Maier, C.; Sowers, K.; Burns, K.D.; Batlle, D. Regulation of urinary ACE2 in diabetic mice. *Am. J. Physiol. Ren. Physiol.* **2013**, *305*, F600–F611. [CrossRef] [PubMed]
13. Wysocki, J.; Ye, M.; Khattab, A.M.; Fogo, A.; Martin, A.; David, N.V.; Kanwar, Y.; Osborn, M.; Batlle, D. Angiotensin-converting enzyme 2 amplification limited to the circulation does not protect mice from development of diabetic nephropathy. *Kidney Int.* **2017**, *91*, 1336–1346. [CrossRef] [PubMed]
14. Haber, P.K.; Ye, M.; Wysocki, J.; Maier, C.; Haque, S.K.; Batlle, D. Angiotensin-converting enzyme 2-independent action of presumed angiotensin-converting enzyme 2 activators: Studies in vivo, ex vivo, and in vitro. *Hypertension* **2014**, *63*, 774–782. [CrossRef] [PubMed]
15. Liu, P.; Wysocki, J.; Souma, T.; Ye, M.; Ramirez, V.; Zhou, B.; Wilsbacher, L.D.; Quaggin, S.E.; Batlle, D.; Jin, J. Novel ACE2-Fc chimeric fusion provides long-lasting hypertension control and organ protection in mouse models of systemic renin angiotensin system activation. *Kidney Int.* **2018**, *94*, 114–125. [CrossRef]
16. Wysocki, J.; Goodling, A.; Burgaya, M.; Whitlock, K.; Ruzinski, J.; Batlle, D.; Afkarian, M. Urine RAS components in mice and people with type 1 diabetes and chronic kidney disease. *Am. J. Physiol. Ren. Physiol.* **2017**, *313*, F487–F494. [CrossRef]
17. Wysocki, J.; Ye, M.; Batlle, D. Plasma and Kidney Angiotensin Peptides: Importance of the Aminopeptidase A/Angiotensin III Axis. *Am. J. Hypertens.* **2015**, *28*, 1418–1426. [CrossRef]
18. Xiao, F.; Hiremath, S.; Knoll, G.; Zimpelmann, J.; Srivaratharajah, K.; Jadhav, D.; Fergusson, D.; Kennedy, C.R.; Burns, K.D. Increased urinary angiotensin-converting enzyme 2 in renal transplant patients with diabetes. *PLoS ONE* **2012**, *7*, e37649. [CrossRef]
19. Lew, R.A.; Warner, F.J.; Hanchapola, I.; Smith, A.I. Characterization of angiotensin converting enzyme-2 (ACE2) in human urine. *Int. J. Pept. Res.* **2006**, *12*, 283–289. [CrossRef]
20. Xiao, F.; Zimpelmann, J.; Agaybi, S.; Gurley, S.B.; Puente, L.; Burns, K.D. Characterization of angiotensin-converting enzyme 2 ectodomain shedding from mouse proximal tubular cells. *PLoS ONE* **2014**, *9*, e85958. [CrossRef]
21. Mizuiri, S.; Aoki, T.; Hemmi, H.; Arita, M.; Sakai, K.; Aikawa, A. Urinary ACE2 in patients with CKD. *Nephrology* **2011**. [CrossRef] [PubMed]
22. Ye, M.; Wysocki, J.; William, J.; Soler, M.J.; Cokic, I.; Batlle, D. Glomerular localization and expression of Angiotensin-converting enzyme 2 and Angiotensin-converting enzyme: Implications for albuminuria in diabetes. *J. Am. Soc. Nephrol.* **2006**, *17*, 3067–3075. [CrossRef] [PubMed]
23. Wysocki, J.; Ye, M.; Soler, M.J.; Gurley, S.B.; Xiao, H.D.; Bernstein, K.E.; Coffman, T.M.; Chen, S.; Batlle, D. ACE and ACE2 activity in diabetic mice. *Diabetes* **2006**, *55*, 2132–2139. [CrossRef] [PubMed]
24. Ye, M.; Wysocki, J.; Naaz, P.; Salabat, M.R.; LaPointe, M.S.; Batlle, D. Increased ACE 2 and decreased ACE protein in renal tubules from diabetic mice: A renoprotective combination? *Hypertension* **2004**, *43*, 1120–1125. [CrossRef]
25. Liu, P.; Wysocki, J.; Serfozo, P.; Ye, M.; Souma, T.; Batlle, D.; Jin, J. A Fluorometric Method of Measuring Carboxypeptidase Activities for Angiotensin II and Apelin 13. *Sci. Rep.* **2017**, *7*, 45473. [CrossRef]
26. Maier, C.; Schadock, I.; Haber, P.K.; Wysocki, J.; Ye, M.; Kanwar, Y.; Flask, C.A.; Yu, X.; Hoit, B.D.; Adams, G.N.; et al. Prolylcarboxypeptidase deficiency is associated with increased blood pressure, glomerular lesions, and cardiac dysfunction independent of altered circulating and cardiac angiotensin II. *J. Mol. Med.* **2017**, *95*, 473–486. [CrossRef]
27. Gurley, S.B.; Allred, A.; Le, T.H.; Griffiths, R.; Mao, L.; Philip, N.; Haystead, T.A.; Donoghue, M.; Breitbart, R.E.; Acton, S.L.; et al. Altered blood pressure responses and normal cardiac phenotype in ACE2-null mice. *J. Clin. Investig.* **2006**, *116*, 2218–2225. [CrossRef]

28. Thelle, K.; Christensen, E.I.; Vorum, H.; Orskov, H.; Birn, H. Characterization of proteinuria and tubular protein uptake in a new model of oral L-lysine administration in rats. *Kidney Int.* **2006**, *69*, 1333–1340. [CrossRef]
29. Tang, J.; Wysocki, J.; Ye, M.; Valles, P.G.; Rein, J.; Shirazi, M.; Bader, M.; Gomez, R.A.; Sequeira-Lopez, M.S.; Afkarian, M.; et al. Urinary Renin in Patients and Mice With Diabetic Kidney Disease. *Hypertension* **2019**, *74*, 83–94. [CrossRef]
30. Lambert, D.W.; Yarski, M.; Warner, F.J.; Thornhill, P.; Parkin, E.T.; Smith, A.I.; Hooper, N.M.; Turner, A.J. Tumor necrosis factor-alpha convertase (ADAM17) mediates regulated ectodomain shedding of the severe-acute respiratory syndrome-coronavirus (SARS-CoV) receptor, angiotensin-converting enzyme-2 (ACE2). *J. Biol. Chem.* **2005**, *280*, 30113–30119. [CrossRef]
31. Salem, E.S.; Grobe, N.; Elased, K.M. Insulin treatment attenuates renal ADAM17 and ACE2 shedding in diabetic Akita mice. *Am. J. Physiol. Ren. Physiol.* **2014**, *306*, F629–F639. [CrossRef] [PubMed]
32. Donoghue, M.; Hsieh, F.; Baronas, E.; Godbout, K.; Gosselin, M.; Stagliano, N.; Donovan, M.; Woolf, B.; Robison, K.; Jeyaseelan, R.; et al. A novel angiotensin-converting enzyme-related carboxypeptidase (ACE2) converts angiotensin I to angiotensin 1-9. *Circ. Res.* **2000**, *87*, E1–E9. [CrossRef] [PubMed]
33. Durvasula, R.V.; Petermann, A.T.; Hiromura, K.; Blonski, M.; Pippin, J.; Mundel, P.; Pichler, R.; Griffin, S.; Couser, W.G.; Shankland, S.J. Activation of a local tissue angiotensin system in podocytes by mechanical strain. *Kidney Int.* **2004**, *65*, 30–39. [CrossRef] [PubMed]
34. Durvasula, R.V.; Shankland, S.J. Activation of a local renin angiotensin system in podocytes by glucose. *Am. J. Physiol. Ren. Physiol.* **2008**, *294*, F830–F839. [CrossRef]
35. Ingelfinger, J.R.; Zuo, W.M.; Fon, E.A.; Ellison, K.E.; Dzau, V.J. In situ hybridization evidence for angiotensinogen messenger RNA in the rat proximal tubule. An hypothesis for the intrarenal renin angiotensin system. *J. Clin. Investig.* **1990**, *85*, 417–423. [CrossRef]
36. Ba Aqeel, S.; Ye, M.; Wysocki, J.; Sanchez, A.; Khattab, A.; Lores, E.; Rademaker, A.; Gao, X.; Bebu, I.; Nelson, R.G.; et al. Urinary angiotensinogen antedates the development of stage 3 CKD in patients with type 1 diabetes mellitus. *Physiol. Rep.* **2019**, *7*, e14242. [CrossRef]
37. Mills, K.T.; Kobori, H.; Hamm, L.L.; Alper, A.B.; Khan, I.E.; Rahman, M.; Navar, L.G.; Liu, Y.; Browne, G.M.; Batuman, V.; et al. Increased urinary excretion of angiotensinogen is associated with risk of chronic kidney disease. *Nephrol. Dial. Transplant.* **2012**, *27*, 3176–3181. [CrossRef]
38. Urushihara, M.; Kagami, S. Role of the intrarenal renin-angiotensin system in the progression of renal disease. *Pediatr. Nephrol.* **2017**, *32*, 1471–1479. [CrossRef]
39. Kobori, H.; Urushihara, M. Augmented intrarenal and urinary angiotensinogen in hypertension and chronic kidney disease. *Pflug. Arch. Eur. J. Physiol.* **2013**, *465*, 3–12. [CrossRef]
40. Vickers, C.; Hales, P.; Kaushik, V.; Dick, L.; Gavin, J.; Tang, J.; Godbout, K.; Parsons, T.; Baronas, E.; Hsieh, F.; et al. Hydrolysis of biological peptides by human angiotensin-converting enzyme-related carboxypeptidase. *J. Biol. Chem.* **2002**, *277*, 14838–14843. [CrossRef]
41. Mehta, R.L.; Pascual, M.T.; Soroko, S.; Savage, B.R.; Himmelfarb, J.; Ikizler, T.A.; Paganini, E.P.; Chertow, G.M. Program to Improve Care in Acute Renal, D. Spectrum of acute renal failure in the intensive care unit: The PICARD experience. *Kidney Int.* **2004**, *66*, 1613–1621. [CrossRef] [PubMed]
42. Liano, F.; Pascual, J. Outcomes in acute renal failure. *Semin. Nephrol.* **1998**, *18*, 541–550. [PubMed]
43. Basile, D.P.; Anderson, M.D.; Sutton, T.A. Pathophysiology of acute kidney injury. *Compr. Physiol.* **2012**, *2*, 1303–1353. [CrossRef] [PubMed]
44. Star, R.A. Treatment of acute renal failure. *Kidney Int.* **1998**, *54*, 1817–1831. [CrossRef]
45. Kontogiannis, J.; Burns, K.D. Role of AT1 angiotensin II receptors in renal ischemic injury. *Am. J. Physiol.* **1998**, *274*, F79–F90. [CrossRef]
46. Da Silveira, K.D.; Pompermayer Bosco, K.S.; Diniz, L.R.; Carmona, A.K.; Cassali, G.D.; Bruna-Romero, O.; de Sousa, L.P.; Teixeira, M.M.; Santos, R.A.; Simoes e Silva, A.C.; et al. ACE2-angiotensin-(1-7)-Mas axis in renal ischaemia/reperfusion injury in rats. *Clin. Sci.* **2010**, *119*, 385–394. [CrossRef]
47. Allred, A.J.; Chappell, M.C.; Ferrario, C.M.; Diz, D.I. Differential actions of renal ischemic injury on the intrarenal angiotensin system. *Am. J. Physiol. Ren. Physiol.* **2000**, *279*, F636–F645. [CrossRef]
48. Ba Aqeel, S.H.; Sanchez, A.; Batlle, D. Angiotensinogen as a biomarker of acute kidney injury. *Clin. Kidney J.* **2017**, *10*, 759–768. [CrossRef]
49. Bellomo, R.; Kellum, J.A.; Ronco, C. Acute kidney injury. *Lancet* **2012**, *380*, 756–766. [CrossRef]

50. Mackie, F.E.; Campbell, D.J.; Meyer, T.W. Intrarenal angiotensin and bradykinin peptide levels in the remnant kidney model of renal insufficiency. *Kidney Int.* **2001**, *59*, 1458–1465. [CrossRef]
51. Okui, S.; Yamamoto, H.; Li, W.; Gamachi, N.; Fujita, Y.; Kashiwamura, S.; Miura, D.; Takai, S.; Miyazaki, M.; Urade, M.; et al. Cisplatin-induced acute renal failure in mice is mediated by chymase-activated angiotensin-aldosterone system and interleukin-18. *Eur. J. Pharmacol.* **2012**, *685*, 149–155. [CrossRef] [PubMed]
52. Fang, F.; Liu, G.C.; Zhou, X.; Yang, S.; Reich, H.N.; Williams, V.; Hu, A.; Pan, J.; Konvalinka, A.; Oudit, G.Y.; et al. Loss of ACE2 exacerbates murine renal ischemia-reperfusion injury. *PLoS ONE* **2013**, *8*, e71433. [CrossRef] [PubMed]
53. Saleh, S.; Ain-Shoka, A.A.; El-Demerdash, E.; Khalef, M.M. Protective effects of the angiotensin II receptor blocker losartan on cisplatin-induced kidney injury. *Chemotherapy* **2009**, *55*, 399–406. [CrossRef]
54. El-Sayed el, S.M.; Abd-Ellah, M.F.; Attia, S.M. Protective effect of captopril against cisplatin-induced nephrotoxicity in rats. *Pak. J. Pharm. Sci.* **2008**, *21*, 255–261.
55. Zhang, J.; Rudemiller, N.P.; Patel, M.B.; Wei, Q.; Karlovich, N.S.; Jeffs, A.D.; Wu, M.; Sparks, M.A.; Privratsky, J.R.; Herrera, M.; et al. Competing Actions of Type 1 Angiotensin II Receptors Expressed on T Lymphocytes and Kidney Epithelium during Cisplatin-Induced AKI. *J. Am. Soc. Nephrol.* **2016**. [CrossRef] [PubMed]
56. Deegan, P.M.; Nolan, C.; Ryan, M.P.; Basinger, M.A.; Jones, M.M.; Hande, K.R. The role of the renin-angiotensin system in cisplatin nephrotoxicity. *Ren. Fail.* **1995**, *17*, 665–674. [CrossRef]
57. Efrati, S.; Berman, S.; Hamad, R.A.; Siman-Tov, Y.; Ilgiyaev, E.; Maslyakov, I.; Weissgarten, J. Effect of captopril treatment on recuperation from ischemia/reperfusion-induced acute renal injury. *Nephrol. Dial. Transplant.* **2012**, *27*, 136–145. [CrossRef]
58. Kocak, C.; Kocak, F.E.; Akcilar, R.; Bayat, Z.; Aras, B.; Metineren, M.H.; Yucel, M.; Simsek, H. Effects of captopril, telmisartan and bardoxolone methyl (CDDO-Me) in ischemia-reperfusion-induced acute kidney injury in rats: An experimental comparative study. *Clin. Exp. Pharmacol. Physiol.* **2016**, *43*, 230–241. [CrossRef]
59. Mehrotra, P.; Patel, J.B.; Ivancic, C.M.; Collett, J.A.; Basile, D.P. Th-17 cell activation in response to high salt following acute kidney injury is associated with progressive fibrosis and attenuated by AT-1R antagonism. *Kidney Int.* **2015**, *88*, 776–784. [CrossRef]
60. Cho, J.H.; Choi, S.Y.; Ryu, H.M.; Oh, E.J.; Yook, J.M.; Ahn, J.S.; Jung, H.Y.; Choi, J.Y.; Park, S.H.; Kim, C.D.; et al. Fimasartan attenuates renal ischemia-reperfusion injury by modulating inflammation-related apoptosis. *Korean J. Physiol. Pharm.* **2018**, *22*, 661–670. [CrossRef]
61. Rafiq, K.; Hitomi, H.; Nakano, D.; Nishiyama, A. Pathophysiological roles of aldosterone and mineralocorticoid receptor in the kidney. *J. Pharmacol. Sci.* **2011**, *115*, 1–7. [CrossRef] [PubMed]
62. Chrysostomou, A.; Pedagogos, E.; MacGregor, L.; Becker, G.J. Double-blind, placebo-controlled study on the effect of the aldosterone receptor antagonist spironolactone in patients who have persistent proteinuria and are on long-term angiotensin-converting enzyme inhibitor therapy, with or without an angiotensin II receptor blocker. *Clin. J. Am. Soc. Nephrol. CJASN* **2006**, *1*, 256–262. [CrossRef] [PubMed]
63. Zhou, X.; Ono, H.; Ono, Y.; Frohlich, E.D. Aldosterone antagonism ameliorates proteinuria and nephrosclerosis independent of glomerular dynamics in L-NAME/SHR model. *Am. J. Nephrol.* **2004**, *24*, 242–249. [CrossRef] [PubMed]

5

Protective Effects of Simvastatin on Endotoxin-Induced Acute Kidney Injury through Activation of Tubular Epithelial Cells' Survival and Hindering Cytochrome C-Mediated Apoptosis

Lana Nežić [1,*,†], Ranko Škrbić [1], Ljiljana Amidžić [2], Radoslav Gajanin [3], Zoran Milovanović [4], Eugenie Nepovimova [5], Kamil Kuča [5,6,*] and Vesna Jaćević [5,7,8,†]

1 Department of Pharmacology, Toxicology and Clinical Pharmacology, School of Medicine, University of Banja Luka, 14 Save Mrkalja St, 78000 Banja Luka, Bosnia and Herzegovina; ranko.skrbic@med.unibl.org
2 Center for Biomedical Research, School of Medicine, University of Banja Luka, 14 Save Mrkalja St, 78000 Banja Luka, Bosnia and Herzegovina; ljiljana.amidzic@med.unibl.org
3 Institute of Pathology, University Clinical Center of Republic of Srpska, School of Medicine, University of Banja Luka, 12 Beba St, 78000 Banja Luka, Bosnia and Herzegovina; radoslav.gajanin@med.unibl.org
4 Special Police Unit, Police Department of the City of Belgrade, Ministry of Interior, Trebevićka 12/A, 11030 Belgrade, Serbia; tinahoks41@gmail.com
5 Department of Chemistry, Faculty of Science, University of Hradec Kralove, Rokitanského 62, 500 03 Hradec Králové, Czech Republic; evzenie.n@seznam.cz (E.N.); v_jacevic@yahoo.com (V.J.)
6 Biomedical Research Center, University Hospital Hradec Kralove, 500 02 Hradec Kralove, Czech Republic
7 Department for Experimental Toxicology and Pharmacology, National Poison Control Centre, Military Medical Academy, 11 Crnotravska St, 11000 Belgrade, Serbia
8 Department of Pharmacological Sciences, Medical Faculty of the Military Medical Academy, the University of Defence in Belgrade, 17 Crnotravska St, 11000 Belgrade, Serbia
* Correspondence: lana.nezic@med.unibl.org (L.N.); kamil.kuca@uhk.cz (K.K.)

† These authors contributed equally to this work.

Abstract: Increasing evidence suggests that apoptosis of tubular cells and renal inflammation mainly determine the outcome of sepsis-associated acute kidney injury (AKI). The study aim was to investigate the molecular mechanism involved in the renoprotective effects of simvastatin in endotoxin (lipopolysaccharide, LSP)-induced AKI. A sepsis model was established by intraperitoneal injection of a single non-lethal LPS dose after short-term simvastatin pretreatment. The severity of the inflammatory injury was expressed as renal damage scores (RDS). Apoptosis of tubular cells was detected by Terminal deoxynucleotidyl transferase-mediated dUTP Nick End Labeling (TUNEL assay) (apoptotic DNA fragmentation, expressed as an apoptotic index, AI) and immunohistochemical staining for cleaved caspase-3, cytochrome C, and anti-apoptotic Bcl-xL and survivin. We found that endotoxin induced severe renal inflammatory injury (RDS = 3.58 ± 0.50), whereas simvastatin dose-dependently prevented structural changes induced by LPS. Furthermore, simvastatin 40 mg/kg most profoundly attenuated tubular apoptosis, determined as a decrease of cytochrome C, caspase-3 expression, and AIs ($p < 0.01$ vs. LPS). Conversely, simvastatin induced a significant increase of Bcl-XL and survivin, both in the strong inverse correlations with cleaved caspase-3 and cytochrome C. Our study indicates that simvastatin has cytoprotective effects against LPS-induced tubular apoptosis, seemingly mediated by upregulation of cell-survival molecules, such as Bcl-XL and survivin, and inhibition of the mitochondrial cytochrome C and downstream caspase-3 activation.

Keywords: simvastatin; endotoxin; tubular apoptosis; cytochrome C; Bcl-XL; survivin

1. Introduction

Acute kidney injury (AKI) is one of the major complications of sepsis-induced multiple organ failure and is accompanied by high mortality [1]. During sepsis, a major mechanism of AKI includes severe inflammation in the renal parenchyma, heterogeneous distortion of microvascular flow at the peritubular and glomerular levels, and severe tubular epithelial injury and apoptosis [1,2].

Lipopolysaccharide (LPS), an endotoxin from the Gram-negative bacteria, has been identified as the major factor associated with the development of sepsis-associated AKI [3]. Proinflammatory cytokine, tumor necrosis factor-α (TNF-α), has a crucial role in the pathogenesis of the AKI caused by endotoxemia, leading to renal inflammatory injury, and acute tubular cell apoptosis presumably by activation of the extrinsic apoptotic pathway [1,4]. The pleiotropic cytokine TNF-α has a particular role in the initiation of cell-survival signaling molecules such as upregulation of anti-apoptotic molecules Bcl-2, and survivin (an inhibitor of apoptosis—IAP) through activation of nuclear factor-kappa (NF-κB) [5]. In addition to the severe inflammatory syndrome, LPS activates Toll-like receptor 4 (TLR4) that is present in the membrane of immune cells and renal tubular epithelial cells, triggering the excessive release of proinflammatory cytokines, oxidative stress, and tubular cell apoptosis [3,6]. Severe tubular cell apoptosis plays an important role in LPS-induced AKI, showing caspase-3-positivity in tubular epithelial cells even at the early phase of AKI [3,7].

Mitochondrial dysfunction and damage are confirmed in the LPS and cecal ligation puncture (CLP) model of septic AKI. Oxidative stress has also been known to contribute to the overproduction of mitochondrial reactive oxygen species (ROS) and early mitochondrial dysfunction after the LPS challenge, which triggers intrinsic apoptosis through the release of pro-apoptotic cytochrome C into the cytosol and activating the caspase cascade. Importantly, antiapoptotic Bcl-2 members, such as Bcl-XL, inhibit cell death by blocking of the cytochrome C release from mitochondria and thereby prevent downstream caspases' (caspase-9, -3, -7) activation [1,2,8,9].

Consistent with these results, LPS-induced AKI and renal tubular cells apoptosis were ameliorated by novel potential agents, such as a pluripotent autocrine growth factor progranulin, an anion transporter uncoupling protein 2 [10], the bee venom [11], and peroxiredoxin protein DJ-1 (Parkinson disease protein 7, Park7) [12], as well as by vitamin D that suppressed p53-upregulated modulator of apoptosis (PUMA) and upregulated expression of a Bcl-2 family antiapoptotic protein [13]. Thus, an LPS-induced AKI model has been commonly recognized to study the pathophysiology of renal tissue injury and tubular cell apoptosis and to evaluate potential new therapeutic agents for this medical condition [2,3].

Numerous experimental studies demonstrated that statins, well-known lipid-lowering drugs, improved survival, and prevent tissue and organ injuries in local inflammation [14] or sepsis induced by LPS or CLP [15,16]. By inhibition of hydroxy-3-methylglutaryl-CoA (HMG-CoA), reductase statins block the mevalonate pathway and activation of intermediate products involved in cell signaling pathways, such as apoptosis or cell survival. One previous study showed that atorvastatin ameliorated contrast-induced nephropathy and reduced the extent of renal tubular cell apoptosis that is associated with the decreased expression of proapoptotic Bax/caspase-3 and increased Bcl-2 [17]. Another study that demonstrated the renoprotective effects of pitavastatin on cisplatin-induced AKI pointed to suppression of the mitogen-activated protein kinase (MAPK)/NF-kB/inflammation axis and intrinsic apoptotic pathway [18].

In the context of the experimental sepsis, we have previously shown that simvastatin improved survival rate and significantly suppressed LPS-induced over-production of proinflammatory cytokines, TNFα and interleukin (IL)-1β [19]. Furthermore, the cell-protective effect of simvastatin pretreatment against LPS has been confirmed on cardiomyocytes [20], hepatocytes, and spleen lymphocytes [21]. These results showed that pretreatment with simvastatin mitigated myocardial, liver, and spleen tissue injuries, and decreased activation of the cleaved caspase-3 along to the reduced apoptotic-cell death in the parenchyma. Simvastatin targets the cell-survival signaling pathway survivin/NF-κB/p65 and anti-apoptotic Bcl-XL in these cells, which appears a protective mechanism in response to LPS-induced tissue injury and programmed cell death [20,21].

Therefore, the present study was designed to determine whether pretreatment with simvastatin (1) ameliorates LPS-induced AKI, and, if it does, (2) to elucidate its role in hindering apoptotic death-inducing pathways in the tubular epithelial cells, and (3) subsequent upregulation of cell-survival mechanisms like survivin and Bcl-XL.

2. Results

2.1. Protective Effects of Simvastatin on the LPS-Induced Acute Renal Injury

Renal specimens taken from the control rats revealed the normal histological structure of the glomeruli and renal tubules (Figure 1A). Treatment with LPS only (Figure 1B) induced congestion and small multifocal hemorrhages in the cortical and interstitial blood vessels with the presence of polymorphonuclear leukocytes (PMNL) infiltrate. Glomerular lesions were characterized by increased numbers of epithelial cells and pericapilar infiltration by PMNL and erythrocytes, predominantly. Both proximal and distal convoluted tubules showed diffuse epithelial cell swelling, loss of brush border, vacuolar degeneration, and focal necrosis. These changes were correlated with the RDS of 3.58 ± 0.50 confirming the LPS-induced severe renal damage (Table 1). Pretreatment with simvastatin 10 mg/kg reduced histopathological changes (RDS = 2.67 ± 0.48, not significantly vs. LPS group). Renal histopathological examination in the simvastatin 20 group (Figure 1C) showed the decreased intensity of tissue damage with the distinct renal tubular epithelial cell swelling and degeneration. Only individual glomeruli showed hypercellularity, with increased numbers of both resident cells and infiltrating leukocytes, indicative of the significantly lower RDS of 2.33 ± 0.47 ($p < 0.05$ vs. control and vs. LPS group, respectively). Renal histology in the simvastatin 40 group was mostly unchanged and showed mild edema and hyperemia, rare small hemorrhages, and a single PNML infiltration throughout the cortex with irregular swelling of renal tubular cells. A mean RDS was minimal, 1.42 ± 0.50, in comparison to the LPS ($p < 0.01$). Semiquantitative assessment of renal tissue lesions reveals that simvastatin ameliorated LPS-induced histopathological changes in a dose-dependent manner (Figure 1C,D).

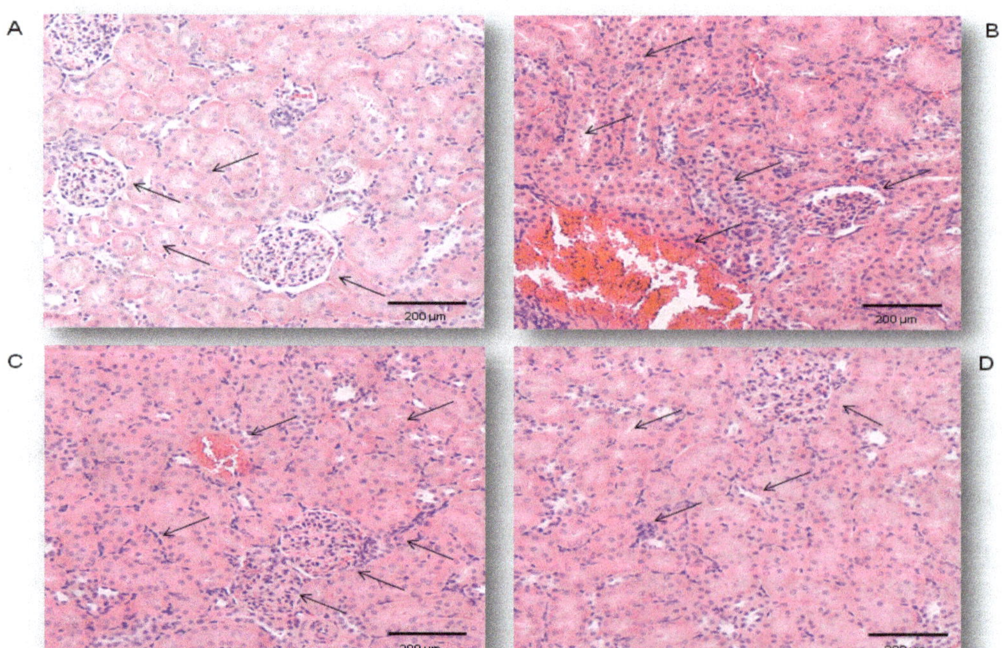

Figure 1. Protective effects of simvastatin pretreatment against LPS-induced acute renal damages, Hematoxylin and Eosin (H&E) method, 200× magnified images, black arrows indicates the gromeruls

and tubules. (**A**) Appearance of renal tissue of control animals, (**B**) renal tissue challenged with LPS, (**C**) renal tissue from simvastatin 20 group, (**D**) renal tissue from simvastatin 40 group. Histopathological analysis revealed decreased renal inflammatory damages in both simvastatin-treated groups, while severe alterations persisted only in the LPS-treated group.

Table 1. The effects of different treatments on the degree of renal alterations—Renal Damage Score (RDS)

Treatment (mg/kg)	Renal Damage Score (6 Kidneys/Group × 6 Slices/Kidney)					$\overline{X}$ ± S.D.
	0	1	2	3	4	
Control	30	6	0	0	0	0.67 ± 0.48
LPS	0	0	0	15	21	3.58 ± 0.50 a^3
Simvastatin 10 group	0	0	12	24	0	2.67 ± 0.48 a^1
Simvastatin 20 group	0	0	24	12	0	2.33 ± 0.47 a^1
Simvastatin 40 group	0	21	15	0	0	1.42 ± 0.50 b^2

Statistical analysis was performed using the Kruskal–Wallis test. a^1, a^3—$p < 0.05$, 0.001 in comparison to the control group, b^2—$p < 0.01$ in comparison to the LPS-only treated group. ($\overline{X}$—mean value, S.D—standard deviation).

2.2. Simvastatin Inhibited Cleaved Caspase-3 Expression and Apoptotic Cell Death of Renal Tubular Epithelial Cells Induced by LPS

Occurrence and the extent of apoptosis of the renal tubular epithelium was assessed based on the expression of cleaved caspase-3 and confirmed by the TUNEL assay with quantification of apoptotic index (AIs, see Methods and Materials Section) (Figure 2A–D and Figure 3A–D). We analyzed tissue sections challenged with simvastatin of 20 and 40 mg/kg, as the dose of 10 mg/kg did not show a significant protective effect on RDS. LPS induced cleavage of caspase-3 (active molecule) predominantly in the renal tubular epithelial cells, characteristically localized in the cytoplasm and perinuclear region of apoptotic cells. As shown in Figure 2, a substantial increase of cleaved caspase-3 expression in the LPS group (43.6% ± 4.4%, $p < 0.01$ vs. control group), was the most profoundly reduced with simvastatin 40 mg/kg (17.2% ± 2.9%, $p < 0.01$ vs. LPS group, and $p < 0.05$ vs. simvastatin 20 group), showing also and dose-dependent efficacy (Figures 2 and 3E).

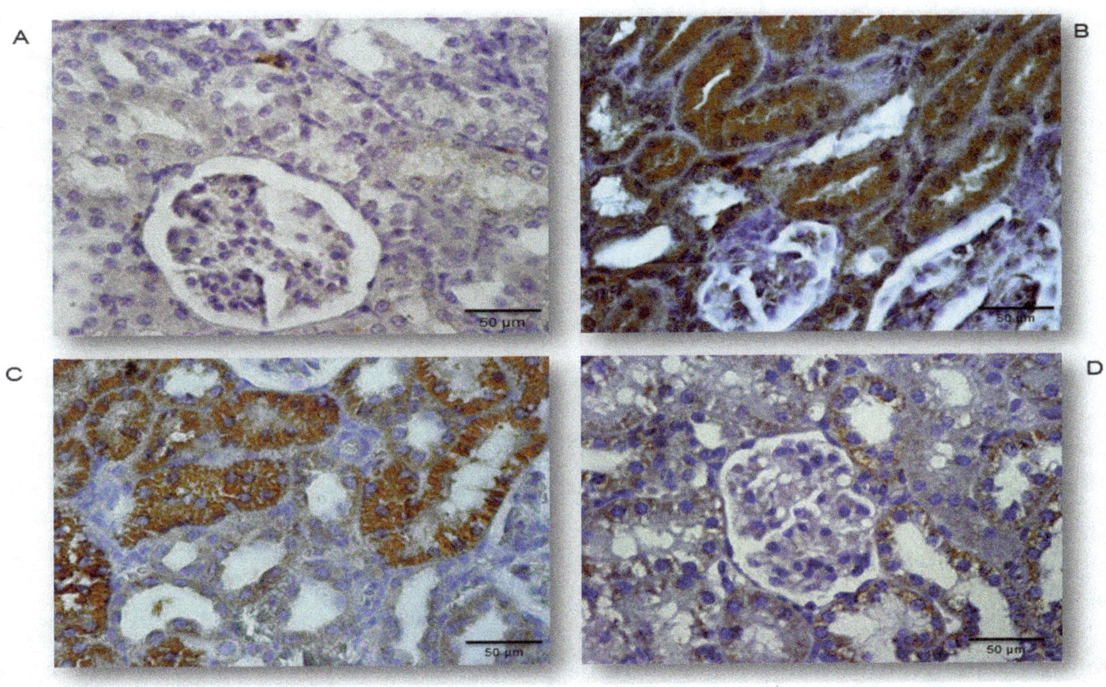

Figure 2. Representative images of apoptotic renal tubular epithelial cells that were challenged with

LPS or pretreated with simvastatin prior to LPS, simvastatin 20 mg/kg or 40 mg/kg, respectively. Attenuation of the renal apoptosis induced by LPS shown as decreased cleaved caspase-3 expression in the tubular epithelial cells, assessed by immunohistochemistry, magnification 400×. (**A**) The control group, (**B**) intense cytoplasmic staining of cleaved caspase 3 in the tubular epithelium in the LPS group, as one of the feature of apoptotic cell, significant reduction of apoptotic cells in the groups treated with simvastatin 20 mg/kg (**C**) and 40 mg/kg, respectively (**D**).

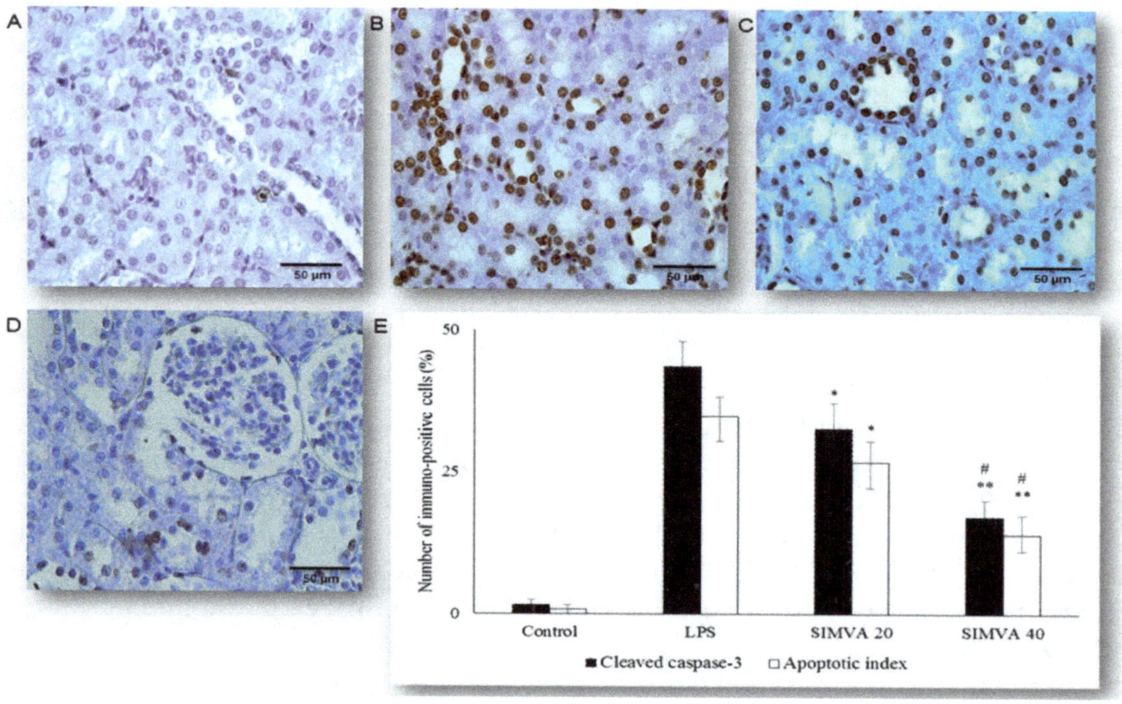

Figure 3. Simvastatin inhibited apoptosis of renal tubular epithelial cells in inflammatory injury induced by LPS, confirmed by TUNEL assay, magnification 400×. The apoptotic indices (AI) are based on the relative number of brown stained nuclei (TUNEL-positive renal tubular epithelial cells) and showed significant increase in the LPS group (**B**), simvastatin 20 mg/kg (**C**), and 40 mg/kg group (**D**) respectively, compared with the control group (**A**). LPS challenge led to a marked increase of TUNEL-positive tubular epithelial cells (shown as AIs in white columns AIs) while the AIs were significantly decreased in the simvastatin groups. Quantitative comparison of the immunohistochemically stained renal tissue for cleaved caspase 3 and the TUNEL-positive tubular epithelial cells expressed as AIs (* $p < 0.05$ vs. LPS group, ** $p < 0.05$ vs. simvastatin 20 group, # $p < 0.01$ vs. LPS group) (**E**).

Definite apoptosis was confirmed with the TUNEL assay that detected chromatin condensation and DNA fragmentation, with the main features of apoptosis shown as dark brown nuclei (Figure 3). The apoptotic indices, as the degrees of apoptosis in renal tissue, significantly increased after LPS administration (in all experimental treated groups) compared with the control ($p < 0.01$), but they were markedly decreased in the group with simvastatin 20 (AI = 26.7% ± 3.7%, $p < 0.05$) and simvastatin 40 group (AI = 14.0% ± 3.3%, $p < 0.01$) in respect to the LPS group (AI = 34.8% ± 3.6%) (Figure 3). Immunohistochemical staining and TUNEL assay revealed insignificant differences in the cleaved caspase-3 expression (total number of immuno-positive cells) compared to the AIs, that were strongly positively correlated across the experimental groups ($p < 0.05$) (Figure 3E). This could be explained by the fact that cytoplasmic immune-positivity of cleaved caspase-3 represents both apoptotic and the cells in pre-apoptosis without condensation of chromatin (TUNEL-positive cells) and with preserved cellular morphology.

2.3. *Simvastatin Attenuated Expression of Pro-Apoptotic Cytochrome C in Renal Tubular Epithelial Cells after LPS Administration*

To further investigate an apoptotic pathway targeted by simvastatin in LPS-induced AKI, we assessed mitochondrial pro-apoptotic marker, cytochrome C. The control group showed minimal immunostaining in the sporadic tubular epithelial cells. LPS administration increased expression of cytochrome C, quantified as the intense brown cytoplasmic staining in the affected tubular cells (45.11% ± 4.14%). Conversely, simvastatin markedly mitigated LPS-induced cytochrome C expression in comparison to the LPS group (Figure 4A–D). Consistently, quantitative analysis of cytochrome C immunopositivity showed a significant difference among groups ($p < 0.05$ in simvastatin 20 group and $p < 0.01$ in simvastatin 40 group vs. LPS, respectively), while very strong positive correlations between apoptotic markers, cleaved caspase-3, and cytochrome C were determined across the groups ($p = 0.01$).

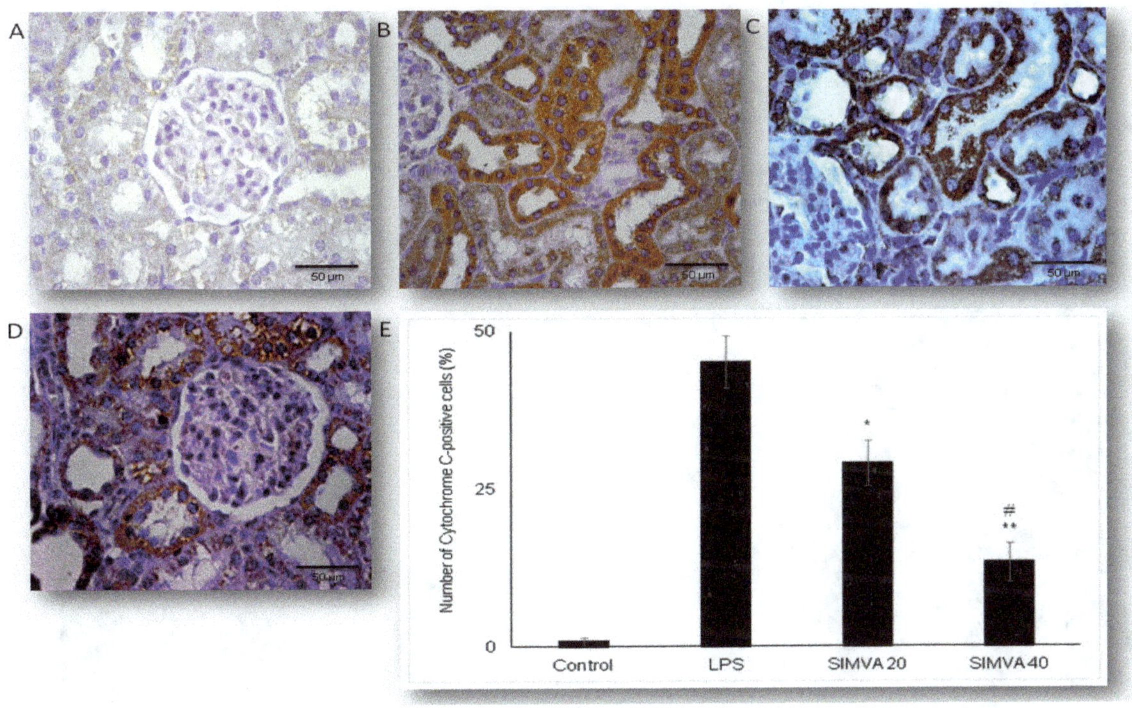

Figure 4. Simvastatin attenuated cytochrome C expression in renal tubular epithelial cells after LPS-administration. The expression of cytochrome C in rat renal tissue examined by immunohistochemical staining, magnification 400×, (**A**) negative immunostaining in the control group, (**B**) intense brown cytoplasmic staining in the tubular epithelium in the LPS group indicates increased expression of the pro-apoptotic protein cytochrome C. A significant decrease of cytochrome C-positive cells in the groups pretreated with simvastatin 20 mg/kg (**C**) and 40 mg/kg group (**D**), respectively. A quantitative analysis of cytochrome C-positive renal tubular epithelial cells assessed in the immunohistochemically stained sections in the renal tissue (* $p < 0.05$ vs. LPS group, ** $p < 0.01$ vs. simvastatin 20 group, # $p < 0.01$ vs. LPS group) (**E**).

2.4. *Expression of Anti-Apoptotic Bcl-XL in Renal Tubular Epithelial Cells after Simvastatin and LPS Administration*

Expression of anti-apoptotic Bcl-xL in renal tubular epithelial cells significantly differed among LPS and simvastatin groups (Figure 5). Immuno-positive Bcl-XL renal tubular cells were sporadically determined in the control, and significantly in the LPS groups (36.4%, $p < 0.05$ vs. control) (Figure 5A,B). Upregulation of Bcl-XL implied that LPS might trigger a potential cell self-protective mechanism against the intrinsic apoptotic pathway. Pretreatment with simvastatin 20 mg/kg and simvastatin 40 mg/kg produced a gradual and significant increase in Bcl-xL expression in the tubular cells compared to the LPS group (56.4% ± 4.8%, $p < 0.05$ and 71.6% ;± 4.9%, $p < 0.01$, respectively), showing intensive brown cytoplasmic staining (Figure 5A–E). To compare the expression of key apoptotic proteins and Bcl-XL in tubular cells in the treated groups, we analyzed their correlations (Figure 6). The result showed the strong inverse correlation between Bcl-XL and cleaved caspase-3-positive cells in the simvastatin 20 group ($R^2 = 0.61$, $p < 0.05$) and simvastatin 40 group ($R^2 = 0.78$, $p < 0.05$) group. As it is shown (Figure 7), Bcl-XL expression is in a very strong negative correlation with cytochrome C in the simvastatin 40 group ($R^2 = 0.81$, $p < 0.05$), similarly as in the simvastatin 20 group, suggesting that through induction of anti-apoptotic Bcl-XL, simvastatin might express a cell-protective mechanism.

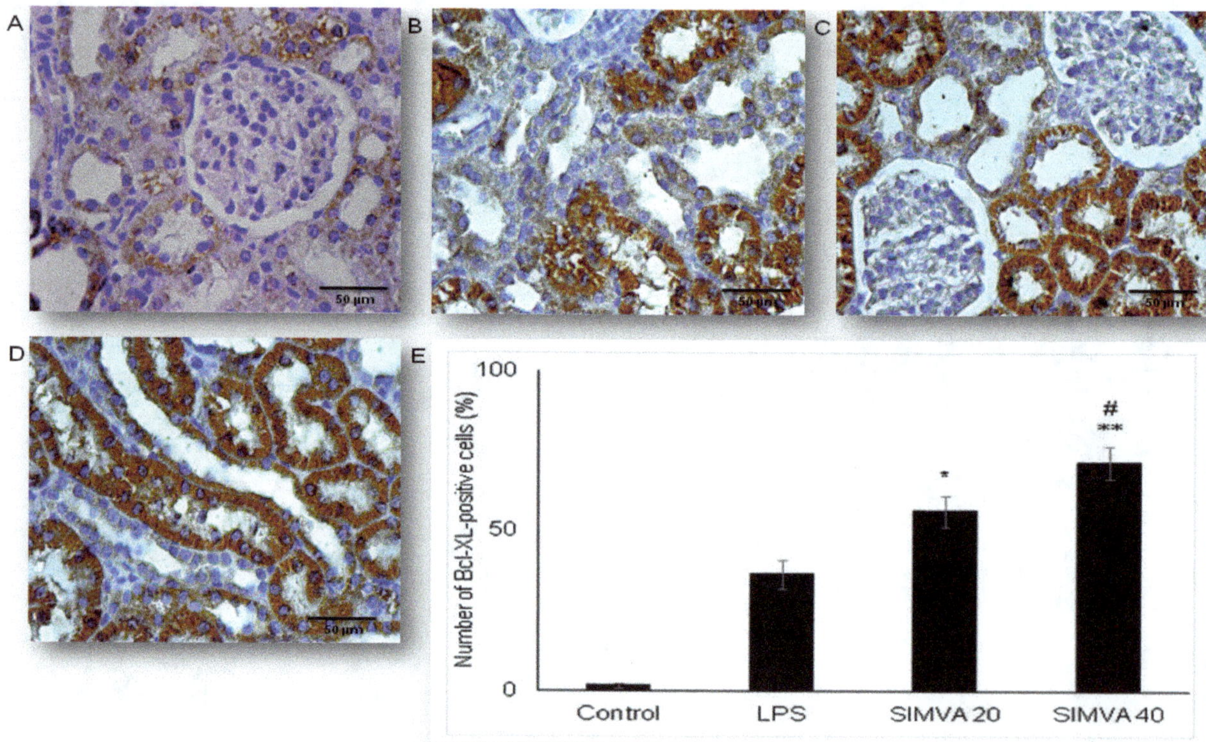

Figure 5. Simvastatin increased Bcl-XL expression in renal tubular epithelial cells after LPS administration. The expression of Bcl-XL in renal tissue was examined by immunohistochemical staining, magnification 400×, (**A**) the control group showed rare immuno-positive cells, (**B**) note Bcl-XL-expression in the tubular epithelial cells in the LPS group, in simvastatin 20 mg/kg (**C**) and 40 mg/kg group (**D**), respectively. Bcl-XL expression significantly increased, and it is determined as intensive brown cytoplasmic staining widely distributed in renal tubular epithelial cells. (**E**) A quantitative analysis of Bcl-XL-positive renal tubular epithelial cells assessed in immunohistochemically stained sections of the renal tissue (* $p < 0.05$ vs. LPS group, ** $p < 0.05$ vs. simvastatin 20 group, # $p < 0.01$ vs. LPS group).

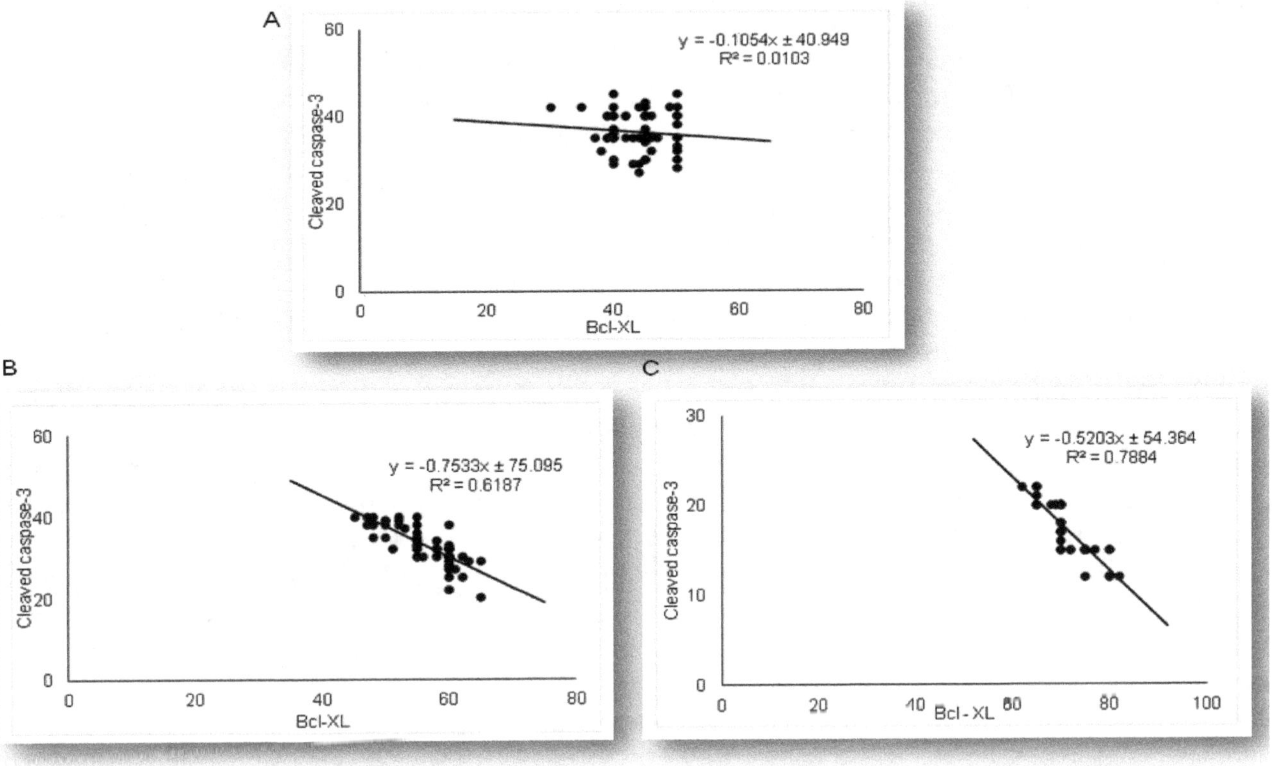

Figure 6. The correlations are shown for Bcl-XL and cleaved-caspase-3 in the renal tubular epithelial cells: (**A**) LPS group only, (**B**) simvastatin 20 mg/kg group, (**C**) simvastatin 40 mg/kg group.

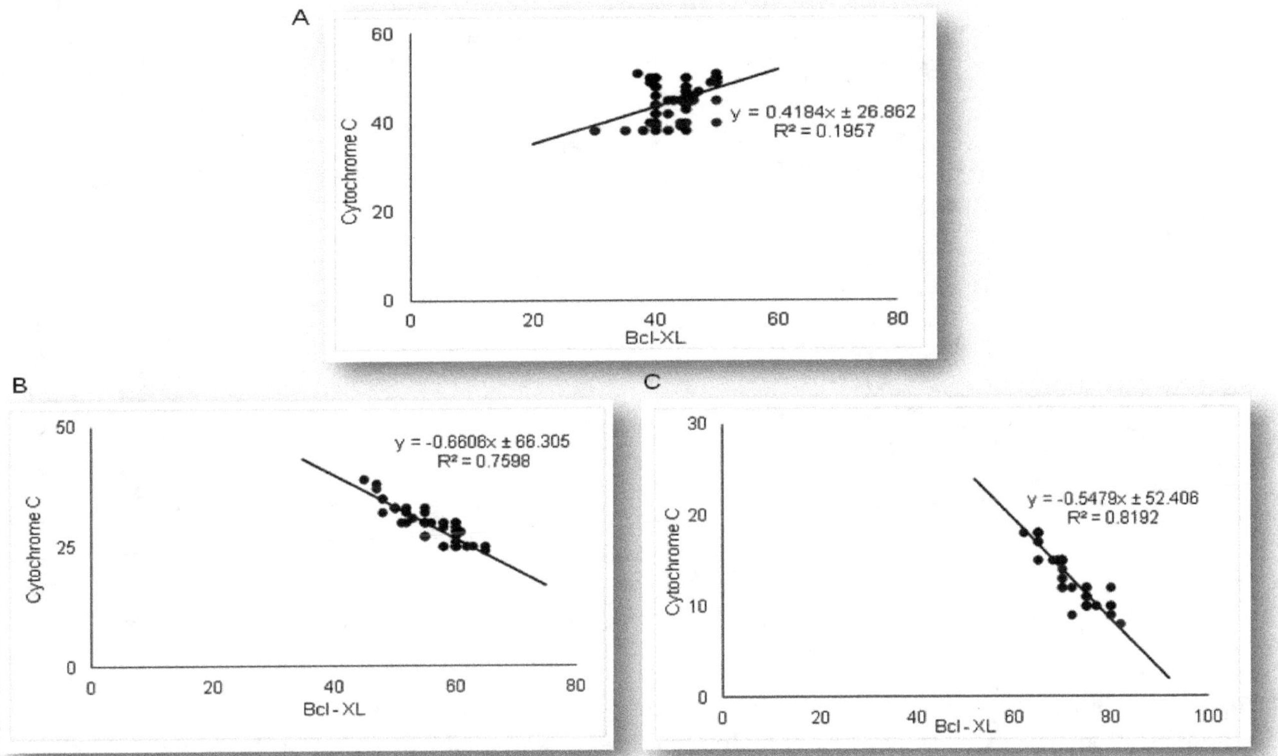

Figure 7. The correlations are shown for Bcl-XL and cytochrome C in the renal tubular epithelial cells: (**A**) LPS group only, (**B**) simvastatin 20 mg/kg group, (**C**) simvastatin 40 mg/kg group.

2.5. Simvastatin Enhanced Survivin Expression in Renal Tubular Epithelial Cells after LPS Administration

As the results demonstrated that simvastatin enhanced Bcl-XL expression in renal tubular epithelial cells after LPS administration, we further analyzed if simvastatin upregulates expression of a downstream inhibitor of apoptosis, survivin (Figure 8). Weak cytoplasmic staining assessed as positive survivin expression in the control was considered as its basal expression (Figure 8A). The LPS challenge resulted in a marked increase of survivin expression in tubular cells ($p < 0.05$ vs. control group), suggesting that survivin itself presents a cell-protective mechanism in LPS injury (Figure 8B). Further results demonstrated that simvastatin induced cell survival pathways, showing a dose-dependent increase in strong cytoplasmic expression of survivin (Figure 8C,D). Quantitative analysis revealed that pretreatment in simvastatin 20 and 40 groups led to a striking increase of survivin expression (49.5% ± 4.7% and 73.3% ± 5.3% vs. LPS group, $p < 0.01$, respectively) (Figure 8E). As survivin is one of the IAPs, we tested its correlation with cleaved caspase-3 and cytochrome C. As illustrated in Figure 9, strong inverse correlations were determined between survivin and cleaved caspase-3 in simvastatin 20 and 40 groups ($R^2 = 0.71$ and $R^2 = 0.83$, $p < 0.01$, respectively). Consistently, Pearson's correlation analysis revealed a strong inverse correlation of survivin with cytochrome C-positive tubular cells in simvastatin 20 and 40 groups ($R^2 = 0.69$ and $R^2 = 0.85$, $p < 0.01$, respectively) (Figure 10), suggesting that simvastatin protects tubular cells in LPS-induced AKI by inhibiting key apoptotic proteins of the intrinsic pathway and activates cell-survival mechanisms.

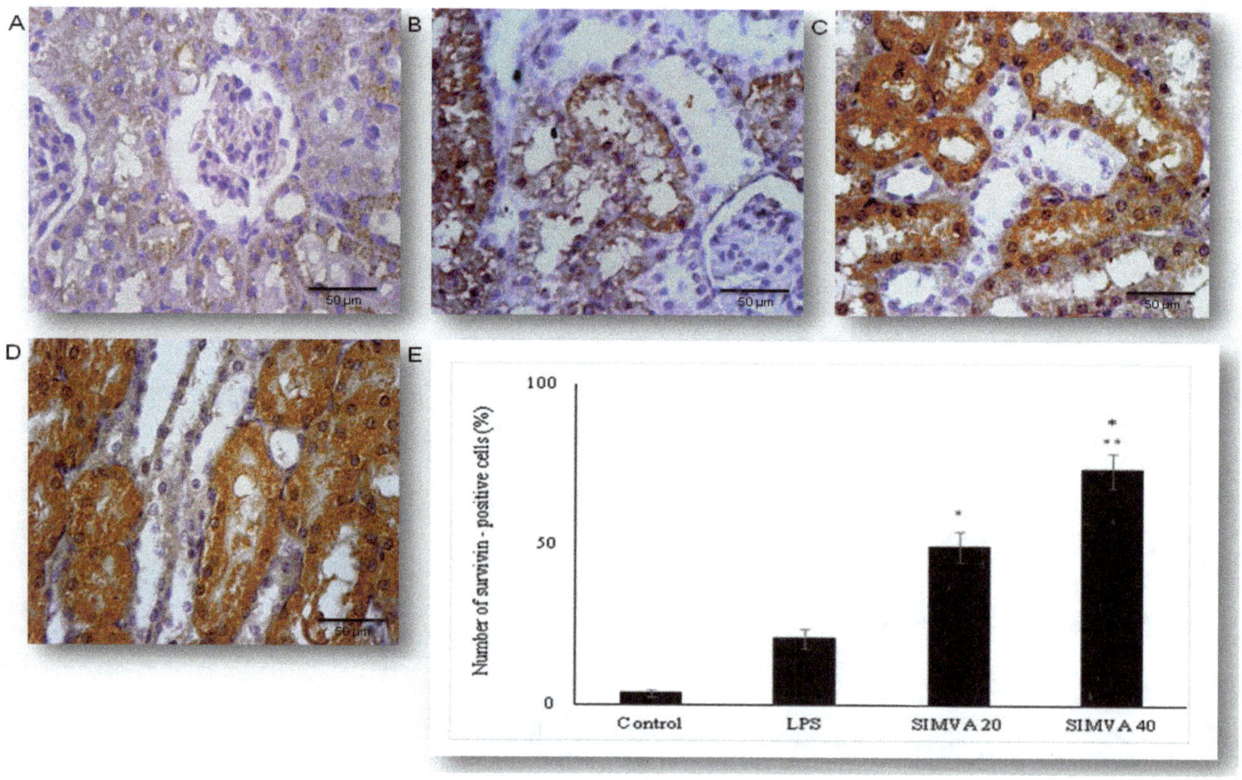

Figure 8. Simvastatin increased survivin expression in renal tubular epithelial cells after LPS administration. The expression of survivin in renal tissue examined by immunohistochemical staining, magnification 400×, (**A**) the control group showed rare immuno-positive cell, (**B**) note immuno-positive survivin cells in the LPS group, in simvastatin 20 group (**C**), and simvastatin 40 group (**D**), survivin expression significantly increased, and it is determined as intensive brown cytoplasmic staining widely distributed in renal tubular epithelial cells. (**E**) A quantitative analysis of survivin-positive renal tubular epithelial cells assessed in immunohistochemically stained sections of the renal tissue (* $p < 0.01$ vs. LPS group, ** $p < 0.05$ vs. simvastatin 20 group).

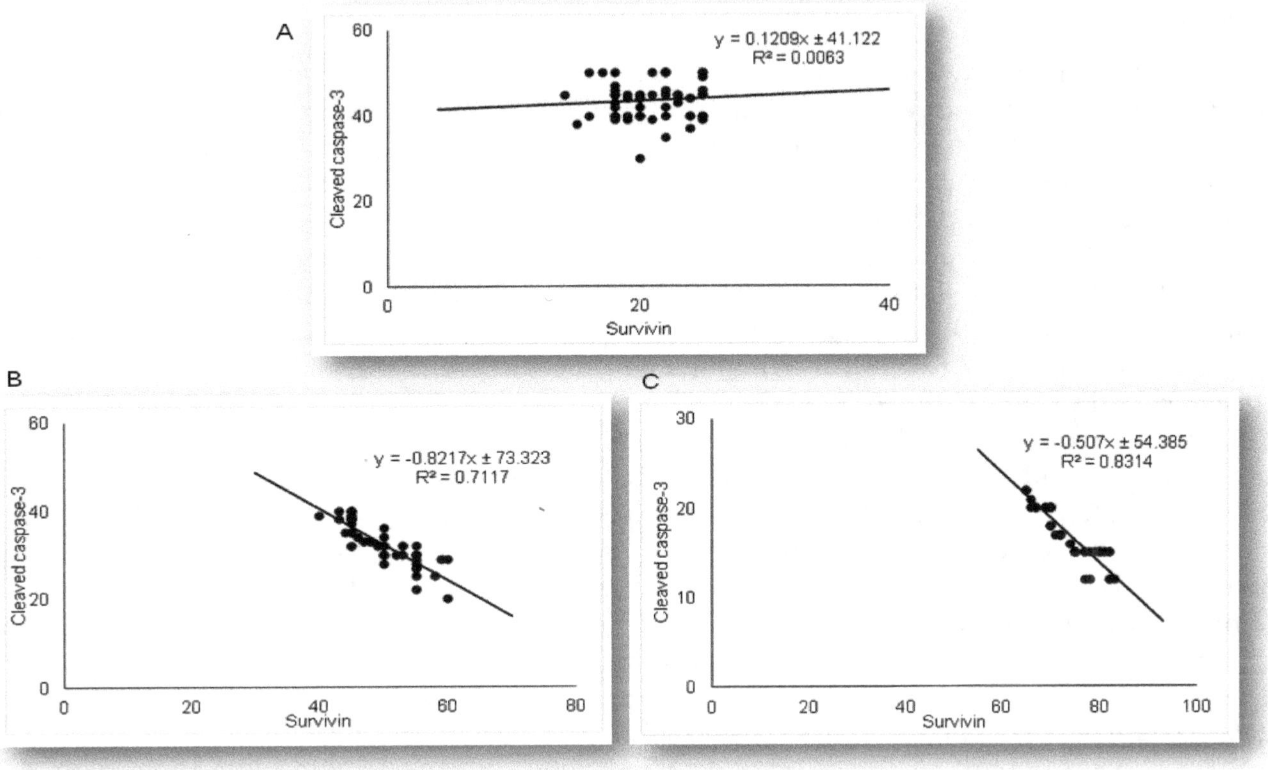

Figure 9. The correlations are shown for survivin and cleaved-caspase-3 in the renal tubular epithelial cells: (**A**) LPS group only, (**B**) simvastatin 20 mg/kg group, (**C**) simvastatin 40 mg/kg group.

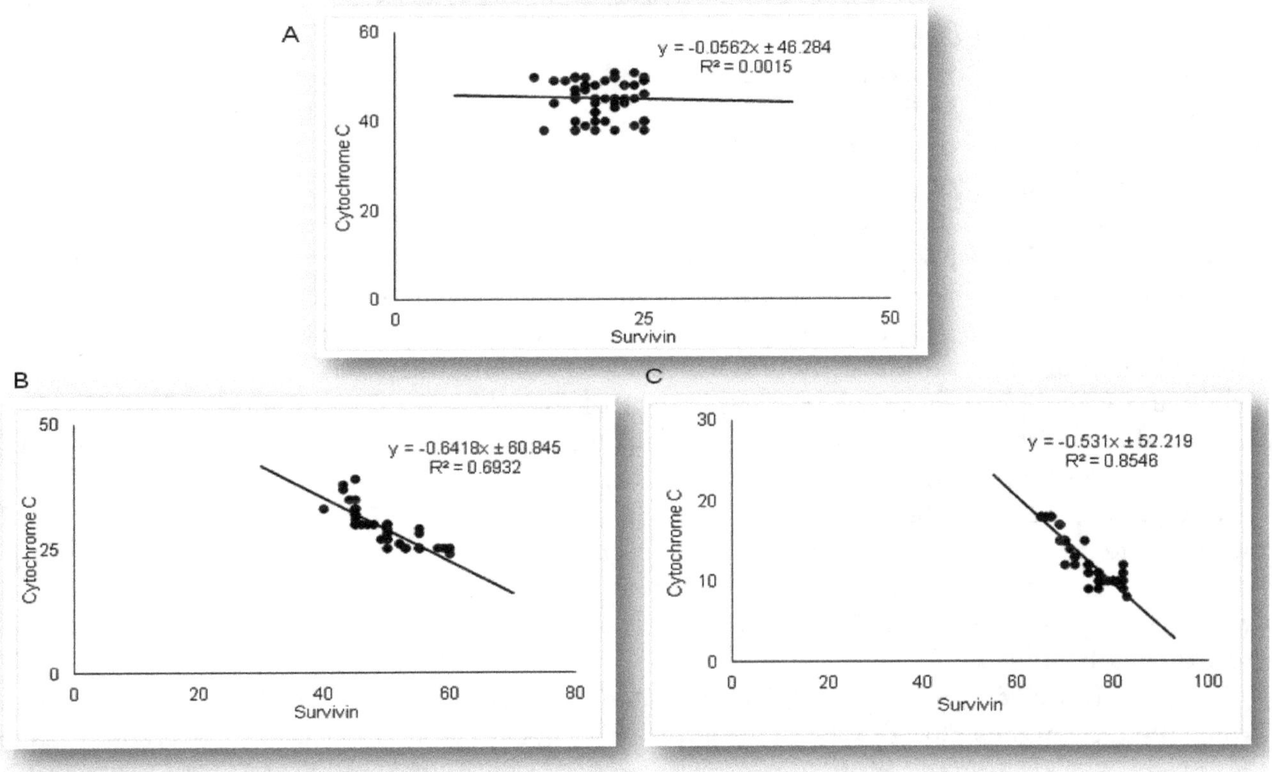

Figure 10. The correlations are shown for survivin and cytochrome C in the renal tubular epithelial cells: (**A**) LPS, (**B**) simvastatin 20 mg/kg group, (**C**) simvastatin 40 mg/kg group.

3. Discussion

In the present study, a standard model of AKI induced by LPS was used to investigate the renoprotective effects of simvastatin on apoptotic signaling molecules in the development of AKI. The main findings indicate that without simvastatin, LPS severely damaged renal tissue, mainly due to induction of glomerular cell proliferation and tubular epithelial cell apoptosis mediated by a mitochondrial apoptotic pathway leading to caspase-3 cleavage. In contrast, with simvastatin pretreatment, the rats were protected against LPS-induced renal inflammatory injury, that is confirmed by attenuated apoptosis of tubular epithelial cells, and significantly increased expression of anti-apoptotic molecules, Bcl-XL and survivin. These results demonstrate that inhibition of cytochrome C apoptotic cascade and activation of IAP might be a mechanism of simvastatin cell-protective effects against bacterial toxin-associated AKI.

Growing experimental evidence has shown that pretreatment with statins prevents tissue injuries induced by bacterial toxins [20–24]. Consistently, our work and the studies by Apaya et al. [25] and Ozkok et al. [26] demonstrated that simvastatin attenuated LPS-induced renal injury, seen as a significantly reduced amount of infiltrating leukocytes associated with minimal histopathological features. It has been known that LPS/TLR4 signaling triggers systemic inflammation but also local renal inflammatory injury and apoptosis through the proinflammatory cytokines TNF-α release, to induce AKI [13]. Our previous results showed that simvastatin dose-dependently decreased overproduction of TNF-α and IL-1β in endotoxemia [19], therefore it is conceivable that in this study, simvastatin targets both inflammatory pathways to protect renal tubules against LPS.

Statins are known to have potent renoprotective effects in gentamicin-, cisplatin-, and cyclosporine-induced nephrotoxicity by a variety of mechanisms, ranging from antioxidant, anti-inflammatory, and anti-apoptotic effects [27]. However, to our knowledge, simvastatin suppression of tubular cell apoptosis in AKI associated with a septic condition has not been reported. Here, we showed that one of the potential protective mechanisms of simvastatin against AKI is blockade of renal tubular cell apoptosis, confirmed by reduced cytochrome C and cleaved caspase-3 expression and corresponding DNA fragmentation. Interestingly, results of antiapoptotic actions of simvastatin through inhibition of pro-apoptotic Bim/Bax and effectors caspases have been well documented in hepatocytes and lymphocytes, and cardiomyocyte in other's and our previous studies [20,21,28,29].

Ultrastructural changes and dysfunctions of renal epithelial mitochondria appear to be an underlying mechanism in septic AKI, similarly to other sepsis-induced multi-organ failure [1,8]. A recent study by Liu et al. [9] showed dominant mitochondrial-mediated apoptosis in CLP-induced AKI with notable leakage of cytochrome C, followed by activation of downstream caspase-9 and -3, and disturbance of mitochondrial dynamics. In the present study, we observed that simvastatin abolished an LPS-induced significant increase of cytochrome C in renal tubular cells. This observation tightly correlates with a marked inhibition of cleaved caspase-3 in simvastatin groups, indicating its cell-protective mechanism against LPS.

Importantly, Bcl-2-related antiapoptotic protein such as Bcl-XL, control outer mitochondrial membrane integrity, bind to proapoptotic Bim/Bax proteins, and inhibit cell-death by preventing the release of pro-apoptotic factors such as cytochrome C or apoptosis-inducing factor [8,30]. Our results showed overexpression of Bcl-XL in tubular cells in simvastatin groups, accompanied by significantly decreased cytochrome C.

Consistently, our previous studies demonstrated that simvastatin upregulated Bcl-XL expression in LPS-challenged organs [20,21], while vitamin D or glycyrrhizin acid, an active ingredient of licorice, by targeting Bcl-2, suppressed tubular apoptosis, and markedly prevented LPS-induced AKI [13,31]. As Bcl-XL is one of the key anti-apoptotic proteins in renal tubular cells, our findings strongly suggest that simvastatin controls apoptosis by targeting Bcl-2 proteins and inhibiting cytochrome C.

Survivin, the unique member of the IAPs family, has a dual cellular role in the regulation of mitosis and inhibition of apoptosis. Biological functions of survivin depend on localization, so that in the cytosol (mitochondrial survivin), it initiates anti-apoptotic activity by blockade caspase cascade, while nuclear localization enables cell division. Cytoprotection by survivin is more selective and appears to target the cascade of mitochondrial cytochrome C-mediated apoptosis in order to prevent caspase-9 and downstream caspase-3 activation [5,32,33]. Previous studies have demonstrated that survivin, expressed dominantly in the proximal tubular cells, prevents development of AKI and renal apoptosis induced by various nephrotoxins (such as folic acid, cisplatin) by suppression of expression of the p53 gene [34,35] and in ischemia/reperfusion (I/R) injury through activation of the Notch-2 intracellular signaling pathway [36]. Our results have demonstrated increased cytoplasmic survivin expression in renal tubular cells in response to LPS that we assumed as induction of a cell-protection mechanism. Further, simvastatin induced intense and dose-dependent expression of survivin in the tubular epithelium that is inversely correlated with cytochrome C and cleaved caspase-3 respectively, and indicates its evident anti-apoptotic effects. Because our previous studies indicated an important role of survivin/NF-κB/p65 pathway activation in cytoprotection against LPS-injury [20,21], similar to Wilson et al. [37], in CLP-induced cardiomyopathy, we hypothesized that simvastatin has significant cell-protective effects in septic AKI but not only by inhibiting of apoptotic cell death but through induction of the important intracellular survival pathways in renal tubular epithelium.

4. Materials and Methods

4.1. Experimental Animals

Adult Wistar rats, 6–8 weeks old (200–220 g), raised at the Institute for Biomedical Researches, Military Medical Academy, Belgrade, Republic of Serbia, were used in this trial.

A typical macrolon plastic cage (Bioscape, Castrop-Rauxel, Germany) filled with clear sawdust (Versele-Laga, Deinze, Belgium) was used for experimental animals' housing. Ambient conditions, the temperature of 22 ± 2 °C, the humidity of 55% ± 15%, air changes/h of 15–20, and the light/dark cycle of 12/12 h, in the animal housing room were centrally regulated. A commercial diet mixture for rats (Veterinary Institute Subotica, Subotica, Republic of Serbia) and tap water ad libitum were applied for animals' feeding.

Before the start of the study, the experimental design, laboratory protocol, and welfare of the experimental animals were approved by the Ethics Committee of Experimental Animals of the Military Medical Academy, Belgrade, Serbia (No. 282-12/2002). This decision confirmed that in the complete experimental study, animal care and all treatments throughout the research are in compliance with Directive 2010/63/EU on the protection of animals used for scientific purposes and the Guidelines for Animal Welfare adopted by the Republic of Serbia (No. 323-07-04943/2014-05/1).

4.2. Drugs

The drug used in the experiment, simvastatin (donation for research purposes only, from pharmaceutical company Krka, Novo Mesto, Slovenia), was prepared in 0.5% methylcellulose as 10 or 20 mg/mL stocks.

Lipopolysaccharide (LPS, endotoxin, producer Sigma Aldrich, Munich, Germany), serotype 0127:B8 *Escherichia coli* was dissolved with sterile pyrogen-free physiologic saline and administered intraperitoneally (i.p.) immediately after dilution.

Each invasive procedure in animals was operated under aseptic conditions.

4.3. Experimental Design

In the model of experimental sepsis, we used endotoxin, and challenged the experimental animals with a non-lethal single dose of LPS i.p. (0.25 LD_{50}/kg). This experimental sepsis is a widely accepted model that is featured with high-grade acute systemic inflammation, inflammatory infiltration, increased oxidative stress, and apoptosis of organ tissues [14,38,39]. Simvastatin was administered in the three different dose regimens (10, 20, and 40 mg/kg p.o.), that was confirmed in our previous experiments as the doses that completely protect the animals against the single median lethal dose

(LD_{50}) of 22.15 mg/kg i.p. of LPS in rats (95% CI 16.5–29.1) [19]. The dose selection of simvastatin was based on the previous rat/murine in vivo studies where the dose range was 10–100 mg/kg/day, considering a rapid upregulation (3- to 10-fold) of HMG-CoA reductase's activity induced by statin treatment or other inhibitors in rodents. Therefore, the simvastatin doses in this experiment were higher compared to those recommended in clinical medicines [14,40,41].

A total of 30 animals were divided into five experimental groups and received the following treatments: (1) Control group (0.5% methylcellulose 1 mL/kg i.p.), (2) LPS group (non-lethal dose as 0.25 LD_{50}/kg i.p., that is equal to 5.5 mg/kg of LPS i.p.), (3) Simvastatin 10 group (simvastatin 10 mg/kg p.o. + 0.25 LD_{50}/kg LPS i.p.), (4) Simvastatin 20 group (simvastatin 20 mg/kg p.o. + 0.25 LD_{50}/kg LPS i.p.), and (5) Simvastatin 40 group (simvastatin 40 mg/kg p.o. + 0.25 LD_{50}/kg LPS i.p.).

After dissolution, simvastatin was given per os via oral gavage in the short-term treatment of 5 days, and the single non-lethal dose of LPS was administered 1.5 h after the simvastatin pretreatment. In the LPS group, animals received the same vehicle (1 mL/kg) of 0.5% methylcellulose for the same period as the simvastatin treatment, prior to LPS injection. The control group received an identical volume of vehicle only. After LPS administration, the animals were monitored continuously for 48 h and then sacrificed.

4.4. Histopathological Examination and Semiquantitative Analysis of Renal Damage Score

The renal protective effect of simvastatin was evaluated after receiving the last treatment. Before sacrification, all animals were immobilized in a dorsal position and euthanized by using sodium pentobarbital in a single dose of 30 mg/kg i.p. (Hemofarm AD, Vršac, Republic of Serbia). Shortly after the autopsy, a renal tissue sample from each animal was fixed in 10% neutral solution during the one-week period. Then, fixed renal tissue samples were divided into six equal sections, which were dehydrated in a series of alcohol (70%, 96%, and 100%) and xylene. After fitting into paraffin blocks, each 2 μm thick renal tissue section was stained using the hematoxylin and eosin (H&E) method.

The whole visual field from each renal slice was analyzed and photographed at magnification 200×, by using a light microscope connected with a digital camera (BX-45, Olympus, Tokyo, Japan) for histopathological examination, as per our method previously published in the literature [42–48]. To assess the degree of renal damages, which consists of edema, hyperemia, neutrophils infiltration, glomerular cells' proliferation, and renal hemorrhages, a semi-quantitative 5-point scale was applied as previously described [43]. The severity of renal impairment expressed as Renal Damage Score (RDS) is shown in Table 2. The exact method for RDS calculation is presented in Table 1.

Table 2. Tissue scoring scale for renal alterations—Renal Damage Score (RDS).

Degree	Description
0	Normal finding.
1	Mild damage: Single glomerular cells slightly enlarged. Mild dilatation of small blood vessels. A few foci of inflammatory cell infiltrates.
2	Moderate damage: < 50% glomerular cells with proliferation. Severe vasodilatation associated with hyperemia and edema. Various numbers of inflammatory cells infiltrates.
3	Severe and focal damage: > 50% glomerular cells with proliferation. Transmural rupture of the blood vessels (up to 50%) associated with an accumulation of inflammatory cells.
4	Severe and diffuse damage: Complete loss of the normal glomerular architecture, and the basal membrane and endothelial cells of the blood vessels (>50%). High-intensity hemorrhages and diffuse accumulation of inflammatory cells.

4.5. Detection and Quantification of Tubular Cell Apoptosis in Situ by TUNEL Method

The TUNEL (Terminal deoxynucleotidyl transferase-mediated dUTP Nick End Labeling) assay was used to assess the apoptosis of renal tubular cells. To perform TUNEL staining on paraffin-embedded sections (4–6 μm thickness), we used the In-Situ Cell Death Detection Kit POD (Roche Molecular Biochemicals, Basel, Switzerland, Cat. No 11 684 817 910) according to the manufacturer's instructions. Renal tissue slides were incubated with anti-fluorescein antibody conjugated with horseradish peroxidase (POD), and then color development was performed using diaminobenzidine (DAB) substrate. According to these instructions, negative (incubation with Label Solution, instead of TUNEL reaction) and positive controls (incubation with DNase I recombinant, grade I) were performed.

Two blinded pathologists assessed TUNEL cells (immuno-positive reaction). The slides were examined under a light microscope (Olympus Plaza, Tokyo, Japan) at 400× magnifications. Twenty non-successive fields per sample were counted for the number of TUNEL-positive tubular cells. Apoptotic index (AI) defined as the percentage (%) of apoptotic tubular cells was calculated according to the formula (1):

$$\text{AI (\% of apoptotic cells)} = \frac{\text{the number of TUNEL} - \text{positive tubular cells} \times 100}{\text{total number of tubular cells}} \tag{1}$$

4.6. Detection and Quantification of Apoptosis Regulating Molecules by Immunohistochemistry

Paraffin-embedded sections of kidney tissues were stained with polyclonal rabbit antibodies for cleaved caspase-3 (Asp 175, Cat. 9661, Cell Signaling Technology, Frankfurt, Germany), monoclonal mouse antibody for Cytochrome C, clone 7H8.2C12 (Cat. MA5-11674, Invitrogen, Thermo Fisher Scientific, Walthman, MA, United States), polyclonal rabbit antibody for anti-apoptotic Bcl-XL (Cat. PA1-37161, Invitrogen, Thermo Fisher Scientific, Walthman, MA, United States), and monoclonal mouse antibody for survivin, clone 8E2 (Cat. MS-1201-P1 NeoMarkers Inc., Fremont, CA, The United States), according to the manufacturer's instructions.

The standard protocol was followed for the immunohistochemistry staining on 3–4 μm deparaffinized and rehydrated tissue sections. Slides were then boiled for 20 min in a microwave oven with a citric acid buffer solution (0.01 mol/L citrate buffer, pH 6.0.). To reduce nonspecific background staining, slides were incubated in 3% hydrogen peroxide for 10 min. Primary antibodies for cleaved caspase-3 (1:300), Cytochrome C (1:100), Bcl-XL (RTU), and survivin (1:50) were applied according to the manufacturer's recommended protocol. The slides were washed thoroughly with phosphate-buffered saline, pH 7.4, between the steps. 3,3′-Diaminobenzidine (DAB) (TL-015-HDJ, Thermo Scientific Lab Vision UltraVision ONE Detection System) was used as chromogen, to develop the antigen-antibody complex, and all slides were then counterstained with H&E, dehydrated, and mounted. Appropriate positive and negative controls were processed in parallel.

The slides were analyzed with a microscope (Olympus, Tokyo, Japan) at 400× magnification. For these sections, the average number of immune-positive cells (tubular cells with intensive optical density expression of cleaved caspase-3, Cytochrome C, BCL-XL, and survivin) across twenty non-successive fields was calculated by two independent pathologists in a blinded manner, using ImageJ software 1.50 (National Institute of Health, Bethesda, Rockville, MD, United States).

Quantitative measurement of the immuno-positive tubular cells was expressed according to this formula (2):

$$\text{\% of positively stained cells} = \frac{\text{the number of positively stained tubular cells} \times 100}{\text{total number of tubular cells}} \tag{2}$$

Survivin expression was evaluated qualitatively, where tubular cells positive for cytoplasmic staining were considered immuno-positive and taken into account [33,49,50].

4.7. Statistical Analysis

The statistical software package SPSS 19.0. (IBM Corporation, New York, NY, The United States) was used to analyze the results which were presented as mean value ($\overline{\mathbf{X}}$) ± standard deviation (SD). To differentiate the renal damage score (RDS) as well as the expression of biomarkers among the groups, we used the Kruskal–Wallis rank test and analysis of variance (one-way ANOVA) followed by the Tamhane's T2 post hoc test, respectively. Correlation analysis was presented as Pearson's correlation coefficient. $p < 0.05$ was considered statistically significant.

5. Conclusions

This study broadened the current understanding of simvastatin anti-apoptotic and cytoprotective effects against LPS-induced AKI. Mechanistically, it seems that simvastatin inhibits the mitochondrial release of cytochrome C and consequent cleavage of the effector caspase-3, resulting in the blockade of tubular cells' apoptosis. Moreover, simvastatin promotes cell-survival by enhancing Bcl-XL and survivin expression, signaling molecules are known that inhibit the intrinsic apoptotic pathway mediated by cytochrome C and directly block caspase-3 respectively, and in turn, inhibits apoptosis in tubular epithelium. Based on our findings in the AKI model reported here, we suggest that using simvastatin for the prevention of AKI in septic conditions is a promising therapeutic option in targeting apoptosis, and more preclinical and clinical studies should be encouraged in this regard.

Author Contributions: Conceptualization, L.N., R.Š., L.A., and V.J.; methodology, L.N., L.A., Z.M., and V.J.; software, L.N., L.A., and V.J.; validation, L.N., R.Š., E.N., and V.J.; formal analysis, L.N., L.A., and V.J.; investigation, L.N., Z.M., and V.J.; resources, L.N., R.Š., R.G., E.N., K.K., and V.J.; writing—original draft preparation, L.N. and V.J.; writing—review and editing, L.N., E.N., K.K., and V.J.; visualization, L.N., L.A., and V.J.; supervision, K.K.; project administration, E.N.; funding acquisition, L.N., R.Š., E.N., K.K., and V.J. All authors have read and agreed to the published version of the manuscript.

Acknowledgments: The research was conducted by the support given from the Ministry of Science and Technology, Republic of Srpska, Bosnia and Herzegovina. This work also supported by the University of Hradec Kralove (Faculty of Science VT2019-2021) and FNHK (UHHK, 00179906), Hradec Kralove, Czech Republic. The Medical Faculty of the Military Medical Academy, the University of Defence in Belgrade, Republic of Serbia (MFVMA/04/20-22) also took part in support of this work.

References

1. Gomez, H.; Kellum, J.A. Sepsis-induced acute kidney injury. *Curr. Opin. Crit. Care.* **2016**, *22*, 546–553. [CrossRef]
2. Plotnikov, E.Y.; Brezgunova, A.A.; Pevzner, I.B.; Zorova, L.D.; Manskikh, V.N.; Popkov, V.A.; Silachev, D.N.; Zorov, D.B. Mechanisms of LPS-Induced acute kidney injury in neonatal and adult rats. *Antioxidants* **2018**, *7*, 105. [CrossRef] [PubMed]
3. Stasi, A.; Intini, A.; Divella, C.; Franzin, R.; Montemurno, E.; Grandaliano, G.; Ronco, C.; Fiaccadori, E.; Pertosa, G.B.; Gesualdo, L.; et al. Emerging role of Lipopolysaccharide binding protein in sepsis-induced acute kidney injury. *Nephrol. Dial. Transpl.* **2017**, *32*, 24–31. [CrossRef] [PubMed]
4. Jo, S.K.; Cha, D.R.; Cho, W.Y.; Kim, H.K.; Chang, K.H.; Yun, S.Y.; Won, N.H. Inflammatory cytokines and lipopolysaccharide induce Fas-mediated apoptosis in renal tubular cells. *Nephron* **2002**, *91*, 406–415. [CrossRef]
5. Flusberg, D.A.; Sorger, P.K. Surviving apoptosis: Life-death signalling in single cells. *Trends Cell. Biol.* **2015**, *25*, 446–458. [CrossRef] [PubMed]
6. Zhang, S.; Li, R.; Dong, W.; Yang, H.; Zhang, L.; Chen, Y.; Wang, W.; Li, C.; Wu, Y.; Ye, Z.; et al. RIPK3 mediates renal tubular epithelial cell apoptosis in endotoxin-induced acute kidney injury. *Mol. Med. Rep.* **2019**, *20*, 1613–1620. [CrossRef]

7. Jacobs, R.; Honore, P.M.; Joannes-Boyau, O.; Boer, W.; De Regt, J.; De Waele, E.; Collin, V.; Spapen, H.D. Septic acute kidney injury: The culprit is inflammatory apoptosis rather than ischemic necrosis. *Blood Purif.* **2011**, *32*, 262–265. [CrossRef]
8. Parikh, S.M.; Yang, Y.; He, L.; Tang, C.; Zhan, M.; Dong, Z. Mitochondrial function and disturbances in the septic kidney. *Semin. Nephrol.* **2015**, *35*, 108–119. [CrossRef]
9. Liu, J.X.; Yang, C.; Zhang, W.H.; Su, H.Y.; Liu, Z.J.; Pan, Q.; Liu, H.F. Disturbance of mitochondrial dynamics and mitophagy in sepsis-induced acute kidney injury. *Life Sci.* **2019**, *235*, 116828. [CrossRef]
10. Zhong, X.; He, J.; Zhang, X.; Li, C.; Tian, X.; Xia, W.; Gan, H.; Xia, Y. UCP2 alleviates tubular epithelial cell apoptosis in lipopolysaccharide-induced acute kidney injury by decreasing ROS production. *Biomed. Pharm.* **2019**, *115*, 108914. [CrossRef]
11. Kim, J.Y.; Lee, S.J.; Maeng, Y.I.; Leem, J.; Park, K.K. Protective Effects of Bee Venom against Endotoxemia-Related Acute Kidney Injury in Mice. *Biology* **2020**, *9*, 154. [CrossRef] [PubMed]
12. Leeds, J.; Scindia, Y.; Loi, V.; Wlazlo, E.; Ghias, E.; Cechova, S.; Portilla, D.; Ledesma, J.; Swaminathan, S. Protective Role of DJ-1 in Endotoxin-induced Acute Kidney Injury. *Am. J. Physiol. Renal. Physiol* **2020**. [CrossRef] [PubMed]
13. Du., J.; Jiang, S.; Hu, Z.; Tang, S.; Sun, Y.; He, J.; Li, Z.; Yi, B.; Wang, I.; Zhang, H.; et al. Vitamin D receptor activation protects against lipopolysaccharide-induced acute kidney injury through suppression of tubular cell apoptosis. *Am. J. Physiol. Ren. Physiol.* **2019**, *316*, F1068–F1077. [CrossRef] [PubMed]
14. Nežić, L.; Škrbić, R.; Dobrić, S.; Stojiljković, M.P.; jaćevič, V.; Stoisavljević, S.; Milovanović, Z.A.; Stojaković, N. Simvastatin and indomethacin have similar anti-inflammatory activity in a rat model of acute local inflammation. *Basic Clin. Pharm. Toxicol.* **2009**, *104*, 185–191. [CrossRef]
15. Zhao, G.; Yu, Y.M.; Kaneki, M.; Bonab, A.A.; Tompkins, R.G.; Fischman, A.J. Simvastatin reduces burn injury-induced splenic apoptosis via down-regulation of the TNF-α/ NF-κB pathway. *Ann. Surg.* **2015**, *261*, 1006–1012. [CrossRef]
16. Wang, Y.; Yang, W.; Zhao, X.; Zhang, R. Experimental study of the protective effect of simvastatin on lung injury in rats with sepsis. *Inflammation* **2018**, *41*, 104–113. [CrossRef]
17. He, X.; Yang, J.; Li, L.; Tan, H.; Wu, Y.; Ran, P.; Sun, S.; Chen, J.; Zhou, Y. Atorvastatin protects against contrast-induced nephropathy via anti-apoptosis by the upregulation of Hsp27 in vivo and in vitro. *Mol. Med. Rep.* **2017**, *15*, 1963–1972. [CrossRef] [PubMed]
18. Kaushik, S.; Tomar, A.; Puthanmadhom Narayanan, S.; Nag, T.C.; Arya, D.C.; Bhatia, J. Pitavastatin attenuates cisplatin–induced renal injury by targeting MAPK and apoptotic pathways. *J. Pharm. Pharm.* **2019**, *71*, 1072–1081. [CrossRef]
19. Nežić, L.; Škrbić, R.; Dobrić, S.; Stojiljković, M.P.; Šatara, S.S.; Milovanović, Z.A.; Stojaković, N. Effect of simvastatin on proinflammatory cytokines production during lipopolysaccharide-induced inflammation in rats. *Gen. Physiol. Biophys.* **2009**, *28*, 119–126.
20. Nežić, L.; Škrbić, R.; Amidžić, L.j.; Gajanin, R.; Kuča, K.; Jaćević, V. Simvastatin protects cardiomyocytes against endotoxin-induced apoptosis and up-regulates survivin/NF-κB/p65 expression. *Sci. Rep.* **2018**, *8*, 14652. [CrossRef]
21. Nežić, L.; Amidžić, L.j.; Škrbić, R.; Gajanin, R.; Nepovimova, E.; Vališ, M.; Kuča, K.; Jaćević, V. Simvastatin inhibits endotoxin-induced apoptosis in liver and spleen through up-regulation of survivin/NF-kB/p65 expression. *Front. Pharm.* **2019**, *10*, 54. [CrossRef] [PubMed]
22. Yasuda, H.; Yuen, P.S.; Hu, X.; Zhou, H.; Star, R.A. Simvastatin improves sepsis-induced mortality and acute kidney injury via renal vascular effects. *Kidn. Int.* **2006**, *69*, 1535–1542. [CrossRef]
23. Chen, C.H.; Lee, R.P.; Wu, W.T.; Liao, K.W.; Hsu, N.; Hsu, B.G. Fluvastatin ameliorates endotoxin-induced multiple organ failure in conscious rats. *Resuscitation* **2007**, *74*, 166–174. [CrossRef]
24. Wang, Y.; Zhang, L.; Zhao, X.; Yang, W.; Zhang, R. An experimental study of the protective effect of simvastatin on sepsis-induced myocardial depression in rats. *Biomed. Pharm.* **2017**, *94*, 705–711. [CrossRef]
25. Apaya, M.K.; Lin, C.Y.; Chiou, C.Y.; Yang, C.C.; Ting, C.Y.; Shyur, L.F. Simvastatin and a plant galactolipid protect animals from septic shock by regulating oxylipin mediator dynamics through the MAPK-cPLA2 signalling pathway. *Mol. Med.* **2016**, *21*, 988–1001. [CrossRef]
26. Özkök, E.; Yorulmaz, H.; Ateş, G.; Aydın, I.; Ergüven, M.; Tamer, Ş. The impact of pretreatment with simvastatin on kidney tissue of rats with acute sepsis. *Physiol. Int.* **2017**, *104*, 158–170. [CrossRef] [PubMed]

27. Yang, Y.; Song, M.; Liu, Y.; Liu, H.; Sun, L.; Peng, Y.; Liu, F.; Venkatachalam, M.A.; Dong, Z. Renoprotective approaches and strategies in acute kidney injury. *Pharm. Ther.* **2016**, *163*, 58–73. [CrossRef] [PubMed]
28. Shinozaki, S.; Inoue, Y.; Yang, W.; Fukaya, M.; Carter, E.A.; Yu, Y.; Fishman, A.; Tompkins, R.; Kanrki, M. Farnesyltransferase inhibitor improved survival following endotoxin challenge in mice. *Biochem. Biophys. Res. Commun.* **2010**, *391*, 1459–1464. [CrossRef]
29. Slotta, J.E.; Laschke, M.W.; Schilling, M.K.; Menger, M.D.; Jeppsson, B.; Thorlacius, H. Simvastatin attenuate hepatic sensitization to lipopolysaccharide after partial hepatectomy. *J. Surg. Res.* **2010**, *162*, 184–192. [CrossRef]
30. Lee, E.F.; Fairlie, W.D. The Structural Biology of Bcl-xL. *Int. J. Mol. Sci.* **2019**, *20*, 2234. [CrossRef]
31. Zhao, H.; Liu, Z.; Shen, H.; Jin, S.; Zhang, S. Glycyrrhizic acid pretreatment prevents sepsis-induced acute kidney injury via suppressing inflammation, apoptosis and oxidative stress. *Eur. J. Pharm.* **2016**, *781*, 92–99. [CrossRef]
32. Dohi, T.; Beltrami, E.; Wall, N.R.; Plescia, J.; Altieri, D.C. Mitochondrial survivin inhibits apoptosis and promotes tumorigenesis. *J. Clin. Inv.* **2004**, *114*, 1117–1127. [CrossRef]
33. Tsang, T.J.; Hsueh, Y.C.; Wei, E.I.; Lundy, D.J.; Cheng, B.; Chen, Y.T.; Wang, S.S.; Hsieh, P.C.H. Subcellular localization of survivin determines its function in cardiomyocytes. *Theranostics* **2017**, *7*, 4577–4590. [CrossRef] [PubMed]
34. Kindt, N.; Menzebach, A.; Van de Wouwer, M.; Betz, I.; De Vriese, A.; Conway, E.M. Protective role of the inhibitor of apoptosis protein, survivin, in toxin-induced acute renal failure. *Faseb. J.* **2008**, *22*, 510–521. [CrossRef] [PubMed]
35. Yang, C.; Guo, Y.; Huang, T.S.; Zhao, J.; Huang, X.J.; Tang, H.X.; An, N.; Pan, Q.; Xu, Y.-Z.; Liu, H.-F. Asiatic acid protects against cisplatin-induced acute kidney injury via anti-apoptosis and anti-inflammation. *Biomed. Pharmacother.* **2018**, *107*, 1354–1362. [CrossRef]
36. Chen, J.; Chen, J.K.; Conway, E.M.; Harris, R.S. Survivin mediates renal proximal tubule recovery from AKI. J. *Am. Soc. Nephrol.* **2013**, *24*, 2023–2033. [CrossRef]
37. Wilson, R.L.; Selvaraju, V.; Lakshmanan, R.; Thirunavukkarasu, M.; Campbell, J.; McFadden, D.W.; Maulik, D.W. Thioredoxin-1 attenuates sepsis-induced cardiomyopathy after cecal ligation and puncture in mice. *J. Surg. Res.* **2017**, *220*, 68–78. [CrossRef]
38. Seemann, S.; Zohles, F.; Lupp, A. Comprehensive comparison of three different animal models for systemic inflammation. *J. Biomed. Sci.* **2017**, *24*, 60. [CrossRef]
39. Kosaka, J.; Lankadeva, Y.R.; May, C.N.; Bellomo, R. Histopathology of septic acute kidney injury: A systematic review of experimental data. *Crit. Care Med.* **2016**, *44*, e897–e903. [CrossRef]
40. Kita, T.; Brown, M.S.; Goldstein, J.L. Feedback regulation of 3-hydroxy-3-methylglutaryl coenzyme A reductase in livers of mice treated with mevinolin, a competitive inhibitor of the reductase. *J. Clin. Inv.* **1980**, *66*, 1094–1100. [CrossRef]
41. Morel, J.; Hargreaves, I.; Brealey, D.; Neergheen, V.; Backman, J.T.; Lindig, S.; Bläss, M.; Bauer, M.; McAuley, D.F.; Singer, M. Simvastatin pre-treatment improves survival and mitochondrial function in a 3-day fluid-resuscitated rat model of sepsis. *Clin. Sci.* **2017**, *131*, 747–758. [CrossRef] [PubMed]
42. Jaćević, V.; Jovic, D.; Kuča, K.; Dragojevic-Simic, V.; Dobric, S.; Trajkovic, S.; Borisev, I.; Segrt, Z.; Milovanovic, Z.; Bokonjic, D.; et al. Effects of Fullerenol nanoparticles and Amifostine on radiation-induced tissue damages: Histopathological analysis. *J. Appl. Biomed.* **2016**, *14*, 285–297. [CrossRef]
43. Jaćević, V.; Djordjevic, A.; Srdjenovic, B.; Milic-Tores, V.; Segrt, Z.; Dragojevic-Simic, V.; Kuca, K. Fullerenol nanoparticles prevent doxorubicin-induced acute hepatotoxicity in rats. *Exp. Mol. Pathol.* **2017**, *102*, 360–369. [CrossRef]
44. Jaćević, V.; Dragojević-Simić, V.; Tatomirović, Ž.; Dobrić, S.; Bokonjić, D.; Kovačević, A.; Nepovimova, E.; Vališ, M.; Kuča, K. The efficacy of amifostine against multiple-dose doxorubicin-induced toxicity in rats. *Int. J. Mol. Sci.* **2018**, *19*, 2370. [CrossRef] [PubMed]
45. Jaćević, V.; Nepovimova, E.; Kuča, K. Toxic injury to the muscle tissue of rats following acute oximes exposure. *Sci. Rep.* **2019**, *9*, 1457. [CrossRef]
46. Jaćević, V.; Nepovimova, E.; Kuča, K. Acute toxic injuries of rat's visceral tissues induced by different oximes. *Sci. Rep.* **2019**, *9*, 16425. [CrossRef]
47. Jaćević, V.; Wu, Q.; Nepovimova, E.; Kuča, K. Efficacy of methylprednisolone on T-2 toxin-induced cardiotoxicity in vivo: A pathohistological study. *Environ. Toxicol. Pharm.* **2019**, *71*, 103221. [CrossRef]

48. Jaćević, V.; Wu, Q.; Nepovimova, E.; Kuča, K. Cardiomiopythy induced by T-2 toxin. *Food Chem. Toxicol.* **2020**, *137*, 111138. [CrossRef]
49. Wang, K.; Brems, J.J.; Gamelli, R.L.; Holterman, X.A. Survivin signalling is regulated through the nuclear factor-kappa B pathway during glycochenodeoxycholate-induced hepatocyte apoptosis. *Biochim. Biophys. Acta* **2010**, *1803*, 1368–1375. [CrossRef]
50. Scheer, A.; Knauer, S.K.; Verhaegh, R. Survivin expression pattern in the intestine of normoxic and ischemic rats. *BMC Gastroenterol.* **2017**, *17*, 76. [CrossRef]

6

Growth Differentiation Factor 15 Ameliorates Anti-Glomerular Basement Membrane Glomerulonephritis in Mice

Foteini Moschovaki-Filippidou [1], Stefanie Steiger [1], Georg Lorenz [2], Christoph Schmaderer [2], Andrea Ribeiro [1], Ekaterina von Rauchhaupt [1], Clemens D. Cohen [1], Hans-Joachim Anders [1], Maja Lindenmeyer [3] and Maciej Lech [1,*]

1 LMU Klinikum, Medizinische Klinik und Poliklinik IV, Ludwig-Maximilians-Universität Munich, 80336 München, Germany; foteini.moschovaki@gmail.com (F.M.-F.); stefanie.steiger@med.uni-muenchen.de (S.S.); andrea.sof@gmail.com (A.R.); katjats95@gmail.com (E.v.R.); C.Cohen@med.uni-muenchen.de (C.D.C.); hjanders@med.uni-muenchen.de (H.-J.A.)

2 Klinikum rechts der Isar, Department of Nephrology, Technical University Munich, 81675 München, Germany; georg.lorenz.gl@googlemail.com (G.L.); christoph.schmaderer@mri.tum.de (C.S.)

3 III. Department of Medicine, University Medical Center Hamburg-Eppendorf, 20246 Hamburg, Germany; m.lindenmeyer@uke.de

* Correspondence: maciej.lech@med.uni-muenchen.de

Abstract: Growth differentiation factor 15 (GDF15) is a member of the transforming growth factor-β (TGF-β) cytokine family and an inflammation-associated protein. Here, we investigated the role of GDF15 in murine anti-glomerular basement membrane (GBM) glomerulonephritis. Glomerulonephritis induction in mice induced systemic expression of GDF15. Moreover, we demonstrate the protective effects for GDF15, as GDF15-deficient mice exhibited increased proteinuria with an aggravated crescent formation and mesangial expansion in anti-GBM nephritis. Herein, GDF15 was required for the regulation of T-cell chemotactic chemokines in the kidney. In addition, we found the upregulation of the CXCR3 receptor in activated T-cells in GDF15-deficient mice. These data indicate that CXCL10/CXCR3-dependent-signaling promotes the infiltration of T cells into the organ during acute inflammation controlled by GDF15. Together, these results reveal a novel mechanism limiting the migration of lymphocytes to the site of inflammation during glomerulonephritis.

Keywords: inflammation; T cells; glomerulonephritis; innate immunity; chemokines

1. Introduction

Anti-glomerular basement membrane glomerulonephritis (anti-GBM nephritis) is a severe acute kidney disease characterized by a variety of lesion patterns, including crescents, vascular loop necrosis, and mesangial expansion, suggesting multiple pathogenic mechanisms [1–4]. The upstream role of the adaptive immune system in failing to maintain immune tolerance and its downstream role in causing antigen-specific immunopathology in the glomerular compartment of the kidney has been widely recognized [3,5–7]. Experimental and clinical studies confirmed that various pro-inflammatory mediators are involved in this process [8–10]. For example, chemokines and transforming growth factor-β (TGF-β) family members regulate the inflammatory process and determine the progression and outcome of anti-GBM nephritis [11–14].

Growth differentiation factor 15 (GDF15, also known as macrophage inhibitory cytokine-1, MIC-1) is produced as a 35 kDa full-length form, cleaved in the N-terminus and secreted as a 25 kDa mature form [15]. GDF15 is a divergent member of the TGF- β superfamily and shows several structural differences compared to the rest of the superfamily. GDF15 is a regulator of inflammatory response dendritic cells maturation [16] and peripheral blood mononuclear proliferation [17]. Moreover, its role was suggested in cervical cancer, glioblastoma, cardiovascular ischemic stress, obesity, and metabolic disease, such as mitochondrial myopathies [18–24]. However, the knowledge of its role in progression of glomerulonephritis (GN) and mechanisms of function is still limited and requires further investigation. T cell-driven effector mechanisms play an important role, particularly in crescentic GN [25], and understanding the function of T-cells in the disease can be beneficial in future therapies for glomerular injury. Some studies showed a functional role for CD4+ T cells as effector cells participating in the development of crescentic GN by executing delayed-type hypersensitivity [26]. Others identified CD4+ cells but not CD8+ cells as crucial for the development of crescentic GN in mice [27]. By contrast, some findings suggest that glomerular injury in anti-GBM GN is driven by macrophage recruitment, which depends on both CD4+ and CD8+ T cells, and that T cell cytotoxicity does not play a role in the progression of the disease [28]. However, an anti-CD8 monoclonal antibody therapy was effective in both the prevention and treatment of experimental autoimmune glomerulonephritis [29], which could be associated with the effects of CD8+ cells on ICAM-1 and cytokine expression in crescentic glomerulonephritis [30]. Until now, systemic GDF15 levels have been shown to correlate with the progression of chronic kidney disease (CKD). Recombinant GDF15 protein reduced fibroblast activation and interstitial fibrosis in a model of unilateral ureter obstruction (UUO), possibly by blocking the TGF-β receptor and N-Myc signaling pathways [31]. Moreover, GDF15 reduces the expression of MHC class II and co-stimulatory molecules, as well as NF-kB family members Rel A and Rel B, IL-2, IFN-γ, and IL-12p40, and increases expression of TGF-β, and IL-10 [32]. In general, GDF15 is believed to be associated with stress responses, but its precise biological functions remain to be elucidated. Although GDF15 has been shown to affect aspects of chronic diseases (both inflammation and fibrosis), whether it controls glomerular disease progression is unclear [31,33,34].

In the present study, we used GDF15-deficient mice to investigate the role of GDF15 in anti-GBM nephritis. We hypothesized that GDF15 ameliorates the anti-Glomerular Basement Membrane (GBM) glomerulonephritis by limiting the inflammation and infiltration of the immune cells into the kidney.

2. Results

2.1. Experimental Anti-GBM Nephritis Is Associated with Higher Systemic and Intrarenal Expression of GDF15

We first asked if we could detect increased levels of GDF15 in mice following anti-GBM nephritis. To develop a reliable model, we tested several protocols and chose one with significant proteinuria and histopathological changes (Figure 1A). The nephrotoxic potential of the GBM antiserum in C57BL/6 mice (without pre-immunization) was previously assessed [35]. To implement the autologous adaptive immune response, we immunized mice with sheep-IgG 7 days prior to anti-GBM serum injection. We compared the development of albuminuria from day 0 to 21 in order to define the time-point with stable glomerular injury (Figure 1A). Moreover, we compared the amount of albuminuria of pre-immunized mice with mice without pre-immunization (heterologous model). Pre-immunization and the administration of anti-GBM serum resulted in a significant increase in albuminuria at 7 and 14 days. RT-PCR analysis of *Gdf15* and serum analysis of the protein revealed a low basal expression level, which was significantly upregulated 14 days upon anti-GBM serum injection (Figure 1B,C). We conclude that GDF15 is induced anti-GBM nephritis and that our protocol (7 + 14 days) of autologous anti-GBM nephritis is suitable to study the role of GDF15 in glomerular inflammation.

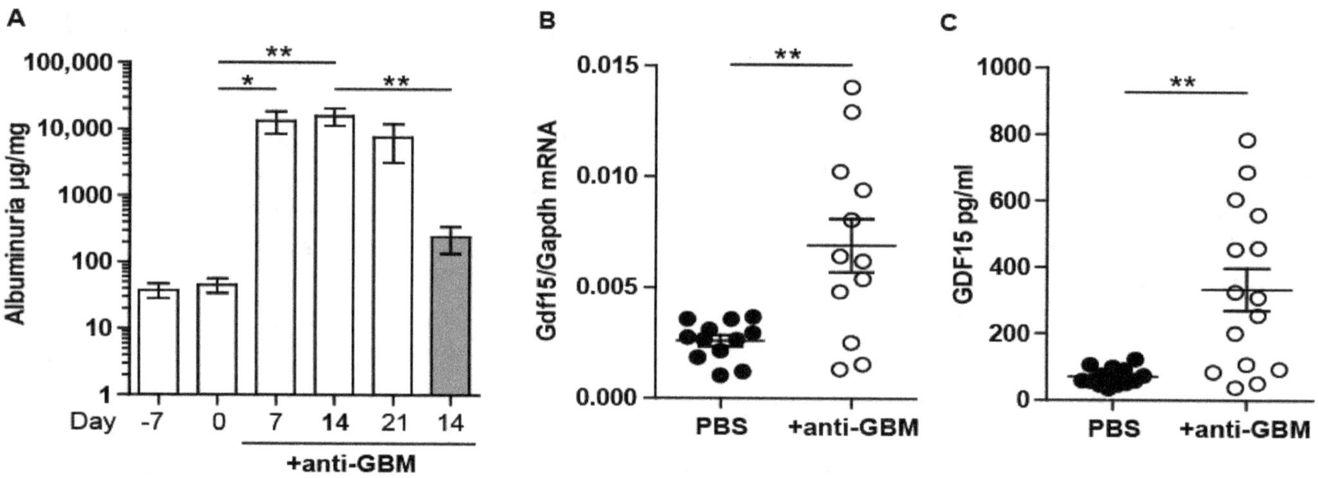

Figure 1. Evaluation of the anti-GBM model and expression of GDF15. (**A**) We used the commercially available GBM antiserum that was raised in sheep against rat GBM. We first examined its nephritogenic potential in C57BL/6 mice by assessing albuminuria 7, 14, and 21 days after a single intravenous injection of antiserum in pre-immunized mice, as well as in mice without pre-immunization (gray bar, 14 days). ($n = 5$, one-way ANOVA). (**B**) Total RNA isolated from kidneys of saline- or antiserum-injected C57BL/6 mice underwent quantitative real-time RT-PCR analysis and revealed significantly higher expression of Gdf15 in treated mice. (**C**) Serum GDF15 level was significantly increased in antiserum-injected C57BL/6 mice ($n = 12$, Student's *t*-Test). Data are mean ± SEM. * $p < 0.05$; ** $p < 0.01$.

2.2. GDF15 Deficiency Aggravates Albuminuria, Kidney Function Loss, and More Severe Tubular and Glomerular Injury in Anti-GBM Nephritis

In order to address the role of GDF15 in glomerular inflammation, we applied the same protocol to C57BL/6 mice and *Gdf15-/-* mice. Plasma levels of multiple cytokines revealed an increased pro-inflammatory systemic signature. We detected significantly increased levels of IL-6, IL-12, TNF-α, and IFN-γ in the serum of GDF15-deficient mice (Figure 2A). Significantly increased glomerular filtration markers such as serum creatinine and blood urea nitrogen, glomerular injury markers-i.e., albuminuria (albumin/urine creatinine ratio), and tubular injury markers-i.e., urinary lipocalin-2 (NGAL) were noted in *Gdf15-/-* mice compared with wild type controls, which indicates more severe kidney disease in knockout mice (Figure 2B).

Based on these data, we assumed that GDF15 might play a protective role in anti-GBM nephritis. Both ongoing inflammation and severe glomerular injury can cause tubular injury. As expected, kidney sections stained with Periodic acid Schiff (PAS) reagent revealed increased tubular cast formation and tubular atrophy (scored as tubular injury TI) in nephritic GDF15-deficient animals compared to nephritic wild type animals (Figure 2D). These results demonstrate that the systemic deletion of *Gdf15* ameliorates proteinuria and renal tubular injury in anti-GBM nephritis. We did not observe any significant differences in total IgG levels in the blood of wild type and knockout mice. Consequently, the whole IgG staining of renal tissue did not reveal significant differences between the two treated groups (Figure 2C).

Because the majority of patients with an anti-GBM disease develop widespread glomerular crescent formation followed by features of rapidly progressive glomerulonephritis, we quantified the number of glomerular crescents of $n = 8$ mice per group. We showed that GDF15-deficient mice displayed enhanced crescent formation (Figure 3A). As endothelial cells (ECs) are involved in the inflammatory process in glomeruli and the progression of glomerulonephritis, we investigated by immunohistochemistry the expression of CD31. Glomerular endothelial injury leads to podocyte loss and proteinuria. A cross-sectional evaluation revealed that the glomeruli of *Gdf15-/-* mice strongly expressed the CD31 marker (Figure 3B). Importantly, we observed the differences in glomerular architecture between wild type and knockout mice, indicating distinct stages of glomerulonephritis. To assess the cellular (including endothelial cell) proliferative responses, we stained renal sections with the antibody against Ki67. We observed increased proliferation of the cells in glomeruli as in the other renal compartments. This indicates the higher rearrangement (triggered by higher injury) of the tissue of knockout mice compared to wild types (Figure 3C). Furthermore, *Gdf15-/-* mice with anti-GBM nephritis exhibited a decreased number of WT1 positive podocytes in the glomeruli (Figure 3D). These pathological features explained massive albuminuria, increased BUN, and serum creatinine observed (Figure 2B). Together, lack of GDF15 induces severe renal disease upon anti-GBM serum treatment, whereas control mice (WT anti-GBM) displayed a less severe phenotype. These data emphasize an indispensable role for GDF15 in kidney disease.

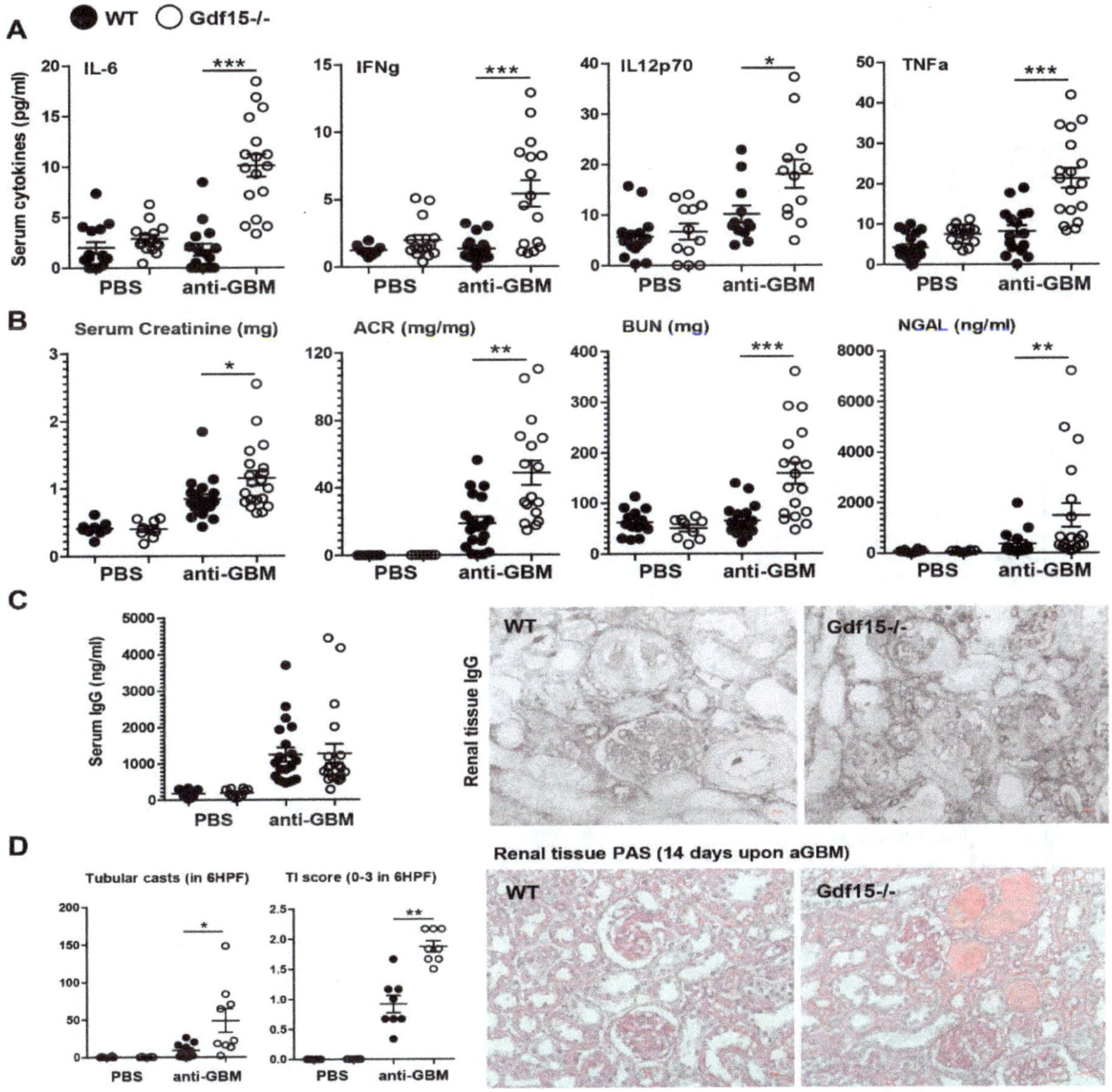

Figure 2. Systemic inflammation, kidney function, and histopathology of anti-GBM nephritis. (**A**) Sera were obtained from wild type or GDF15-deficient C57BL/6 mice on day 14 after saline or antiserum (anti-GBM) injection. Cytokine levels were quantified by flow cytometry ($n = 15$–17, one-way ANOVA). (**B**) Renal function parameter ($n = 15$–17, one-way ANOVA). (**C**) Serum IgG levels ($n = 15$–17, one-way ANOVA) and immunohistochemistry staining for IgG on kidney sections were quantified. (**D**) Kidneys from WT or KO mice were paraffin-embedded, stained with Periodic acid-Schiff (PAS) reagent, and quantified to assess tubular casts formation and tubular injury score ($n = 8$ mice per group, one-way ANOVA). Representative images of renal sections (original magnification 400×). Data are mean ± SEM. * $p < 0.05$; ** $p < 0.01$; *** $p < 0.001$.

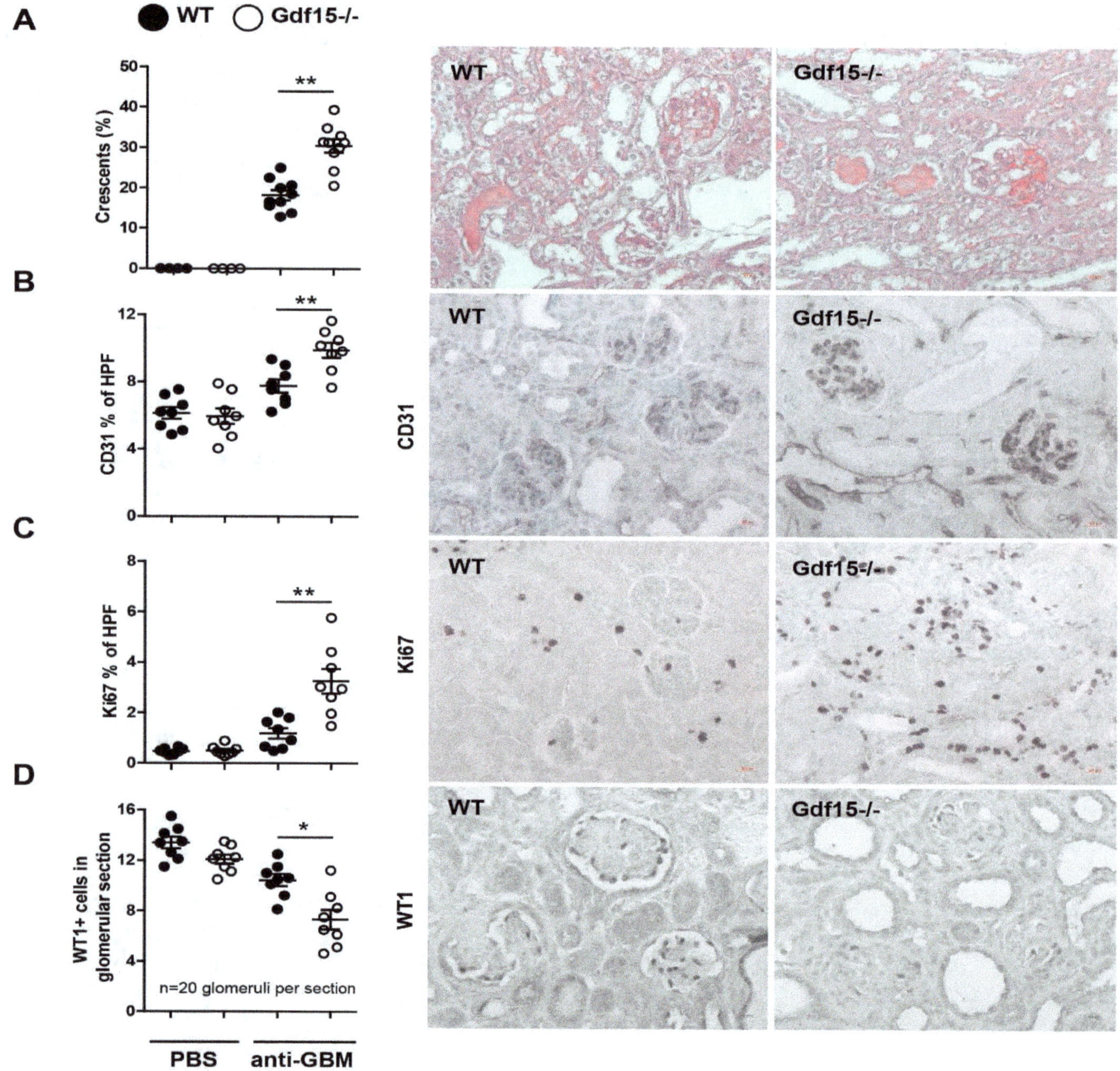

Figure 3. Kidney histopathology of anti-GBM nephritis. Sections were obtained from wild type or GDF15-deficient C57BL/6 mice on day 14 after saline or antiserum (anti-GBM) injection. Kidneys from WT or KO mice were paraffin-embedded and stained either with (**A**) PAS, (**B**) anti-CD31 antibody, (**C**) anti-ki67 antibody and (**D**) anti-WT1 antibody, and quantified (n = 8 mice per group, one-way ANOVA). Representative images of renal sections (original magnification 400×). Data are mean ± SEM. * $p < 0.05$; ** $p < 0.01$.

2.3. Gdf15-Deficient Mice Exhibit Increased Renal Inflammation in Anti-GBM Nephritis Model

Further, we investigated the impact of GDF15 on renal inflammation as one of the key determinants of glomerular damage and albuminuria in the early phase of anti-GBM nephritis. We hypothesized that the mechanism underlying severe glomerulonephritis in *Gdf15-/-* mice could be associated with T cells. T-cells play a crucial role in proliferative and crescentic glomerulonephritis and can be a trigger of severe and rapid damage even in the absence of glomerular antibody deposition [3,8,36]. Indeed, we observed a significant increase in the number of CD3+ T cells, neutrophils, and macrophages on kidney sections from anti-GBM-treated *Gdf15-/-* mice compared with WT mice (Figure 4A). At the preselected mRNA level, the expression of the glomerular extracellular matrix proteins, matrix remodeling enzymes matrix metalloproteinase-7 and matrix metalloproteinase-9, as well as inflammation markers, was higher in anti-GBM-treated *Gdf15-/-* mice compared with WT mice on day 14 (Figure 4B). However, the further quantification of samples revealed that the expression of chemokines/cytokines *Ccl2, Ccl5, Cxcl1, Cxcl10, Ctgf, and Il2*, as well as adhesion molecules *Icam1* and *Vcam1*, were significantly more expressed in GDF15-deficient mice compared to wild type mice upon anti-GBM serum treatment. Together, the systemic lack of GDF15 leads to an increased progression of renal disease by orchestrating inflammation and immune cell influx.

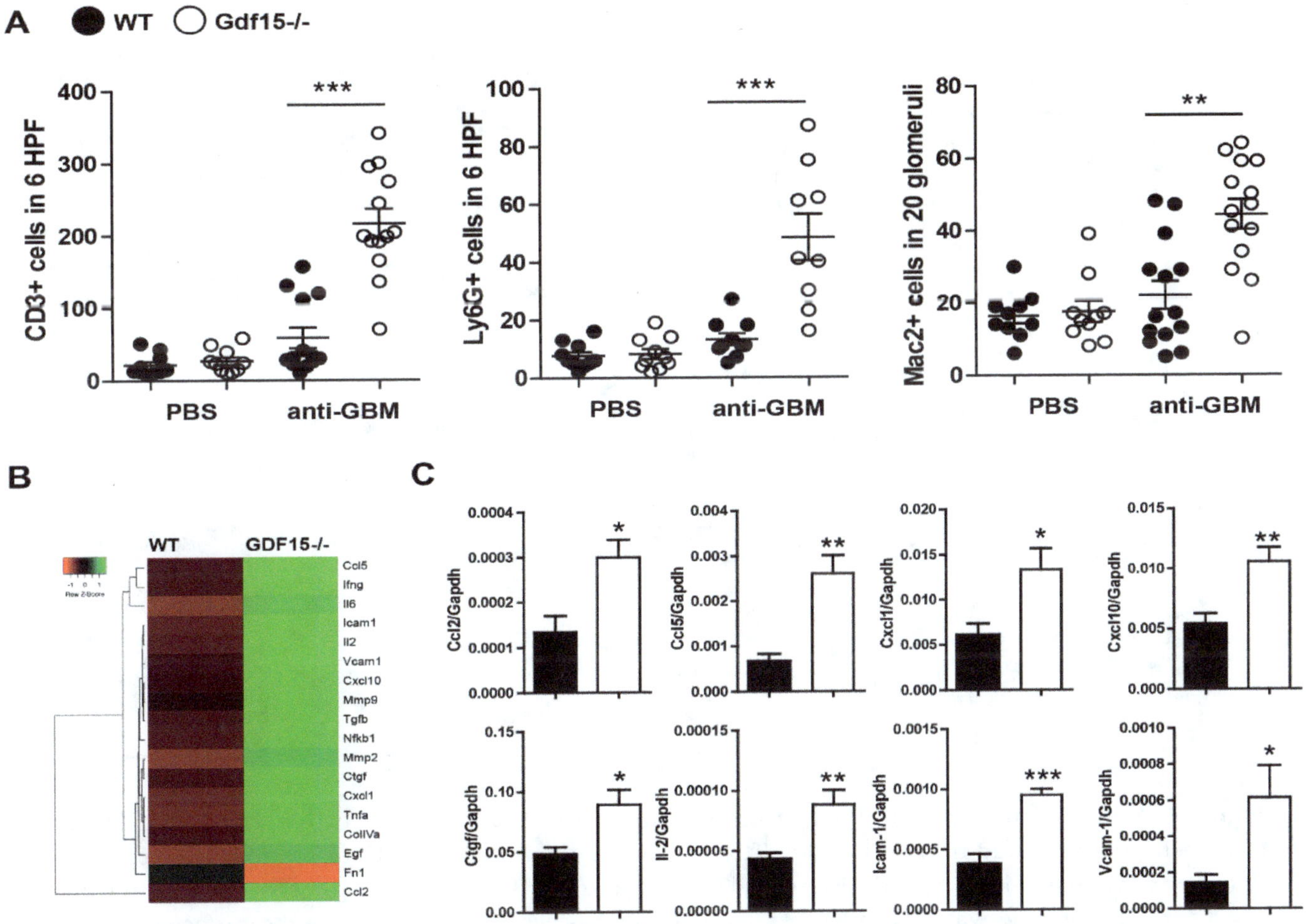

Figure 4. Kidney inflammation in wild type and *Gdf15* KO mice with anti-GBM nephritis. (**A**) Kidney sections were stained with anti- CD3, Ly6G, or Mac2 antibodies and quantified by counting, as indicated on graphs and in material and methods (n = 9–15 mice per group, one-way ANOVA). (**B**) Heat map depicting kidney expression of pre-selected genes of wild type and GDF15-deficient mice upon anti-GBM serum treatment. (**C**) Gene expression levels in kidneys were quantified by real-time PCR. Data are shown as means of the ratio of the specific mRNA vs. that of *Gapdh* mRNA (n = 6–8 samples per group, Student's t-Test). Data are mean ± SEM. * $p < 0.05$; ** $p < 0.01$; *** $p < 0.001$ versus control mice.

2.4. *T Cells from Wild Type and Knockout Mice Display No Differences in Expression of Adhesions Markers*

Due to the observed kidney influx of CD3+ cells and the increased IL-2 expression (crucial T-cell cytokine), we hypothesized that T cells from *Gdf15-/-* mice could also have an adhesion associated phenotype. To evaluate the effect of GDF15-deficiency on the adhesive capacity of T cells, we established an in vitro system in order to analyze the expression of several adhesion markers on T cells isolated from spleens. After the activation of naïve T cells with LPS, we did not observe increased expression of

CD28, CD154, CD62L, and CD11a/CD18 in CD4+ T cells (Figure 5B) nor CD8+ T cells (Figure 5C) in comparison with unprimed vehicle-treated cells. We did not see any significant differences between WT and KO cells. After in vitro stimulation, T cells from wild type and *Gdf15-/-* mice showed no differences in TCR internalization, evidenced by the reduction in CD3 MFI (data not shown). Interestingly, we observed a shift towards CD8+ cytotoxic T cells in primed GDF15-deficient cells (Figure 5A). The accumulation of effector CD8+ T lymphocytes may suggest increased damage to the surrounding tissue.

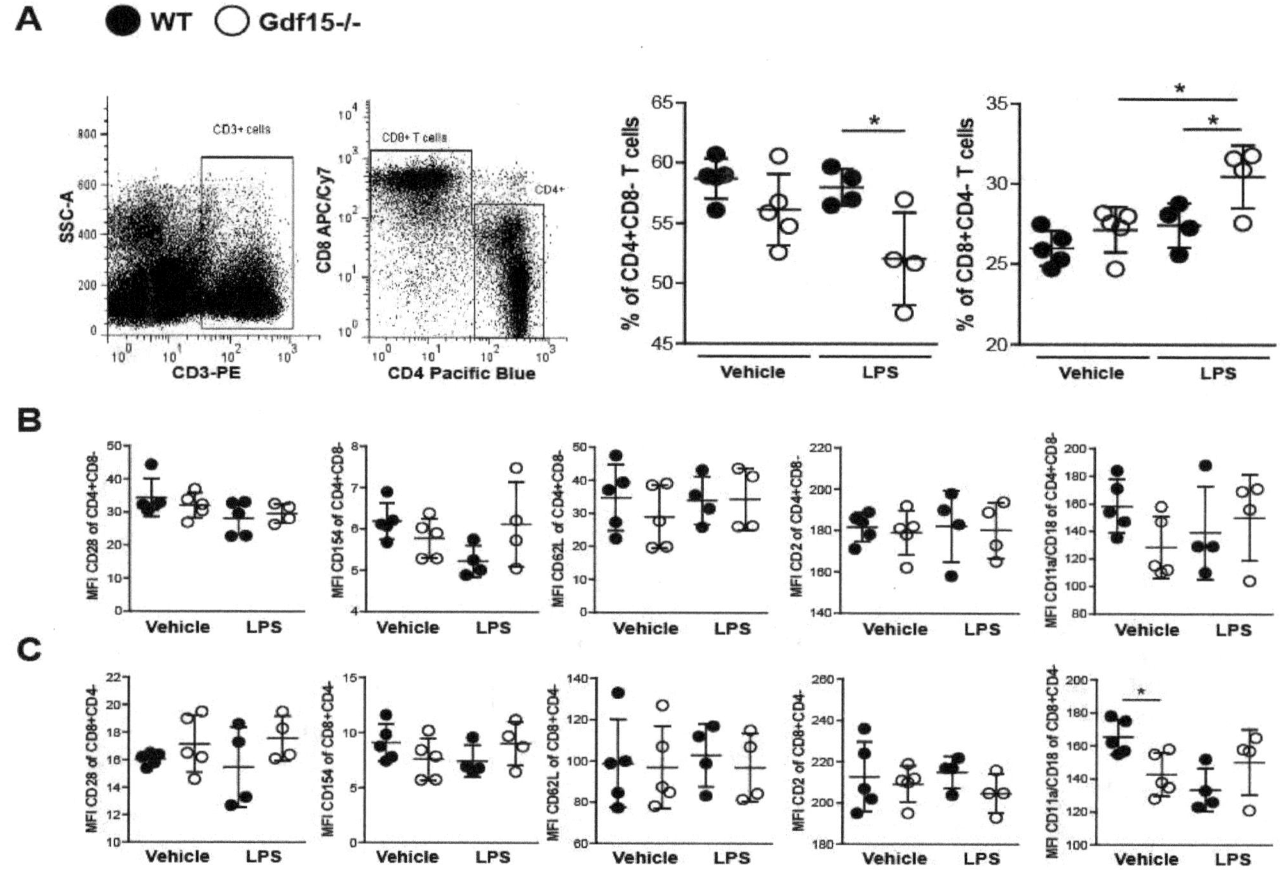

Figure 5. Stimulation of splenic T cells from WT and *Gdf15* KO mice with or without LPS ex vivo. (**A**) T cells were isolated from WT and *Gdf15* KO mice and stimulated with or without LPS for 24 h. The percentage of CD4+CD8- and CD8+CD4- T cells was quantified by flow cytometry (gating strategy, $n = 4$–5 per group, one-way ANOVA). (**B**,**C**) Mean fluorescence intensity (MFI) of the surface markers CD28, CD154, CD62L, CD2, and CD11a/CD18 on LPS-stimulated or untreated CD4+CD8- T cells (**B**) and CD8+CD4- T cells (**C**) ($n = 4$–5 per group, one-way ANOVA). Data are mean ± SD. * $p < 0.05$.

As the trafficking of T cells to tissues mainly depends on the tissue microenvironment, we decided to investigate the effect of chemokines that were highly expressed during anti-GBM nephritis on the migratory potential of T cells. We used both naïve and activated T cells (interaction with APC upon LPS treatment), and analyzed their migration towards the chemokines CXCL1, CXCL10, and CCL5 using migration chambers with micro-channels for 24 h. We observed a significant increase in the percentage of T cells from GDF15-deficient mice that migrated towards CXCL10 but not CXCL1 and CCL5 (Figure 6A). CXCL10 is known to be highly expressed during kidney disease [37–39]. Its receptor CXCR3 is expressed on effector T cells and crucial in T cell trafficking and function [40,41]. Moreover, IFNγ activates the Stat-dependent pathway in tissue-resident cells to enhance the production of CXCL10 during tissue injury. We previously observed high Cxcl10 expression in kidney tissue and high systemic levels of IFN-γ in treated *Gdf15* KO mice. We hypothesized that the elevated number of effector T cells might not only be associated with the CXCR3 receptor. Therefore, we looked at the level of Cxcr3 in naïve and activated T cells. Indeed, we found a significantly higher mRNA and protein levels of CXCR3 in T cells from GDF15-deficient mice upon activation (Figure 6B,C). Taken together, these data indicate that GDF15 plays a role in the migration of T cells to the side of inflammation via a CXCL10-CXCR3 dependent mechanism.

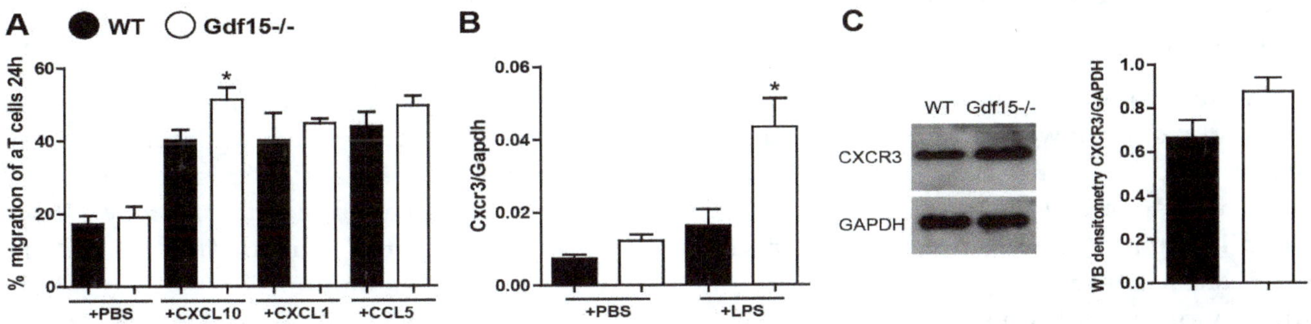

Figure 6. Quantification of T cell migration and CXCR3 expression. (**A**) T cells from the spleens of WT and GDF15-deficient mice were isolated and migration assays were performed. The percentage of migrated T cells towards the chemokines CXCL10, CXCL1, and CCL5 was quantified after 24 h ($n = 4$ per group, one-way ANOVA, * $p < 0.05$). (**B**) Cxcr3 expression levels in LPS-stimulated or untreated T cells were quantified by real-time PCR. Data are shown as means of the ratio of the Cxcr3 mRNA vs. Gapdh mRNA ($n = 4$ per group, one-way ANOVA, * $p < 0.05$). (**C**) CXCR3 protein expression levels in LPS-activated T cells were quantified by Western blot. The histogram shows the densitometry of two independent experiments; no statistical analysis was performed. Data are mean ± SEM.

2.5. *Gene Expression Analysis of GDF15, CXCL10 and CXCR3 in Patients with RPGN*

In order to estimate the transferability of our results to human disease, we assessed transcriptional levels of *GDF15*, *CXCL10*, and *CXCR3* in the glomerular and tubular compartment from human renal biopsy specimens using Affymetrix microarray expression data. For this project, we used biopsies of individuals with rapidly progressive glomerulonephritis (RPGN) versus living donor (LD) biopsy specimens (Figure 7). In both, the glomerular and the tubular compartment of the patient cohort, *GDF15* was significantly downregulated in patients with RPGN compared with controls. At the same time, the *CXCL10* and its receptor *CXCR3* were significantly upregulated it both the glomerular and tubular compartment. Together, genes that seem to be regulated by GDF15 in the experimental mouse model of anti-GBM were induced during rapidly progressive glomerulonephritis in the glomerular and tubular compartment of the kidney.

A

		Glom_LD7_RPGN7		
Entrez Gene	Gene Symbol	Fold change	Log Fold Change	q-value (%)
2833	CXCR3	1.133	0.180	4.322
3627	CXCL10	4.377	2.130	0.013
9518	GDF15	0.392	-1.351	1.343

B

		Tub_LD7_RPGN7		
Entrez Gene	Gene Symbol	Fold change	Log Fold Change	q-value (%)
2833	CXCR3	1.082	0.114	4.917
3627	CXCL10	5.509	2.462	0.000
9518	GDF15	0.652	-0.618	0.446

Figure 7. Gene expression analysis of *GDF15*, *CXCL10*, and *CXCR3* genes in (**A**) glomerular and (**B**) tubular

compartment of manually microdissected kidney biopsies from patients with RPGN. Values are expressed as a log2-fold change compared to controls (living donors, LD). All represented genes are significantly changed ($q < 0.05$). (**A**) Glomerular expression single hybridization (LD: $n = 18$, RPGN: $n = 23$), (**B**) Tubular compartment expression (LD: $n = 18$, RPGN: $n = 21$). Red represents upregulation and blue represents downregulation of the transcript.

3. Discussion

We hypothesized that a GDF-15-associated mechanism is responsible for the development of GBM. Our results now show that the cytokine GDF15 protects from kidney injury and inflammation in a mouse model of anti-GBM nephritis. Furthermore, we demonstrate that Gdf15 is induced locally as well as systemically in the injured kidney and that GDF15 acts as an anti-inflammatory cytokine by regulating systemic cytokine production. GDF15 is involved in the recruitment of T cells into the injured tissue, a phenomenon associated with CXCL10-CXCR3 signaling. This finding is in line with previous reports on the functional role of GDF15 demonstrating that this cytokine can regulate chemokine-triggered β2 integrin activation on myeloid cells [42]. We further expand this knowledge by reporting on the enhanced migratory capability of peripheral blood mononuclear cells towards CXCL10 ex vivo and provide evidence for increased numbers of infiltrating immune cells in kidneys of mice with anti-GBM nephritis. The accumulation of T lymphocytes within the kidney might display a key event contributing to kidney injury. Some of the studies evidenced that anti-GBM GN depends on both CD4 and CD8 T cells without direct T cell-mediated cytotoxicity [28]. Other investigations support the hypothesis that especially CD8+ T cells are important mediators of glomerulonephritis [43]. Nevertheless, chemokines and chemokine receptors play a role in the process of T cell recruitment to the site of inflammation. Here, we show that both CXCL10, as well as its receptor, might be regulated by GDF15. Previous studies highlighted the importance of CXCL10 during inflammation and showed that CXCL10 is critical for the recruitment of CXCR3-expressing effector T cells to the injured tissue [44]. In in vivo models, CXCR3-expressing CD4+ and CD8+ T cells did not migrate efficiently into inflamed tissues of CXCL10-deficient mice compared to wild type, suggesting that CXCR3 expression is crucial for the selection of cells that respond to CXCL10 [44]. Consistent with earlier studies, our data indicate that GDF15 limits the inflammatory response during injury by restricting immune cell infiltration. Kempf et al. showed that GDF15 protects against fatal cardiac rupture by counteracting chemokine-triggered β2 integrin activation on myeloid cells [42]. This, for the first time, implied that GDF15 might be involved in the regulation of cytoskeleton rearrangement. In our experiments, except for changes in inflammation and significant effects of GDF15 on chemokine production, we could observe significant upregulation of *Icam* and *Vcam* adhesion molecules in the injured kidneys of *Gdf15-/-* mice. This suggests pleiotropic effects of GDF15 in the process of progressive GN, whereby GDF15 orchestrates the migration of T cell populations into the kidney. Therefore, treatment with GDF15 seems to be more beneficial than blocking particular chemokines and chemokine receptors to inhibit the selective migration of defined cell populations to the site of inflammation.

Other mechanisms potentially contributing to exaggerated injury in GDF-15-deficient mice include the polarization of cytotoxic CD8 T cells. Although overall surface marker expression upon LPS stimulation was comparable to wild type, we observed a significant decrease in the number of CD4+ T cells but an increase in CD8+ T cells upon activation in knockout cells. This suggests a distinct immune response associated with specific T cell subsets and more severe clinical manifestations in GDF15-deficient mice. CD8+ cytotoxic T cells serve as a potent source of inflammation by producing perforin and granzymes and inducing apoptosis in target cells [45–47]. By contrast, CD4+ helper T cells support the immune responses by promoting the activation and/or proliferation of immune cells [48]. The polarization of T cells towards CD8+ T cells could be an additional explanation for the severe phenotype observed in knockout mice.

In addition, we observed a protective role of GDF15 in both the glomerular and tubular compartment as evidenced by increased macrophage infiltration and expression of inflammatory markers in *Gdf15-/-* mice, indicating that glomerular inflammation in autologous anti-GBM disease involves both innate and adaptive immunity [49,50] and that GDF15 could act as a regulator of both immune responses. Currently, it is unclear whether the injured glomeruli cause tubular damage or whether both processes occur independently of each other due to the accumulation of immunoglobulins and immune complexes in the kidney. In our model, the glomerular damage is accompanied by tubule interstitial damage and both seem to depend on GDF15, because the injury in knockout mice is significantly higher. Therefore, we investigated both the tubular and glomerular compartment of patients with RPGN. RPGN is associated with a high frequency of crescentic glomerulonephritis [51]. Since we observed significant changes in GDF15 in an experimental anti-GBM model, as well as enhanced CXCL10-CXCR3 signaling, we chose to compare the expression of these three transcripts. Our analysis revealed the significant downregulation of GDF15 and at the same time the upregulation of CXCL10 and CXCR3. In support of our experimental findings, the human data suggest that the level of GDF15 affects the infiltration of CXCR3-expressing T cells to the site of injury. For instance, Dai et al. showed that the anti-CXCR3 treatment of mice inhibits autoreactive CD8+ T cells in the skin and peripheral lymphoid tissues [52]. Moreover, in a mouse model of vitiligo, CXCL10-/- unlike CXCL9-/- mice did not develop depigmentation, indicating that the CXCL10-CXCR3 axis is responsible for this disease [53]. In humans, the blockade of CXCL10 showed positive effects on the progression of rheumatoid arthritis, indicating a therapeutic approach in blocking the CXCL10-CXCR3 axis not only in experimental mouse models but also in human disease [54].

Stable and accurate noninvasive markers, as well as a better understanding of the pathophysiology of rapidly progressive GN could enable fast, precise diagnosis and appropriate treatment of the disease. Until now, several studies showed that GDF15 is associated with a rapid decline in kidney function, suggesting that might be a useful predictor for the development of kidney disease. For instance, recent investigations of two independent cohorts showed that systemic GDF15 levels correlate with the intrarenal expression of *GDF15* and are significantly associated with the progression of kidney disease [55]. Enhanced GDF15 levels correlate not only with increased mortality in hemodialysis and diabetic nephropathy (DN) patients [56,57] but also with all-cause mortality [58,59]. Moreover, in DN patients, high levels of GDF15 are associated with a decline in estimated glomerular filtration rate and faster progression to kidney failure [57]. Surely, the enhanced levels of GDF15 can deliver information about the deterioration of kidney function [60–62]. However, the suitability of GDF15 as a precise marker for kidney disease needs further investigation. Moreover, its role as a urinary marker on the progression of kidney disease, as well as the correlation of plasma and urine GDF15 levels, needs to be elucidated [63]. Our experimental study with GDF15-deficient mice proves the strong impact of the protein on the outcome of kidney disease and shows increased systemic and kidney expression of GDF15 during experimental GN. This increase in GDF15 levels during kidney diseases is associated with the increased production of GDF15 in response to stress (unpublished data) rather than with decreased protein clearance from circulation. Collectively, our data suggest that GDF15 reduces the outcome of experimental GN and contributes to pathogenesis by modulating T cell phenotypes and reducing the accumulation of T cells in the kidney. GDF15 may serve as a useful therapeutic molecule that could reduce disease progression by its effect on CXCL10 and CXCR3. The wide range of reported effects is diverse and the inconsistency of the published functions can be referred to by the commercial source of recombinant GDF15, which was contaminated with bioactive concentrations of TGF-β1 [64]. To avoid this issue, we used mice deficient in the GDF15 protein, which consistently proves the immunomodulatory functions of GDF15 in glomerular disease.

4. Materials and Methods

Animal studies: GDF15-deficient mouse strain (MGI: 2386300, *Gdf15tm1Sjl*) were backcrossed to the C57BL/6 strain. Female and male mice were housed in sterile filter top cages with a 12 h dark/light cycle. The study was carried out following the principles of the Directive 2010/63/EU on the Protection of Animals Used for Scientific Purpose and with approval by the local government authorities (27.02.2015; ROB 55.2-1-54-2532-63-12). Induction of anti-GBM nephritis: For the induction of anti-GBM nephritis, mice were pre-immunized subcutaneously with 100 μL of 2 mg/mL sheep IgG (Jackson ImmunoResearch Laboratories Inc., West Grove, PA, USA), dissolved in complete Freund's adjuvant (Sigma-Aldrich, St. Louis, MI, USA). Five days later, sheep anti-rat glomeruli (GBM) serum (Probetex, San Antonio, TX, USA) was injected via the tail vein.

Kidney parameters: Urinary albumin excretion was evaluated by a double-sandwich ELISA. First, 96-well plates were coated with goat anti-mouse albumin antibody A90-13A-5 (Bethyl Laboratories, Montgomery, TX, USA) and plates were incubated overnight at 4 °C. After blocking for half an hour at room temperature in 0.5% BSA in PBS with 0.05% Tween20, urine samples, and mouse albumin standard (Sigma-Aldrich, St. Louis, MI, USA) were added on the plate in triplicates for 2 h. Mouse urine samples were diluted in serial dilutions ranging from $1:10^2$ to $1:10^7$. As a secondary antibody, HRP-conjugated anti-mouse albumin antibody A90-134P-7 (Bethyl Laboratories) was used. Urinary Lipocalin-2/NGAL levels were determined using a commercially available mouse ELISA DuoSet kit (R&D Systems, Park Abingdon, UK), according to manufacturer's recommendations. The samples and standard curve dilutions were added on the plate in triplicates and incubated for two hours. Mouse urine samples were diluted in serial dilutions ranging from $1:10^3$ to $1:10^6$. TMB substrate solution (BD, Franklin Lakes, NJ, USA) was applied and the reaction was stopped after fifteen minutes with 2 M H_2SO_4. OD was measured at 450 nm and the calculation of the final concentrations was performed using a four-parameter logistic curve. Creatinine levels in urine and serum were determined using the creatinine assay DiaSys kit (Diagnostic Systems GmbH, Holzheim, Germany). Urine samples were prepared in dilutions of 1:10, while serum was used undiluted. According to the manufacturer's recommendations, 10 μL of sample or standard was pipetted on 96-well plates in triplicates. Then, 200 μL of prepared reagent provided by the kit was added and absorbance was measure at 492 nm 60 s later. Two more measurements were performed 120 s and 20 min later. Concentrations were calculated using a linear standard curve. Kidney function was determined by measuring serum blood urea nitrogen (DiaSys Diagnostic Systems) and serum creatinine levels determined by the Jaffe method (DiaSys Diagnostic Systems).

Evaluation of kidney histopathology: Organs were fixed in 4% buffered formalin and embedded in paraffin. For quantitative analysis, cells were counted in sections (from at least 8–16 mice per group) or analyzed using Adobe Photoshop CS4Extended (% of stained high power field). The PAS score evaluation was performed following a semi-quantitative scoring system with a scale from 0 to 3. Samples were blinded before evaluation. CD3 positive and Ly6G positive cell quantification was performed by counting the number of positive cells in six adjacent high-power fields (Hpf) of the renal cortex and medulla. For the evaluation of the Mac-2 staining, stained cells in 20 glomeruli per sample were counted.

Mouse IgG detection: The levels of mouse IgG in the serum were determined using the mouse IgG ELISA kit (Bethyl Laboratories), according to the manufacturer's recommendations. Briefly, 96-well plates were coated with coating antibody provided by the kit diluted (1:100) in 0.05 M Carbonate Bicarbonate with pH = 9.6 overnight at 4 °C. After 30 min blocking in 1% BSA in TrisNaCl samples and standard were added on the plate and incubated for one hour. Following five washing steps with TrisNaCl, the detection antibody was added on the plate in a dilution of 1:50,000. After the washing steps, TMB substrate solution (BD) was applied and the reaction was stopped with 2 M H_2SO_4. OD was measured at 450 nm and the calculation of the final concentrations was performed using a four-parameter logistic curve.

Flow cytometry: T cells were isolated from spleens of WT and *Gdf15-/-* mice and stimulated with or without LPS ex vivo for 24 h. After stimulation, T cells were collected, centrifuged, and resuspended in wash buffer (0.1% BSA, 0.01% sodium azide in D-PBS). After blocking the Fc receptor with anti-mouse CD16/32 (2.4G2) for 5 min, cells were stained with the surface antibodies FITC anti-mouse CD28, PacificBlue anti-mouse CD4, APC/Cy7 anti-mouse CD8a, PE anti-mouse CD3, PE/Cy7 anti-mouse CD154, PerCP/Cy5.5 anti-mouse CD2, APC anti-mouse CD11a/CD18, BV510 anti-mouse CD62L (all from BioLegend) for 30 min. After staining, cells were washed with wash buffer and flow cytometry was performed using the BD FACS Canto II (Becton Dickinson, New Jersey, USA). Data were analyzed with the software FlowJo 8.7 (Tree Star Inc., Ashland, OR, USA). For cytokine analysis of serum from mice or cell culture experiments, samples were prepared according to the instruction of the BD Cytometric Bead Array Mouse Inflammation Kit. The concentrations of the cytokines IL-6, IL-10, MCP-1, IFN-γ, TNF, and IL-12p70 in the samples were determined by the software FlowJo 8.7.

Real-time quantitative PCR: SYBR Green Dye detection system was used for quantitative real-time PCR on Light Cycler 480 (Roche, Mannheim, Germany). Gene-specific primers (225 nM, Metabion, Martinsried, Germany) were used. Standard controls for genomic DNA contamination, RNA quality, and general PCR performance were included. RNA was isolated from the samples using the Norgen Biotek Total RNA Purification kit (Thorold, ON, Canada) and MagNA Lyser Green beads (Roche, Basel, Switzerland) according to the manufacturer's instructions. The data were evaluated using the 2ΔΔCT method.

Patients and microarray analysis: Human kidney biopsy specimens and Affymetrix microarray expression data were procured within the framework of the European Renal cDNA Bank–Kröner–Fresenius Biopsy Bank. Biopsies were obtained from patients after informed consent and with the approval of the local ethics committees [65]. Following a renal biopsy, the tissue was transferred to RNase inhibitor and microdissected into glomeruli and tubulointerstitium. Total RNA was isolated from micro-dissected glomeruli, reverse transcribed, and linearly amplified according to a protocol previously reported [66]. CEL file normalization was performed with the Robust Multichip Average method using RMAExpress (Version 1.0.5) and the human Entrez-Gene custom CDF annotation from Brain Array version 18 (http://brainarray.mbni.med.umich.edu/Brainarray/default.asp). To identify differentially expressed genes, the SAM (Significance Analysis of Microarrays) method was applied using TiGR (MeV, Version 4.8.1) [67]. Published gene expression profiles from patients with RPGN as well as controls (living donors (LD)) were used in this study (GSE104954, GSE104948,).

Statistical analysis: Data were expressed as mean ± SEM. Data from wild type and knockout mice were compared with one-way ANOVA on ranks, followed by the Student–Newman–Keuls test using SigmaStat Software (Jandel Scientific, Erkrath, Germany). The student *t*-test was used for direct comparisons between single groups—i.e., wild type and knockout cells/mice in case of normally distributed data or samples size $n > 15$. Mann–Whitney U test was used to analyze data with small sample size and non-parametric distribution of data. We used GraphPad Prism software. A p-value < 0.05 indicated statistical significance. Statistical significance was indicated as follows: p-value of <0.05 (*); p-value of <0.01 (**); p-value of <0.001 (***).

Author Contributions: Conceptualization, F.M.-F. and M.L. (Maciej Lech); formal analysis, F.M.-F., S.S., G.L., A.R., E.v.R., M.L. (Maja Lindenmeyer) and M.L. (Maciej Lech); investigation, F.M.-F., S.S., G.L., A.R., E.v.R. and M.L. (Maciej Lech); resources, H.-J.A., C.D.C. and M.L. (Maciej Lech); writing—original draft preparation, M.L. (Maciej Lech); writing—review and editing, F.M.-F., S.S., G.L., A.R., E.v.R., H.-J.A., C.S., M.L. (Maja Lindenmeyer) and M.L. (Maciej Lech); visualization, F.M.-F., S.S., M.L. (Maja Lindenmeyer) and M.L. (Maciej Lech); supervision, M.L. (Maciej Lech); project administration, M.L. (Maciej Lech); funding acquisition, M.L. (Maciej Lech). All authors have read and agreed to the published version of the manuscript.

Acknowledgments: We thank Karina Adamowicz and Jana Mandelbaum for expert technical support. This work is presented in part in the thesis project of E.vR to the Medical Faculty of the LMU Munich. The ERCB-KFB was supported by the Else Kröner–Fresenius Foundation. We also thank all participating centers of the European Renal cDNA Bank—Kröner–Fresenius biopsy bank (ERCB-KFB) and their patients for their cooperation. For active members at the time of the study see [68].

Abbreviations

MDPI	Multidisciplinary Digital Publishing Institute
DOAJ	Directory of open access journals
TLA	Three letter acronym
LD	Linear dichroism

References

1. McAdoo, S.P.; Pusey, C.D. Anti-Glomerular Basement Membrane Disease. *Clin. J. Am. Soc. Nephrol.* **2017**, *12*, 1162–1172. [CrossRef] [PubMed]
2. Canney, M.; O'Hara, P.V.; McEvoy, C.M.; Medani, S.; Connaughton, D.M.; Abdalla, A.A.; Doyle, R.; Stack, A.G.; O'Seaghdha, C.M.; Clarkson, M.R.; et al. Spatial and Temporal Clustering of Anti-Glomerular Basement Membrane Disease. *Clin. J. Am. Soc. Nephrol.* **2016**, *11*, 1392–1399. [CrossRef] [PubMed]
3. Kurts, C.; Panzer, U.; Anders, H.J.; Rees, A.J. The immune system and kidney disease: Basic concepts and clinical implications. *Nat. Rev. Immunol.* **2013**, *13*, 738–753. [CrossRef] [PubMed]
4. Kumar, S.V.; Kulkarni, O.P.; Mulay, S.R.; Darisipudi, M.N.; Romoli, S.; Thomasova, D.; Scherbaum, C.R.; Hohenstein, B.; Hugo, C.; Muller, S.; et al. Neutrophil Extracellular Trap-Related Extracellular Histones Cause Vascular Necrosis in Severe GN. *J. Am. Soc. Nephrol.* **2015**, *26*, 2399–2413. [CrossRef] [PubMed]
5. Artinger, K.; Kirsch, A.H.; Aringer, I.; Moschovaki-Filippidou, F.; Eller, P.; Rosenkranz, A.R.; Eller, K. Innate and adaptive immunity in experimental glomerulonephritis: A pathfinder tale. *Pediatr. Nephrol.* **2017**, *32*, 943–947. [CrossRef] [PubMed]
6. Suarez-Fueyo, A.; Bradley, S.J.; Klatzmann, D.; Tsokos, G.C. T cells and autoimmune kidney disease. *Nat. Rev. Nephrol.* **2017**, *13*, 329–343. [CrossRef]
7. Krebs, C.F.; Steinmetz, O.M. CD4(+) T Cell Fate in Glomerulonephritis: A Tale of Th1, Th17, and Novel Treg Subtypes. *Mediat. Inflamm.* **2016**, *2016*, 5393894. [CrossRef]
8. Summers, S.A.; Steinmetz, O.M.; Li, M.; Kausman, J.Y.; Semple, T.; Edgtton, K.L.; Borza, D.B.; Braley, H.; Holdsworth, S.R.; Kitching, A.R. Th1 and Th17 cells induce proliferative glomerulonephritis. *J. Am. Soc. Nephrol.* **2009**, *20*, 2518–2524. [CrossRef]
9. Hopfer, H.; Holzer, J.; Hunemorder, S.; Paust, H.J.; Sachs, M.; Meyer-Schwesinger, C.; Turner, J.E.; Panzer, U.; Mittrucker, H.W. Characterization of the renal CD4+ T-cell response in experimental autoimmune glomerulonephritis. *Kidney Int.* **2012**, *82*, 60–71. [CrossRef]
10. Odobasic, D.; Gan, P.Y.; Summers, S.A.; Semple, T.J.; Muljadi, R.C.; Iwakura, Y.; Kitching, A.R.; Holdsworth, S.R. Interleukin-17A promotes early but attenuates established disease in crescentic glomerulonephritis in mice. *Am. J. Pathol.* **2011**, *179*, 1188–1198. [CrossRef]
11. Paust, H.J.; Turner, J.E.; Riedel, J.H.; Disteldorf, E.; Peters, A.; Schmidt, T.; Krebs, C.; Velden, J.; Mittrucker, H.W.; Steinmetz, O.M.; et al. Chemokines play a critical role in the cross-regulation of Th1 and Th17 immune responses in murine crescentic glomerulonephritis. *Kidney Int.* **2012**, *82*, 72–83. [CrossRef] [PubMed]
12. Zhou, A.; Ueno, H.; Shimomura, M.; Tanaka, R.; Shirakawa, T.; Nakamura, H.; Matsuo, M.; Iijima, K. Blockade of TGF-beta action ameliorates renal dysfunction and histologic progression in anti-GBM nephritis. *Kidney Int.* **2003**, *64*, 92–101. [CrossRef] [PubMed]
13. Mesnard, L.; Keller, A.C.; Michel, M.L.; Vandermeersch, S.; Rafat, C.; Letavernier, E.; Tillet, Y.; Rondeau, E.; Leite-de-Moraes, M.C. Invariant natural killer T cells and TGF-beta attenuate anti-GBM glomerulonephritis. *J. Am. Soc. Nephrol.* **2009**, *20*, 1282–1292. [CrossRef] [PubMed]
14. Kanamaru, Y.; Nakao, A.; Mamura, M.; Suzuki, Y.; Shirato, I.; Okumura, K.; Tomino, Y.; Ra, C. Blockade of TGF-beta signaling in T cells prevents the development of experimental glomerulonephritis. *J. Immunol.* **2001**, *166*, 2818–2823. [CrossRef] [PubMed]
15. Bootcov, M.R.; Bauskin, A.R.; Valenzuela, S.M.; Moore, A.G.; Bansal, M.; He, X.Y.; Zhang, H.P.; Donnellan, M.; Mahler, S.; Pryor, K.; et al. MIC-1, a novel macrophage inhibitory cytokine, is a divergent member of the TGF-beta superfamily. *Proc. Natl. Acad. Sci. USA* **1997**, *94*, 11514–11519. [CrossRef]
16. Zhou, Z.; Li, W.; Song, Y.; Wang, L.; Zhang, K.; Yang, J.; Zhang, W.; Su, H.; Zhang, Y. Growth differentiation factor-15 suppresses maturation and function of dendritic cells and inhibits tumor-specific immune response. *PLoS ONE* **2013**, *8*, e78618. [CrossRef] [PubMed]

17. Soucek, K.; Slabakova, E.; Ovesna, P.; Malenovska, A.; Kozubik, A.; Hampl, A. Growth/differentiation factor-15 is an abundant cytokine in human seminal plasma. *Hum. Reprod* **2010**, *25*, 2962–2971. [CrossRef]
18. Rochette, L.; Meloux, A.; Zeller, M.; Cottin, Y.; Vergely, C. Functional roles of GDF15 in modulating microenvironment to promote carcinogenesis. *Biochim. Biophys. Acta Mol. Basis Dis.* **2020**, *1866*, 165798. [CrossRef]
19. Emmerson, P.J.; Wang, F.; Du, Y.; Liu, Q.; Pickard, R.T.; Gonciarz, M.D.; Coskun, T.; Hamang, M.J.; Sindelar, D.K.; Ballman, K.K.; et al. The metabolic effects of GDF15 are mediated by the orphan receptor GFRAL. *Nat. Med.* **2017**, *23*, 1215–1219. [CrossRef]
20. Baek, S.J.; Eling, T. Growth differentiation factor 15 (GDF15): A survival protein with therapeutic potential in metabolic diseases. *Pharmacol. Ther.* **2019**, *198*, 46–58. [CrossRef]
21. Tsai, V.W.W.; Husaini, Y.; Sainsbury, A.; Brown, D.A.; Breit, S.N. The MIC-1/GDF15-GFRAL Pathway in Energy Homeostasis: Implications for Obesity, Cachexia, and Other Associated Diseases. *Cell Metab.* **2018**, *28*, 353–368. [CrossRef] [PubMed]
22. Wang, W.; Yang, X.; Dai, J.; Lu, Y.; Zhang, J.; Keller, E.T. Prostate cancer promotes a vicious cycle of bone metastasis progression through inducing osteocytes to secrete GDF15 that stimulates prostate cancer growth and invasion. *Oncogene* **2019**, *38*, 4540–4559. [CrossRef] [PubMed]
23. Li, S.; Ma, Y.M.; Zheng, P.S.; Zhang, P. GDF15 promotes the proliferation of cervical cancer cells by phosphorylating AKT1 and Erk1/2 through the receptor ErbB2. *J. Exp. Clin. Cancer Res.* **2018**, *37*, 80. [CrossRef] [PubMed]
24. Emmerson, P.J.; Duffin, K.L.; Chintharlapalli, S.; Wu, X. GDF15 and Growth Control. *Front. Physiol.* **2018**, *9*, 1712. [CrossRef]
25. Kalluri, R.; Danoff, T.M.; Okada, H.; Neilson, E.G. Susceptibility to anti-glomerular basement membrane disease and Goodpasture syndrome is linked to MHC class II genes and the emergence of T cell-mediated immunity in mice. *J. Clin. Investig.* **1997**, *100*, 2263–2275. [CrossRef]
26. Huang, X.R.; Holdsworth, S.R.; Tipping, P.G. Evidence for delayed-type hypersensitivity mechanisms in glomerular crescent formation. *Kidney Int.* **1994**, *46*, 69–78. [CrossRef]
27. Tipping, P.G.; Huang, X.R.; Qi, M.; Van, G.Y.; Tang, W.W. Crescentic glomerulonephritis in CD4- and CD8-deficient mice. Requirement for CD4 but not CD8 cells. *Am. J. Pathol.* **1998**, *152*, 1541–1548.
28. Huang, X.R.; Tipping, P.G.; Apostolopoulos, J.; Oettinger, C.; D'Souza, M.; Milton, G.; Holdsworth, S.R. Mechanisms of T cell-induced glomerular injury in anti-glomerular basement membrane (GBM) glomerulonephritis in rats. *Clin. Exp. Immunol.* **1997**, *109*, 134–142. [CrossRef]
29. Reynolds, J.; Norgan, V.A.; Bhambra, U.; Smith, J.; Cook, H.T.; Pusey, C.D. Anti-CD8 monoclonal antibody therapy is effective in the prevention and treatment of experimental autoimmune glomerulonephritis. *J. Am. Soc. Nephrol.* **2002**, *13*, 359–369.
30. Fujinaka, H.; Yamamoto, T.; Feng, L.; Kawasaki, K.; Yaoita, E.; Hirose, S.; Goto, S.; Wilson, C.B.; Uchiyama, M.; Kihara, I. Crucial role of CD8-positive lymphocytes in glomerular expression of ICAM-1 and cytokines in crescentic glomerulonephritis of WKY rats. *J. Immunol.* **1997**, *158*, 4978–4983.
31. Kim, Y.I.; Shin, H.W.; Chun, Y.S.; Park, J.W. CST3 and GDF15 ameliorate renal fibrosis by inhibiting fibroblast growth and activation. *Biochem. Biophys. Res. Commun.* **2018**, *500*, 288–295. [CrossRef] [PubMed]
32. Zhang, Y.; Zhang, G.; Liu, Y.; Chen, R.; Zhao, D.; McAlister, V.; Mele, T.; Liu, K.; Zheng, X. GDF15 Regulates Malat-1 Circular RNA and Inactivates NFkappaB Signaling Leading to Immune Tolerogenic DCs for Preventing Alloimmune Rejection in Heart Transplantation. *Front. Immunol.* **2018**, *9*, 2407. [CrossRef] [PubMed]
33. Zhang, Y.; Jiang, M.; Nouraie, M.; Roth, M.G.; Tabib, T.; Winters, S.; Chen, X.; Sembrat, J.; Chu, Y.; Cardenes, N.; et al. GDF15 is an epithelial-derived biomarker of idiopathic pulmonary fibrosis. *Am. J. Physiol. -Lung Cell. Mol. Physiol.* **2019**, *317*, L510–L521. [CrossRef] [PubMed]
34. Luan, H.H.; Wang, A.; Hilliard, B.K.; Carvalho, F.; Rosen, C.E.; Ahasic, A.M.; Herzog, E.L.; Kang, I.; Pisani, M.A.; Yu, S.; et al. GDF15 Is an Inflammation-Induced Central Mediator of Tissue Tolerance. *Cell* **2019**, *178*, 1231–1244. [CrossRef]
35. Lichtnekert, J.; Kulkarni, O.P.; Mulay, S.R.; Rupanagudi, K.V.; Ryu, M.; Allam, R.; Vielhauer, V.; Muruve, D.; Lindenmeyer, M.T.; Cohen, C.D.; et al. Anti-GBM glomerulonephritis involves IL-1 but is independent of NLRP3/ASC inflammasome-mediated activation of caspase-1. *PLoS ONE* **2011**, *6*, e26778. [CrossRef]

36. Tipping, P.G.; Holdsworth, S.R. T cells in glomerulonephritis. *Springer Semin. Immunopathol.* **2003**, *24*, 377–393. [CrossRef]
37. Zhang, Y.; Thai, K.; Kepecs, D.M.; Winer, D.; Gilbert, R.E. Reversing CXCL10 Deficiency Ameliorates Kidney Disease in Diabetic Mice. *Am. J. Pathol.* **2018**, *188*, 2763–2773. [CrossRef]
38. Gniewkiewicz, M.S.; Czerwinska, M.; Gozdowska, J.; Czerwinska, K.; Sadowska, A.; Deborska-Materkowska, D.; Perkowska-Ptasinska, A.; Kosieradzki, M.; Durlik, M. Urinary levels of CCL2 and CXCL10 chemokines as potential biomarkers of ongoing pathological processes in kidney allograft: An association with BK virus nephropathy. *Pol. Arch. Intern. Med.* **2019**, *129*, 592–597. [CrossRef]
39. Nakaya, I.; Wada, T.; Furuichi, K.; Sakai, N.; Kitagawa, K.; Yokoyama, H.; Ishida, Y.; Kondo, T.; Sugaya, T.; Kawachi, H.; et al. Blockade of IP-10/CXCR3 promotes progressive renal fibrosis. *Nephron Exp. Nephrol.* **2007**, *107*, e12–e21. [CrossRef]
40. Groom, J.R.; Luster, A.D. CXCR3 in T cell function. *Exp. Cell Res.* **2011**, *317*, 620–631. [CrossRef]
41. Groom, J.R.; Luster, A.D. CXCR3 ligands: Redundant, collaborative and antagonistic functions. *Immunol. Cell Biol.* **2011**, *89*, 207–215. [CrossRef] [PubMed]
42. Kempf, T.; Zarbock, A.; Widera, C.; Butz, S.; Stadtmann, A.; Rossaint, J.; Bolomini-Vittori, M.; Korf-Klingebiel, M.; Napp, L.C.; Hansen, B.; et al. GDF-15 is an inhibitor of leukocyte integrin activation required for survival after myocardial infarction in mice. *Nat. Med.* **2011**, *17*, 581–588. [CrossRef] [PubMed]
43. Chang, J.; Eggenhuizen, P.; O'Sullivan, K.M.; Alikhan, M.A.; Holdsworth, S.R.; Ooi, J.D.; Kitching, A.R. CD8+ T Cells Effect Glomerular Injury in Experimental Anti-Myeloperoxidase GN. *J. Am. Soc. Nephrol.* **2017**, *28*, 47–55. [CrossRef]
44. Klein, R.S.; Lin, E.; Zhang, B.; Luster, A.D.; Tollett, J.; Samuel, M.A.; Engle, M.; Diamond, M.S. Neuronal CXCL10 directs CD8+ T-cell recruitment and control of West Nile virus encephalitis. *J. Virol.* **2005**, *79*, 11457–11466. [CrossRef] [PubMed]
45. Trapani, J.A.; Jans, D.A.; Jans, P.J.; Smyth, M.J.; Browne, K.A.; Sutton, V.R. Efficient nuclear targeting of granzyme B and the nuclear consequences of apoptosis induced by granzyme B and perforin are caspase-dependent, but cell death is caspase-independent. *J. Biol. Chem.* **1998**, *273*, 27934–27938. [CrossRef] [PubMed]
46. Trapani, J.A.; Smyth, M.J. Functional significance of the perforin/granzyme cell death pathway. *Nat. Rev. Immunol.* **2002**, *2*, 735–747. [CrossRef]
47. Nagata, S.; Golstein, P. The Fas death factor. *Science* **1995**, *267*, 1449–1456. [CrossRef]
48. Fung-Leung, W.P.; Schilham, M.W.; Rahemtulla, A.; Kundig, T.M.; Vollenweider, M.; Potter, J.; van Ewijk, W.; Mak, T.W. CD8 is needed for development of cytotoxic T cells but not helper T cells. *Cell* **1991**, *65*, 443–449. [CrossRef]
49. Brown, H.J.; Lock, H.R.; Wolfs, T.G.; Buurman, W.A.; Sacks, S.H.; Robson, M.G. Toll-like receptor 4 ligation on intrinsic renal cells contributes to the induction of antibody-mediated glomerulonephritis via CXCL1 and CXCL2. *J. Am. Soc. Nephrol.* **2007**, *18*, 1732–1739. [CrossRef]
50. Allam, R.; Anders, H.J. The role of innate immunity in autoimmune tissue injury. *Curr. Opin. Rheumatol.* **2008**, *20*, 538–544. [CrossRef]
51. Greenhall, G.H.; Salama, A.D. What is new in the management of rapidly progressive glomerulonephritis? *Clin. Kidney J.* **2015**, *8*, 143–150. [CrossRef] [PubMed]
52. Dai, Z.; Xing, L.; Cerise, J.; Wang, E.H.; Jabbari, A.; de Jong, A.; Petukhova, L.; Christiano, A.M.; Clynes, R. CXCR3 Blockade Inhibits T Cell Migration into the Skin and Prevents Development of Alopecia Areata. *J. Immunol.* **2016**, *197*, 1089–1099. [CrossRef] [PubMed]
53. Goebeler, M.; Toksoy, A.; Spandau, U.; Engelhardt, E.; Brocker, E.B.; Gillitzer, R. The C-X-C chemokine Mig is highly expressed in the papillae of psoriatic lesions. *J. Pathol.* **1998**, *184*, 89–95. [CrossRef]
54. Yellin, M.; Paliienko, I.; Balanescu, A.; Ter-Vartanian, S.; Tseluyko, V.; Xu, L.A.; Tao, X.; Cardarelli, P.M.; Leblanc, H.; Nichol, G.; et al. A phase II, randomized, double-blind, placebo-controlled study evaluating the efficacy and safety of MDX-1100, a fully human anti-CXCL10 monoclonal antibody, in combination with methotrexate in patients with rheumatoid arthritis. *Arthritis Rheum.* **2012**, *64*, 1730–1739. [CrossRef] [PubMed]
55. Nair, V.; Robinson-Cohen, C.; Smith, M.R.; Bellovich, K.A.; Bhat, Z.Y.; Bobadilla, M.; Brosius, F.; de Boer, I.H.; Essioux, L.; Formentini, I.; et al. Growth Differentiation Factor-15 and Risk of CKD Progression. *J. Am. Soc. Nephrol.* **2017**, *28*, 2233–2240. [CrossRef] [PubMed]

56. Breit, S.N.; Carrero, J.J.; Tsai, V.W.; Yagoutifam, N.; Luo, W.; Kuffner, T.; Bauskin, A.R.; Wu, L.; Jiang, L.; Barany, P.; et al. Macrophage inhibitory cytokine-1 (MIC-1/GDF15) and mortality in end-stage renal disease. *Nephrol. Dial. Transplant.* **2012**, *27*, 70–75. [CrossRef] [PubMed]
57. Lajer, M.; Jorsal, A.; Tarnow, L.; Parving, H.H.; Rossing, P. Plasma growth differentiation factor-15 independently predicts all-cause and cardiovascular mortality as well as deterioration of kidney function in type 1 diabetic patients with nephropathy. *Diabetes Care* **2010**, *33*, 1567–1572. [CrossRef]
58. Anand, I.S.; Kempf, T.; Rector, T.S.; Tapken, H.; Allhoff, T.; Jantzen, F.; Kuskowski, M.; Cohn, J.N.; Drexler, H.; Wollert, K.C. Serial measurement of growth-differentiation factor-15 in heart failure: Relation to disease severity and prognosis in the Valsartan Heart Failure Trial. *Circulation* **2010**, *122*, 1387–1395. [CrossRef]
59. Eggers, K.M.; Kempf, T.; Wallentin, L.; Wollert, K.C.; Lind, L. Change in growth differentiation factor 15 concentrations over time independently predicts mortality in community-dwelling elderly individuals. *Clin. Chem.* **2013**, *59*, 1091–1098. [CrossRef]
60. Na, K.R.; Kim, Y.H.; Chung, H.K.; Yeo, M.K.; Ham, Y.R.; Jeong, J.Y.; Kim, K.S.; Lee, K.W.; Choi, D.E. Growth differentiation factor 15 as a predictor of adverse renal outcomes in patients with immunoglobulin A nephropathy. *Intern. Med. J.* **2017**, *47*, 1393–1399. [CrossRef]
61. Ham, Y.R.; Song, C.H.; Bae, H.J.; Jeong, J.Y.; Yeo, M.K.; Choi, D.E.; Na, K.R.; Lee, K.W. Growth Differentiation Factor-15 as a Predictor of Idiopathic Membranous Nephropathy Progression: A Retrospective Study. *Dis. Markers* **2018**, *2018*, 1463940. [CrossRef] [PubMed]
62. Carlsson, A.C.; Nowak, C.; Lind, L.; Ostgren, C.J.; Nystrom, F.H.; Sundstrom, J.; Carrero, J.J.; Riserus, U.; Ingelsson, E.; Fall, T.; et al. Growth differentiation factor 15 (GDF-15) is a potential biomarker of both diabetic kidney disease and future cardiovascular events in cohorts of individuals with type 2 diabetes: A proteomics approach. *Upsala J. Med. Sci* **2020**, *125*, 37–43. [CrossRef] [PubMed]
63. Simonson, M.S.; Tiktin, M.; Debanne, S.M.; Rahman, M.; Berger, B.; Hricik, D.; Ismail-Beigi, F. The renal transcriptome of db/db mice identifies putative urinary biomarker proteins in patients with type 2 diabetes: A pilot study. *Am. J. Physiol. Renal Physiol.* **2012**, *302*, F820–F829. [CrossRef] [PubMed]
64. Olsen, O.E.; Skjaervik, A.; Stordal, B.F.; Sundan, A.; Holien, T. TGF-beta contamination of purified recombinant GDF15. *PLoS ONE* **2017**, *12*, e0187349. [CrossRef] [PubMed]
65. Cohen, C.D.; Frach, K.; Schlondorff, D.; Kretzler, M. Quantitative gene expression analysis in renal biopsies: A novel protocol for a high-throughput multicenter application. *Kidney Int.* **2002**, *61*, 133–140. [CrossRef] [PubMed]
66. Cohen, C.D.; Klingenhoff, A.; Boucherot, A.; Nitsche, A.; Henger, A.; Brunner, B.; Schmid, H.; Merkle, M.; Saleem, M.A.; Koller, K.P.; et al. Comparative promoter analysis allows de novo identification of specialized cell junction-associated proteins. *Proc. Natl. Acad. Sci. USA* **2006**, *103*, 5682–5687. [CrossRef]
67. Tusher, V.G.; Tibshirani, R.; Chu, G. Significance analysis of microarrays applied to the ionizing radiation response. *Proc. Natl. Acad. Sci. USA* **2001**, *98*, 5116–5121. [CrossRef]
68. Shved, N.; Warsow, G.; Eichinger, F.; Hoogewijs, D.; Brandt, S.; Wild, P.; Kretzler, M.; Cohen, C.D.; Lindenmeyer, M.T. Transcriptome-based network analysis reveals renal cell type-specific dysregulation of hypoxia-associated transcripts. *Sci. Rep.* **2017**, *7*, 8576. [CrossRef]

7

Podocytes—The Most Vulnerable Renal Cells in Preeclampsia

Ewa Kwiatkowska [1,†], Katarzyna Stefańska [2,†,*], Maciej Zieliński [3,†], Justyna Sakowska [3], Martyna Jankowiak [3], Piotr Trzonkowski [3], Natalia Marek-Trzonkowska [4,5] and Sebastian Kwiatkowski [6]

1 Clinical Department of Nephrology, Transplantology and Internal Medicine, Pomeranian Medical University, 70-111 Szczecin, Poland; ewakwiat@gmail.com
2 Department of Obstetrics, Medical University of Gdańsk, 80-210 Gdańsk, Poland
3 Department of Medical Immunology, Medical University of Gdańsk, 80-210 Gdańsk, Poland; mzielinski@gumed.edu.pl (M.Z.); justynas@gumed.edu.pl (J.S.); martyna830@gumed.edu.pl (M.J.); ptrzon@gumed.edu.pl (P.T.)
4 International Centre for Cancer Vaccine Science Cancer Immunology Group, University of Gdansk, 80-822 Gdańsk, Poland; natalia.marek@gumed.edu.pl
5 Laboratory of Immunoregulation and Cellular Therapies, Department of Family Medicine, Medical University of Gdańsk, 80-210 Gdańsk, Poland
6 Department of Obstetrics and Gynecology, Pomeranian Medical University, 70-111 Szczecin, Poland; kwiatkowskiseba@gmail.com
* Correspondence: kciach@wp.pl
† These authors equally contributed to the study.

Abstract: Preeclampsia (PE) is a disorder that affects 3–5% of normal pregnancies. It was believed for a long time that the kidney, similarly to all vessels in the whole system, only sustained endothelial damage. The current knowledge gives rise to a presumption that the main role in the development of proteinuria is played by damage to the podocytes and their slit diaphragm. The podocyte damage mechanism in preeclampsia is connected to free VEGF and nitric oxide (NO) deficiency, and an increased concentration of endothelin-1 and oxidative stress. From national cohort studies, we know that women who had preeclampsia in at least one pregnancy carried five times the risk of developing end-stage renal disease (ESRD) when compared to women with physiological pregnancies. The focal segmental glomerulosclerosis (FSGS) is the dominant histopathological lesion in women with a history of PE. The kidney's podocytes are not subject to replacement or proliferation. Podocyte depletion exceeding 20% resulted in FSGS, which is a reason for the later development of ESRD. In this review, we present the mechanism of kidney (especially podocytes) injury in preeclampsia. We try to explain how this damage affects further changes in the morphology and function of the kidneys after pregnancy.

Keywords: preeclampsia; podocytes; VEGF; FSGS; proteinuria

1. Preeclampsia

According to state-of-the-art research and current knowledge, generalized endothelial damage caused by factors excreted by the placenta into the maternal circulation is the cause of preeclampsia (PE). Angiogenic imbalance leads to epithelial dysfunction. In turn, the imbalance is caused by decreased concentrations of vascular endothelial growth factor (VEGF) and placental growth factor (PlGF), and increased concentrations of soluble fms-like tyrosine kinase-1 (sFlt-1)—a VEGF receptor, and endoglin [1]. The development of preeclampsia is associated with arterial hypertension, proteinuria—usually nephrotic, and decreased glomerular filtration often meeting the criteria for acute kidney injury.

2. Glomerular Lesions Secondary to Preeclampsia

The most characteristic histopathological lesion observed in the kidneys of preeclamptic patients is glomerular endotheliosis, which is known to include swollen epithelial cells showing fenestration loss, and fibrin deposits in the subendothelial regions, with both lesions leading to the narrowing or even closing of the glomerular capillaries, and the appearance is that of a "bloodless glomerulus" [2]. Based on the histopathological appearance, it was believed for a long time that the kidney, similarly to all vessels in the whole system, only sustained endothelial damage. Proteinuria was thought to be caused by damage to this part of the filtration barrier. In the glomerulus, the filtration membrane has a unique three-layer structure. Its luminal surface consists of the endothelium, the basement membrane constitutes the inner layer, and the third layer is made of podocytes, with the slit diaphragm sealing the spaces between them. In preeclampsia, two of the filtration membrane components—the endothelium and the podocytes—are damaged, thus leading to proteinuria. Podocytes, with their well-developed contractile apparatus, are capable of regulating the filtration area and the hydraulic resistance of the entire filtration barrier [3]. By contracting their processes, they counter the pressure that inflates the capillaries and thus stabilize the structure of the glomerulus [4]. In a mature glomerulus, podocytes are the only cells participating in the metabolic turnover of the basement membrane, synthesizing its components and producing the proteinases that degrade it [4,5]. Additionally, they produce proteins modulating the properties of the capillary endothelium and are thus regulators of both the expression and function of all the filtration barrier elements [6]. The currently accepted knowledge gives rise to a presumption that the main role in the development of proteinuria is played by damage to the podocytes and their slit diaphragm.

3. Podocytes

As mentioned before, podocytes line the external surface of the glomerular basement membrane. Each podocyte is associated with more than one arteriole, and each arteriole is covered by more than one podocyte. Podocytes are composed of the cellular body, primary processes, and foot processes (or pedicels). The foot processes contain a contractile apparatus including actin, myosin, actinin, talin, vinculin, and vimentin, which opposes the hemodynamic forces of the glomerular capillaries. [7,8] Podocytes' main task is to participate in glomerular filtration. The glomerular filtrate flows through endothelial fenestrae, the basement membrane, and the slit diaphragms in the spaces between the foot processes. The slit diaphragms are the most important functional elements of the three-layer filtration membrane. They are anchored in the basolateral region of the foot processes. The pedicels are composed of many proteins that form an interacting complex. Damage to one of its elements disorders the function of the slit diaphragms. One of the main proteins of the complex is nephrin, which has an extracellular domain, a transmembrane domain, and an intracellular domain. The extracellular domain forms a network of connections, thus creating the structure for the slit diaphragm, while the intracellular fragment interacts with other proteins, such as CD2AP and CD2-associated protein, podocin, and kinases, passing information from the slit diaphragms on to the podocyte. [9,10] Neph1, a protein similar to nephrin, joins forces with nephrin in building the slit diaphragm structure. Another membrane protein—podocin—binds with the cytoplasmic domain of nephrin and two other proteins—CD2AP and Neph1 [11]. Podocin stabilizes the interacting complex of nephrin, Neph1, and CD2AP. CD2AP is an adaptor protein. It contains five parts, one of which binds with actin. CD2AP is found in all human tissues, although experiments on murine models have shown that normal function only requires its presence in the kidneys [12,13]. Proper interaction of the nephrin-podocin-CD2AP complex is believed to be essential for the flow of fluids, electrolytes, and proteins through the filtration slit to occur [8]. Neph1 also interacts with the protein zonula occludens-1 (ZO-1) [11]. α-actinin that binds actin is another slit diaphragm protein [14]. It is responsible for the contractility of the podocyte processes and the adhesion of pedicels to the basement membrane. Nephrin is believed to bind with α-actinin through podocin. A genetic defect of the proteins forming the slit diaphragm structure—nephrin and Neph1—leads to massive proteinuria. Defects to the intracellular proteins (CD2AP, podocin, and α-actinin-4) cause less pronounced proteinuria, often in later life [15]. Disordered cooperation between the slit diaphragm structure proteins and the contractile element—actin—of the pedicels leads to atrophy of the pedicels, their detachment from the basement membrane, and proteinuria [11]. Podocytes are damaged by detachment from the basement membrane that is associated with the presence of podocytes and their proteins in the urine, or mitotic catastrophe—podocytes may enter the cell cycle, but they rarely undergo mitosis and cannot complete cytokinesis and may undergo apoptosis for variety of reasons. Such damage to the filtration membrane cause proteinuria [6,16,17]. Understandingly, podocytes include other proteins, as well, such as synaptopodin that cooperates with the contractile apparatus, podocalyxin that covers the surface of podocytes giving them negative electric charge, and integrins that attach the pedicels to the basement membrane. Figure 1 shows the scheme of podocytes foot process and slit diaphragm proteins.

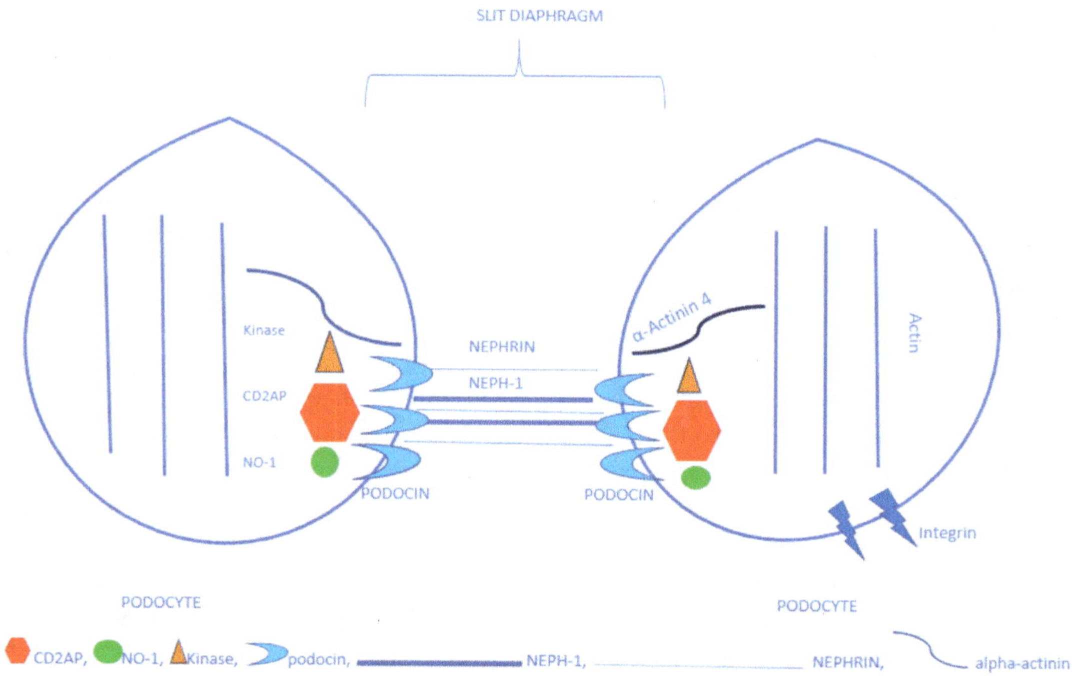

Figure 1. The simplified picture of the construction of a slit diaphragm.

4. Urinary Excretion of Podocytes and Their Proteins Secondary to Preeclampsia

Many reports are pointing to damage to individual elements of podocytes and slit diaphragms in preeclampsia. As mentioned above, the principal building blocks of the slit diaphragm include nephrin, another job of which is to pass the information on to the pedicels. Ozdemir et al. have found increased concentrations of nephrin in the blood and the urine of patients with severe preeclampsia and intrauterine growth restriction (IUGR). In their study, nephrin levels correlated negatively with fetal weight and age, and positively with creatinine concentration and systolic and diastolic pressure [18]. Wang has found that urine nephrin levels correlate with the severity of proteinuria—in other words, the more severe podocyte and slit diaphragm damage the more pronounced the proteinuria [19]. Jung has noticed that increased urine concentrations of nephrin predate the signs of preeclampsia by an average of nine days [20]. Additionally, other authors have observed that urinary levels of nephrin are higher in PE patients than both in control group women and patients with gestational hypertension [21]. Many reports indicate, as well, the presence of podocytes in the urine, which suggests they have lost attachment to the basement membrane and the filtration membrane has been ruptured. The urinary amounts of podocytes correlate with the severity of preeclampsia [19]. Wang et al. have observed decreased nephrin expression in the excreted podocytes. In their study, they encouraged oxidative stress in the incubated healthy podocyte environment and found that nephrin expression went down. In the same podocytes, they also found downregulated expression of superoxide dismutase—an antioxidant enzyme (CuZn-SOD) [22]. Biopsy specimens from PE patients revealed decreased expression of nephrin compared with the control group [23]. In an experiment in which sFlt and anti-VEGF antibodies were administered intraperitoneally to mice, a similar biopsy specimen appearance was observed. Collino et al. noticed that podocyte incubation with plasma from PE patients did not lead to nephrin depletion. In their study, they subsequently incubated glomerular endothelial cells in PE patient plasma and used the resulting environment to incubate podocytes. They found that nephrin was lost as a result of cleavage of its extracellular domain by proteases and its redistribution. Further on, they established that in response to the PE patient serum, the endothelium produced endothelin 1 (ET-1), which, in addition to being the main cause of activation of the proteases that cleaved nephrin's extracellular domain, which is the main protein of slit diaphragm [24,25]. The application of recombinant endothelin on cultured podocytes caused the shedding of nephrin from these cells [24]. The same author blocked the activity of VEGF on the glomerular endothelium to find increased endothelin production [25]. Kerlay has analyzed the available clinical studies that assessed urinary podocyte proteins as markers for the development of preeclampsia [26]. In his study, he found that urinary nephrin had the highest sensitivity (0.81) and specificity (0.84) as a marker for the development of preeclampsia [26]. Podocin stabilizes the nephrin-Neph1-CD2AP complex and binds nephrin to α-actinin. This is a key protein in transmitting information from the slit diaphragm to the inside of the podocyte. In his study, Martineau found that preeclamptic patients had higher urinary podocin concentrations than the control group [27]. These concentrations correlated positively with the severity of albuminuria, proteinuria, and arterial pressure, and negatively with gestational age [27]. In his study, Gialni examined podocin-positive extracellular vesicles in the urine and found there were higher levels in PE patients than in the control group. In his paper, he presented the concept that damage to the podocytes is associated with nephrinuria related to nephrin shedding from these cells. According to his claim, this phenomenon causes decreased expression of nephrin in the renal biopsy specimens and in the urine podocytes. Podocin stays bound to the podocytes and its presence in the urine is associated with podocyturia [28]. In his experiment on murine models in which preeclampsia was caused by the administration of a nitric oxide analog, Baijnath identified the mRNA of podocin and nephrin in the urine [29]. As mentioned above, the adaptor protein CD2AP is part of the nephrin-Neph1-Podocin complex. In his study, Henao experimented with podocytes placed in PE patient sera [30]. He found that the distribution of two proteins—podocin and CD2AP—changed. He also noticed that their changed distribution caused an increase in the tension of the contractile apparatus of the podocyte. Additionally, he studied electrical resistance of the podocyte layer and found that, if increased, it suggested low permeability of the filtration membrane, especially for proteins. Podocytes placed in PE pregnant patient serum had lower electrical resistance. The author believed that the changed podocin and CD2AP distribution disordered the entire complex composed of the slit diaphragm and the inside of the foot process containing the contractile apparatus [30].

5. The Podocyte Damage Mechanism in Preeclampsia

Free VEGF Deficiency

sFlt-1 that is present in preeclampsia binds with the receptor for VEGF and inhibits its impact on various cells in the system. In the podocytes, especially their foot processes, the expression of all the VEGF-A isoforms is observed. Podocytes are the main sources of VEGF in the glomerulus [31]. A study using the electron microscope established the presence of VEGF in the foot process, the basement membrane, and the luminal surface of the endothelium. It was found that VEGF produced by the podocytes moved in the opposite direction to the glomerular filtrate. VEGF receptors were found both on the podocytes and the endothelial cells. VEGF produced by the podocytes has autocrine and paracrine effects on the endothelium [32,33]. In other studies, mice deprived of podocyte-produced VEGF died upon birth due to renal failure. No normally developed filtration membrane was found in the renal specimens. The problem did not only affect the podocytes, though, as the endothelial cells failed to form the fenestration typical of the glomerulus, as well. Such a phenotype is the responsibility of VEGF produced and secreted by podocytes [24]. The lack of VEGF's paracrine effect on the endothelium is believed to be responsible for the typical histopathological appearance of the glomerulus in preeclampsia, i.e., glomerular endotheliosis. This experiment proved the influence of VEGF produced by podocytes on the function of podocytes and the endothelium [34]. Podocyte-produced VEGF is bound by heparan sulfate present in the basement membrane, where it is stored and from where it is transported further on. VEGF is known to be necessary for normal podocyte function. It stimulates phosphorylation of nephrin, which prevents podocyte apoptosis [32]. Moreover, VEGF increases interaction between podocin and CD2AP [35]. Administration of anti-VEGF antibodies or sFlt-1 prevents nephrin expression in the podocytes and damages them [33]. In a study on cancer patients treated with anti-VEGF antibodies, podocyturia was observed [36]. Podocytes have a type 1 receptor for VEGF, i.e., VEGFR1, through which VEGF exerts an autocrine effect. No VEGFR-2 receptor was found on their surface. Preeclampsia is known to be accompanied by increased levels of the soluble form of the VEGF receptor, i.e., fms-like tyrosine kinase-1 (sFlt-1), a compound that competes with VEGFR1 for VEGF, which is why podocytes are so exposed to damage in preeclampsia [37]. Experiments have shown that VEGF is necessary to transmit impulses from nephrin (its extracellular domain) to actin—a component of the contractile elements of the podocyte process [35]. Mature mice deprived of VEGF demonstrated damage to all three layers of the filtration membrane [35].

6. Endothelial Damage-Related Disorders

6.1. *Nitric Oxide (NO) Deficiency*

Excess amounts of antiangiogenic factors sFlt-1 and endolgin, and a deficiency of angiogenic factors VEGF and PlGF, lead to generalized endothelial damage. This is associated with reduced activity of nitric oxide synthase and decreased levels of this vasodilating factor [38]. In his experiment on murine models, Baijnath administered an analog of L-arginine that inhibited nitric oxide synthesis and caused preeclampsia-like symptoms, including podocyturia, defined as the urinary presence of the mRNA of podocin and nephrin. The histopathological appearance mainly included endothelial damage in the form of swelling, loss of fenestration, and the closing of the vascular walls. This experiment proves the interdependence of the endothelium and the podocytes. The lack of endothelial synthesis of NO causes damage to the podocytes. This mechanism is not yet fully understood. In the same experiment, sildenafil citrate, known to increase cGMP levels (the same result as that of NO), eliminated podocyturia, and prevented histopathological lesions in the glomerulus [29]. It was found that the administration of sildenafil citrate decreased the level of sFlt-1 and increased VEGF synthesis.

6.2. *Endothelin-1*

Collino's experiment indicating that the decreased nephrin expression was not caused by the PE patient plasma itself but by endothelin-1, produced by the endothelium under the influence of that plasma, was mentioned above. The application of recombinant endothelin on cultured podocytes caused the shedding of nephrin from the podocytes [24,25]. Preeclamptic patients are observed to have significantly increased plasma concentrations of endothelin-1 [39]. In one study, the administration of blockers of receptors for endothelin-1 before the infusion of sFlt-1 prevented the development of hypertension in murine experiments [40].

6.3. Oxidative Stress

The abnormal placenta of a PE patient is the source of reactive oxygen species, as well as compounds that damage the endothelium, which itself becomes the source of reactive oxygen species [41]. Wang's experiment proved that oxidative stress causes damage to podocytes [22]. The podocytes singled out from PE patient urine were shown to demonstrate no expression of nephrin, and none of the superoxide dismutase (SOD) that is normally present on the surface of the foot processes. The author theorized that at this location the job for superoxide dismutase was to protect nephrin (its extracellular domain) against oxidative stress. To prove his thesis, he subjected cultured podocytes to oxidative stress. He achieved the loss of expression of nephrin and superoxide dismutase. He could not prove the direct interdependence of SOD and nephrin but showed that oxidative stress caused nephrin shedding, which had a damaging effect on the filtration membrane [22]. Another author, Zao, studied biopsy specimens from preeclamptic patients to find their decreased expression of nephrin, which proved damage to the podocytes. He also examined a marker of oxidative stress. He found an increased expression of nitrotyrosine and a decreased expression of CuZn-SOD in the biopsy specimens collected from preeclamptic patients when compared with the control group. Nitrotyrosine is a marker of increased oxidative stress and it is formed when a protein molecule is nitrated by peroxynitrite. Superoxide dismutase is the only antioxidant enzyme to dismutate superoxide radicals generated by living cells [42].

7. Preeclampsia and the Risk of Developing End-Stage Renal Disease (ESRD)

The effect of past preeclampsia on the women's health in later life has long been the subject of much debate. Many authors implicate that a history of PE increases the risk of cardiovascular and renal diseases [43,44]. Other studies have shown a higher incidence of microalbuminuria 5 years after preeclampsia [45]. As it was not certain whether that was the result of PE or perhaps co-morbidities that contributed to PE, national cohort studies were carried out. One such study was a Norwegian research paper published in 2008 that was based on the birth registry for 1967–1991, and the ESRD diagnosis registry for 1980 to date. The research showed a higher incidence of ESRD in former preeclamptic patients [43]. Similarly, Swedish national cohort study results published in 2019 confirmed that women who had preeclampsia in at least one pregnancy carried five-times the risk of developing ESRD when compared to women with physiological pregnancies. This correlation was independent of other factors such as co-morbidities, socioeconomic status, or age [46]. Thought needs to be given as to why this happens. In the above work, it was shown that preeclampsia was associated with damage to the podocytes. Podocytes are terminally differentiated cells that do not proliferate or renew. Their damage decreases their number in the glomerulus and leaves a void instead. Podocytes injury is depicted in the following scheme (Figure 2).

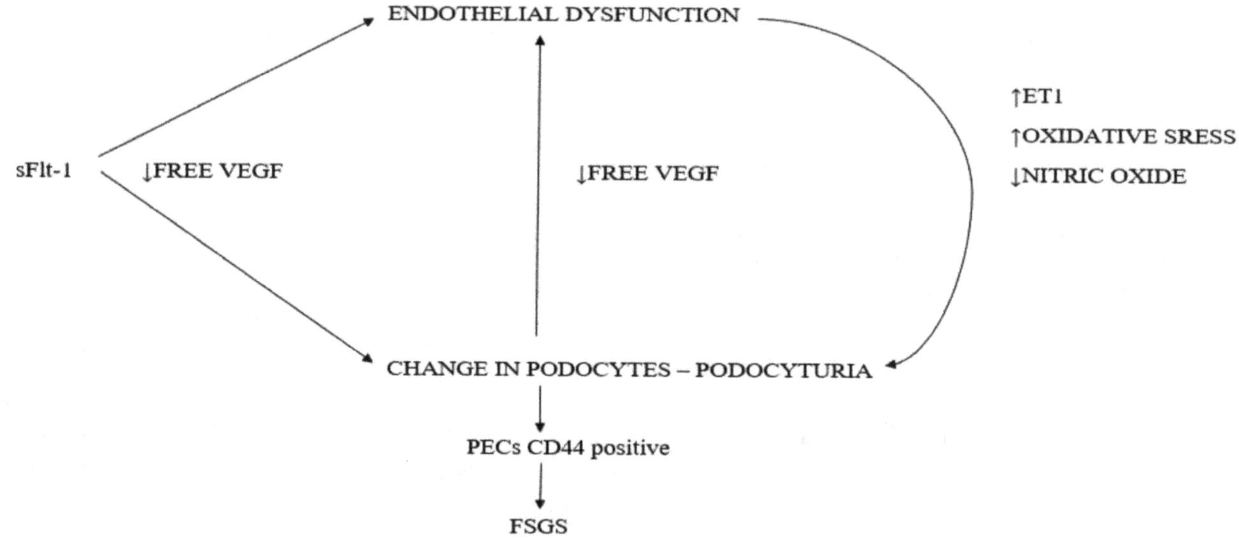

Figure 2. The scheme of podocytes injury in preeclampsia.

8. The Mechanism behind Focal Segmental Glomerulosclerosis (FSGS)

There are very few reports on histopathological lesions in the kidneys of patients with a history of PE, which is linked to the ethical contraindications for such studies. However, even those few existing ones suggest that focal segmental glomerulosclerosis (FSGS) is the dominant histopathological lesion [47–50]. The development of FSGS begins with the loss of podocytes. The kidney of an adult person has approx. 500–600 podocytes per glomerulus, which are not subject to replacement or proliferation. In their study on murine models, Wharram et al. found that podocyte depletion exceeding 20% resulted in FSGS [51]. The development of FSGS because of podocyte depletion has been proven in experimental and clinical studies [52,53]. Podocyte depletion results in a mismatch between the vascular basement membrane area requiring coverage by podocytes and the actual area of the podocytes. The capillaries with the uncovered basement membrane move towards Bowman's capsule to establish a sort of connection (a cell bridge) with its epithelium Parietal Epithelial Cells (PECs) (lining Bowman's capsule). Between these bridges, an extracellular matrix gathers that forms fibrous connections with Bowman's capsule (tuft adhesion). Additionally, after cell bridge formation, PECs de novo express the marker of activation CD44 and start to deposit the Bowman's-type matrix leading in the tuft adhesion. The CD44-positive PECs are found only in the sclerotic region. [54] Recently are more and more information about the role of PECs in the sclerotic process in secondary FSGS even in PE. [55] Instead of moving to the proximal tubule, the filtrate produced here moves—under Bowman's capsule epithelial cells—to the peritubular space thus causing tubular atrophy, which then inflicts irreversible damage on the glomerulus. This filtrate has a large protein content as it is not filtrated by the podocyte layer. A further gathering of the extracellular matrix and hyaline substance at the site of the connection with Bowman's capsule leads to obliteration of the glomerular capillaries. This is where mesangial expansion often occurs [56]. A typical appearance of focal segmental glomerulosclerosis develops. It should be added that proteinuria is not only a sign of filtration membrane damage, as the appearance of proteins in the so-called Bowman's space causes further damage to the podocytes and Bowman's capsule epithelial cells and stimulates their apoptosis. In this way, the segmental lesion leads with time to the development of generalized glomerulosclerosis [57]. Additionally, research on children with idiopathic FSGS has shown that proteinuria stimulates the apoptosis of proximal and distal tubular epithelial cells [58]. This provokes the spread of the lesions beyond the glomerulus and across the entire nephron. Moreover, Matsusaka has proven that damage to one podocyte is carried over to the neighboring healthy podocytes, thus causing the domino effect [59]. As a result of the mismatch between the podocyte area and the glomerular basement membrane area, some endothelial cells are not affected by the paracrine effect of VEGF (which is secreted by the podocyte under normal circumstances). This leads to damage to the endothelium—its typical fenestrated phenotype. The changed endothelium may produce compounds that exacerbate podocyte damage [60]. The process, initiated by primary damage to the podocytes secondary to preeclampsia, continues to develop postpartum when the original damaging factors are no longer present. Initially, this causes FSGS-type lesions, and in the long-term leads to the sclerosis of the entire glomerulus and damage to the entire nephron.

9. Conclusions

In preeclampsia, the angiogenic imbalance leads mainly to podocyte damage. The disordered structure of the podocytes leads to their detachment from the basement membrane and urinary excretion (podocyturia). As podocytes do not undergo replacement or proliferation, their numbers are reduced. If the percentage of the damaged podocytes exceeds 20, FSGS-type lesions set in and, being irreversible and progressive, lead with time to the deterioration of renal function.

A history of preeclampsia is known to be associated with a higher (by five times) probability of developing ESRD, but despite the increased probability, the condition does not affect a large percentage of patients. It is our job as physicians to inform our patients of the need for long-term follow-up monitoring. This should include an albuminuria test, urinalysis, renal function assessment, and arterial pressure measurement on a yearly basis, at least. Patients must be made aware that a past preeclampsia increases the risk of cardiovascular diseases, as well. Apart from reporting for follow-up tests, they could be stimulated to also adopt a healthy lifestyle and avoid any additional risk factors for cardiovascular and renal diseases. The importance of the right diet, exercise, and body weight control, and the need to avoid smoking and alcohol, should be highlighted.

References

1. Tomimatsu, T.; Mimura, K.; Endo, M.; Kumasawa, K.; Kimura, T. Pathophysiology of Preeclampsia: An Angiogenic Imbalance and Long-Lasting Systemic Vascular Dysfunction. *Hypertens. Res.* **2017**, *40*, 305–310. [CrossRef] [PubMed]
2. Hussein, W.; Lafayette, R.A. Renal Function in Normal and Disordered Pregnancy. *Curr. Opin. Nephrol. Hypertens.* **2014**, *23*, 46–53. [CrossRef] [PubMed]
3. Morton, M.J.; Hutchinson, K.; Mathieson, P.W.; Witherden, I.R.; Saleem, M.A.; Hunter, M. Human podocytes possess a stretch-sensitive, Ca_2+-activated K+ channel: Potential implications for the control of glomerular filtration. *J. Am. Soc. Nephrol.* **2004**, *15*, 2981–2987. [CrossRef]
4. Mundel, P.; Kriz, W. Structure and function of podocytes: An update. *Anat. Embryol.* **1995**, *192*, 385–397. [CrossRef]
5. Asanuma, K.; Shirato, I.; Ishidoh, K.; Kominami, E.; Tomino, Y. Selective modulation of the secretion of proteinases and their inhibitors by growth factors in cultured differentiated podocytes. *Kidney Int.* **2002**, *62*, 822–831. [CrossRef]
6. Armaly, Z.; Jadaon, J.E.; Jabbour, A.; Abassi, Z.A. Preeclampsia: Novel Mechanisms and Potential Therapeutic Approaches. *Front. Physiol.* **2018**, *259*, 973. [CrossRef]
7. Humphries, J.D.; Wang, P.; Streuli, C.; Geiger, B.; Humphries, M.J.; Ballestrem, C. Vinculin controls focal adhesion formation by direct interactions with talin and actin. *J. Cell Biol.* **2007**, *179*, 1043–1057. [CrossRef]
8. Ichimura, K.; Kurihara, H.; Sakai, T. Actin filament organization of foot processes in rat podocytes. *J. Histochem. Cytochem.* **2003**, *51*, 1589–1600. [CrossRef]

9. Philippe, A.; Nevo, F.; Esquivel, E.L.; Reklaityte, D.; Gribouval, O.; Tete, M.J.; Loirat, C.; Dantal, J.; Fischbach, M.; Pouteil-Noble, C.; et al. Nephrin mutations can cause childhood-onset steroid-resistant nephrotic syndrome. *J. Am. Soc. Nephrol.* **2008**, *19*, 1871–1878. [CrossRef]
10. Garg, P.; Verma, R.; Nihalani, D.; Johnstone, D.B.; Holzman, L.B. Neph1 cooperates with nephrin to transduce a signal that induces actin polymerization. *Mol. Cell Biol.* **2007**, *27*, 8698–8712. [CrossRef]
11. Jalanko, H. Pathogenesis of proteinuria: Lessons learned from nephrin and podocin. *Pediatr. Nephrol.* **2003**, *18*, 487–491. [CrossRef] [PubMed]
12. Grunkemeyer, J.A.; Kwoh, C.; Huber, T.B.; Shaw, A.S. CD2-associated Protein (CD2AP) Expression in Podocytes Rescues Lethality of CD2AP Deficiency. *J. Biol. Chem.* **2005**, *19*, 29677–29681. [CrossRef] [PubMed]
13. Grahammer, F.; Schell, C.; Huber, T.B. The podocyte slit diaphragm—From a thin grey line to a complex signalling hub. *Nat. Rev. Nephrol.* **2013**, *9*, 587–598. [CrossRef] [PubMed]
14. Kaplan, J.M.; Kim, S.H.; North, K.N.; Rennke, H.; Correia, L.A.; Tong, H.Q.; Mathis, B.J.; Rodríguez-Pérez, J.C.; Allen, P.G.; Beggs, A.H.; et al. Mutations in ACTN4, Encoding alpha-actinin-4, Cause Familial Focal Segmental Glomerulosclerosis. *Nat. Genet.* **2000**, *24*, 251–256. [CrossRef] [PubMed]
15. Meyrier, A. Mechanisms of Disease: Focal Segmental Glomerulosclerosis. *Nat. Clin. Pract. Nephrol.* **2005**, *1*, 44–54. [CrossRef] [PubMed]
16. Craici, I.M.; Wagner, S.J.; Bailey, K.R.; Fitz-Gibbon, P.D.; Wood-Wentz, C.M.; Turner, S.T.; Hayman, S.R.; White, W.M.; Brost, B.C.; Rose, C.H.; et al. Podocyturia predates proteinuria and clinical features of preeclampsia: Longitudinal prospective study. *Hypertension* **2013**, *61*, 1289–1296. [CrossRef] [PubMed]
17. Liapis, H.; Romagnani, P.; Anders, H.J. New Insights into the Pathology of Podocyte Loss: Mitotic catastrophe. *Am. J. Pathol.* **2013**, *183*, 1364–1374. [CrossRef]
18. Ozdemir, F.; Tayyar, A.T.; Acmaz, G.; Aksoy, H.; Erturk, G.; Muhtaroglu, S.; Tayyar, M. Comparison of blood and urine nephrin levels in preeclampsia and intrauterine growth retardation. *Pak. J. Med. Sci.* **2016**, *32*, 40–43. [CrossRef]
19. Wang, Y.; Gu, Y.; Loyd, S.; Jia, X.; Groome, L.J. Increased urinary levels of podocyte glycoproteins, matrix metallopeptidases, inflammatory cytokines, and kidney injury biomarkers in women with preeclampsia. *Am. J. Physiol. Renal Physiol.* **2015**, *309*, 1009–1017. [CrossRef]
20. Jung, Y.J.; Cho, H.Y.; Cho, S.; Kim, Y.H.; Jeon, J.D.; Kim, Y.J.; Lee, S.; Park, J.; Kim, H.Y.; Park, Y.W.; et al. The Level of Serum and Urinary Nephrin in Normal Pregnancy and Pregnancy with Subsequent Preeclampsia. *Yonsei Med. J.* **2017**, *58*, 401–406. [CrossRef]
21. Garovic, V.D.; Wagner, S.J.; Turner, S.T.; Rosenthal, D.W.; Watson, W.J.; Brost, B.C.; Rose, C.H.; Gavrilova, L.; Craigo, P.; Bailey, K.R.; et al. Urinary podocyte excretion as a marker for preeclampsia. *Am. J. Obstet. Gynecol.* **2007**, *196*, 320. [CrossRef] [PubMed]
22. Wang, Y.; Zhao, S.; Gu, Y.; Lewis, D.F. Loss of slit protein nephrin is associated with reduced antioxidant superoxide dismutase expression in podocytes shed from women with preeclampsia. *Physiol. Rep.* **2018**, *6*, 13785. [CrossRef] [PubMed]
23. Konieczny, A.; Ryba, M.; Wartacz, J.; Czyżewska-Buczyńska, A.; Hruby, Z.; Witkiewicz, W. Podocytes in Urine, a Novel Biomarker of Preeclampsia? *Adv. Clin. Exp. Med.* **2013**, *22*, 145–149. [PubMed]
24. Hauser, P.V.; Collino, F.; Bussolati, B.; Camussi, G. Nephrin and endothelial injury. *Curr. Opin. Nephrol. Hypertens.* **2009**, *18*, 3–8. [CrossRef] [PubMed]
25. Collino, F.; Bussolati, B.; Gerbaudo, E.; Marozio, L.; Pelissetto, S.; Benedetto, C.; Camussi, G. Preeclamptic sera induce nephrin shedding from podocytes through endothelin-1 release by endothelial glomerular cells. *Am. J. Physiol. Renal Physiol.* **2008**, *294*, 1185–1194. [CrossRef] [PubMed]
26. Kerley, R.N.; McCarthy, C. Biomarkers of Glomerular Dysfunction in Pre-Eclampsia—A Systematic Review. *Pregnancy Hypertens.* **2018**, *14*, 265–272. [CrossRef]
27. Martineau, T.; Boutin, M.; Côté, A.M.; Maranda, B.; Bichet, D.G.; Auray-Blais, C. Tandem Mass Spectrometry Analysis of Urinary Podocalyxin and Podocin in the Investigation of Podocyturia in Women with Preeclampsia and Fabry Disease Patients. *Clin. Chim. Acta* **2019**, *495*, 67–75. [CrossRef]
28. Gilani, S.I.; Anderson, U.D.; Jayachandran, M.; Weissgerber, T.L.; Zand, L.; White, W.M.; Milic, N.; Gonzalez Suarez, M.L.; Vallapureddy, R.R.; Nääv, A.; et al. Urinary Extracellular Vesicles of Podocyte Origin and Renal Injury in Preeclampsia. *J. Am. Soc. Nephrol.* **2017**, *28*, 3363–3372. [CrossRef]

29. Baijnath, S.; Murugesan, S.; Mackraj, I.; Gathiram, P.; Moodley, J. The effects of sildenafil citrate on urinary podocin and nephrin mRNA expression in an L-NAME model of pre-eclampsia. *Mol. Cell. Biochem.* **2016**, *427*, 59–67. [CrossRef]
30. Henao, D.E.; Arias, L.F.; Mathieson Ni, L.; Welsh, G.I.; Bueno, J.C.; Agudelo, B.; Cadavid, A.P.; Saleem, M.A. Preeclamptic Sera Directly Induce Slit-Diaphragm Protein Redistribution and Alter Podocyte Barrier-Forming Capacity. *Nephron. Exp. Nephrol.* **2008**, *110*, 73–81. [CrossRef]
31. Guan, F.; Villegas, G.; Teichman, J.; Mundel, P.; Tufro, A. Autocrine VEGF-A System in Podocytes Regulates Podocin and Its Interaction with CD2AP. *Am. J. Physiol. Renal Physiol.* **2006**, *291*, 422–428. [CrossRef] [PubMed]
32. Eremina, V.; Quaggin, S.E. The Role of VEGF-A in Glomerular Development and Function. *Curr. Opin. Nephrol. Hypertens.* **2004**, *13*, 9–15. [CrossRef] [PubMed]
33. Wagner, S.J.; Craici, I.M.; Grande, J.P.; Garovic, V.D. From Placenta to Podocyte: Vascular and Podocyte Pathophysiology in Preeclampsia. *Clin. Nephrol.* **2012**, *78*, 241–249. [CrossRef]
34. Eremina, V.; Sood, M.; Haigh, J.; Nagy, A.; Lajoie, G.; Ferrara, N.; Gerber, H.P.; Kikkawa, Y.; Miner, J.H.; Quaggin, S.E. Glomerular-specific alterations of VEGF-A expression lead to distinct congenital and acquired renal diseases. *J. Clin. Invest.* **2003**, *111*, 707–716. [CrossRef] [PubMed]
35. Tufro, A.; Veron, D. VEGF and Podocytes in Diabetic Nephropathy. *Semin. Nephrol.* **2012**, *32*, 385–393. [CrossRef] [PubMed]
36. Müller-Deile, J.; Bröcker, V.; Grünwald, V.; Hiss, M.; Bertram, A.; Kubicka, S.; Ganser, A.; Haller, H.; Schiffer, M. Renal side effects of VEGF-blocking therapy. *NDT Plus* **2010**, *3*, 172–175. [CrossRef]
37. Kwiatkowski, S.; Kwiatkowska, E.; Torbe, A. The role of disordered angiogenesis tissue markers (sflt-1, Plgf) in present day diagnosis of preeclampsia. *Ginekol. Pol.* **2019**, *90*, 173–176. [CrossRef] [PubMed]
38. Sharma, D.; Trivedi, S.S.; Bhattacharjee, J. Oxidative Stress and eNOS (Glu298Asp) Gene Polymorphism in Preeclampsia in Indian Population. *Mol. Cell Biochem.* **2011**, *353*, 189–193. [CrossRef]
39. Saleh, L.; Verdonk, K.; Visser, W.; Meiracker, A.H.; Danser, A.H.J. The Emerging Role of endothelin-1 in the Pathogenesis of Pre-Eclampsia. *Ther. Adv. Cardiovasc. Dis.* **2016**, *10*, 282–293. [CrossRef]
40. Murphy, S.R.; LaMarca, B.B.D.; Cockrell, K.; Granger, J.P. Role of Endothelin in Mediating Soluble Fms-Like Tyrosine Kinase 1-induced Hypertension in Pregnant Rats. *Hypertension* **2010**, *55*, 394–398. [CrossRef]
41. Aouache, R.; Biquard, L.; Vaiman, D.; Miralles, F. Oxidative Stress in Preeclampsia and Placental Diseases. *Int. J. Mol. Sci.* **2018**, *19*, 1496. [CrossRef] [PubMed]
42. Zhao, S.; Gu, X.; Groome, L.J.; Wang, Y. Decreased Nephrin and GLEPP-1, But Increased VEGF, Flt-1, and Nitrotyrosine, Expressions in Kidney Tissue Sections from Women with Preeclampsia. *Reprod. Sci.* **2009**, *16*, 970–979. [CrossRef] [PubMed]
43. Vikse, B.E.; Irgens, M.; Leivestad, T.; Skjaerven, R.; Iversen, B.M. Preeclampsia and the Risk of End-Stage Renal Disease. *N. Engl. J. Med.* **2008**, *359*, 800–809. [CrossRef] [PubMed]
44. Smith, G.C.; Pell, J.P.; Walsh, D. Pregnancy Complications and Maternal Risk of Ischaemic Heart Disease: A Retrospective Cohort Study of 129,290 Births. *Lancet* **2001**, *357*, 2002–2006. [CrossRef]
45. Bar, J.; Kaplan, B.; Wittenberg, C.; Erman, A.; Boner, G.; Ben-Rafael, Z.; Hod, M. Microalbuminuria After Pregnancy Complicated by Pre-Eclampsia. *Nephrol. Dial. Transplant.* **1999**, *14*, 1129–1132. [CrossRef] [PubMed]
46. Khashan, A.S.; Evans, M.; Kublickas, M.; McCarthy, F.P.; Kenny, L.C.; Stenvinkel, P.; Fitzgerald, T.; Kublickiene, K. Preeclampsia and Risk of End Stage Kidney Disease: A Swedish Nationwide Cohort Study. *PLoS Med.* **2019**, *16*, 1002875. [CrossRef]
47. Webster, P.; Webster, L.M.; Cook, H.T.; Horsfield, C.; Seed, P.T.; Vaz, R.; Santos, C.; Lydon, I.; Homsy, M.; Lightstone, L.; et al. A Multicenter Cohort Study of Histologic Findings and Long-Term Outcomes of Kidney Disease in Women Who Have Been Pregnant. *Clin. J. Am. Soc. Nephrol.* **2017**, *12*, 408–416. [CrossRef]
48. Kida, H.; Takeda, S.; Yokoyama, H.; Tomosugi, N.; Abe, T.; Hattori, N. Focal glomerular sclerosis in pre-eclampsia. *Clin. Nephrol.* **1985**, *24*, 221–227. [PubMed]
49. Nochy, D.; Hinglais, N.; Jacquot, C.; Gaudry, C.; Remy, P.; Bariety, J. De novo focal glomerular sclerosis in preeclampsia. *Clin. Nephrol.* **1986**, *25*, 116–121.
50. Nagai, Y.; Arai, H.; Washizawa, Y.; Ger, Y.; Tanaka, M.; Maeda, M.; Kawamura, S. FSGS-like lesions in pre-eclampsia. *Clin. Nephrol.* **1991**, *36*, 134–140.

51. Wharram, B.L.; Goyal, M.; Wiggins, J.E.; Sanden, S.K.; Hussain, S.; Filipiak, W.E.; Saunders, T.L.; Dysko, R.C.; Kohno, K.; Holzman, L.B.; et al. Podocyte Depletion Causes Glomerulosclerosis: Diphtheria Toxin-Induced Podocyte Depletion in Rats Expressing Human Diphtheria Toxin Receptor Transgene. *J. Am. Soc. Nephrol.* **2005**, *16*, 2941–2952. [CrossRef] [PubMed]
52. Fukuda, A.; Wickman, L.T.; Venkatareddy, M.P.; Sato, Y.; Chowdhury, M.A.; Wang, S.Q.; Shedden, K.A.; Dysko, R.C.; Wiggins, J.E.; Wiggins, R.C. Angiotensin II-dependent Persistent Podocyte Loss From Destabilized Glomeruli Causes Progression of End Stage Kidney Disease. *Kidney Int.* **2012**, *81*, 40–55. [CrossRef] [PubMed]
53. Matsusaka, T.; Xin, J.; Niwa, S.; Kobayashi, K.; Akatsuka, A.; Hashizume Wang, Q.C.; Pastan, I.; Fogo, A.G.; Ichikawa, L. Genetic Engineering of Glomerular Sclerosis in the Mouse via Control of Onset and Severity of Podocyte-Specific Injury. *J. Am. Soc. Nephrol.* **2005**, *16*, 1013–1023. [CrossRef] [PubMed]
54. Smeets, B.; Kuppe, C.; Sicking, E.M.; Fuss, A.; Jirak, P.; Kuppevelt, T.H.; Endlich, K.; Wetzels, J.F.M.; Gröne, H.J.; Floege, J.; et al. Parietal Epithelial Cells Participate in the Formation of Sclerotic Lesions in Focal Segmental Glomerulosclerosis. *J. Am. Soc. Nephrol.* **2011**, *22*, 1262–1274. [CrossRef]
55. Saritas, T.; Moeller, M.J. Glomerular Disease: Pre-Eclampsia, Podocyturia and the Role of Parietal Epithelial Cells. *Nat. Rev. Nephrol.* **2014**, *10*, 615–616. [CrossRef]
56. Jefferson, J.A.; Shankland, S.J. The Pathogenesis of Focal Segmental Glomerulosclerosis. *Adv. Chronic Kidney Dis.* **2014**, *21*, 408–416. [CrossRef]
57. Chang, A.M.; Ohse, T.; Krofft, R.D.; Wu, J.S.; Eddy, A.A.; Pippin, J.W.; Shankland, S.J. Albumin-induced Apoptosis of Glomerular Parietal Epithelial Cells Is Modulated by Extracellular Signal-Regulated Kinase $^{1/2}$. *Nephrol. Dial. Transplant.* **2012**, *27*, 1330–1343. [CrossRef]
58. Erkan, E.; Garcia, C.D.; Patterson, L.T.; Mishra, J.; Mitsnefes, M.; Kaskel, F.J.; Devarajan, P. Induction of Renal Tubular Cell Apoptosis in Focal Segmental Glomerulosclerosis: Roles of Proteinuria and Fas-Dependent Pathways. *J. Am. Soc. Nephrol.* **2005**, *16*, 398–407. [CrossRef]
59. Matsusaka, T.; Sandgren, E.; Shintani, A.; Kon, V.; Pastan, I.; Fogo, A.G.; Ichikawa, I. Podocyte Injury Damages Other Podocytes. *J. Am. Soc. Nephrol.* **2011**, *22*, 1275–1285. [CrossRef]
60. Eremina, V.; Jefferson, J.A.; Kowalewska, J.; Hochster, H.; Haas, M.; Weisstuch, J.; Richardson, C.; Kopp, J.B.; Kabir, M.G.; Backx, P.H.; et al. VEGF Inhibition and Renal Thrombotic Microangiopathy. *N. Engl. J. Med.* **2008**, *358*, 1129–1136. [CrossRef]

8

Autophagy Dynamics and Modulation in a Rat Model of Renal Ischemia-Reperfusion Injury

Jean-Paul Decuypere [1,2], Shawn Hutchinson [1,2], Diethard Monbaliu [1,2], Wim Martinet [3], Jacques Pirenne [1,2] and Ina Jochmans [1,2,*]

1 Laboratory of Abdominal Transplantation, Transplantation Research Group, Department of Microbiology and Immunology, KU Leuven, B-3000 Leuven, Belgium; jeanpaul.decuypere@kuleuven.be (J.-P.D.); shawn.hutchinson@uhn.ca (S.H.); diethard.monbaliu@uzleuven.be (D.M.); jacques.pirenne@uzleuven.be (J.P.)
2 Department of Abdominal Transplant Surgery, University Hospitals Leuven, B-3000 Leuven, Belgium
3 Department of Pharmaceutical Sciences, University of Antwerp, B-2610 Antwerp, Belgium; wim.martinet@uantwerpen.be
* Correspondence: ina.jochmans@uzleuven.be

Abstract: Renal ischemia-reperfusion (IR) injury leading to cell death is a major cause of acute kidney injury, contributing to morbidity and mortality. Autophagy counteracts cell death by removing damaged macromolecules and organelles, making it an interesting anchor point for treatment strategies. However, autophagy is also suggested to enhance cell death when the ischemic burden is too strong. To investigate whether the role of autophagy depends on the severity of ischemic stress, we analyzed the dynamics of autophagy and apoptosis in an IR rat model with mild (45 min) or severe (60 min) renal ischemia. Following mild IR, renal injury was associated with reduced autophagy, enhanced mammalian target of rapamycin (mTOR) activity, and apoptosis. Severe IR, on the other hand, was associated with a higher autophagic activity, independent of mTOR, and without affecting apoptosis. Autophagy stimulation by trehalose injected 24 and 48 h prior to onset of severe ischemia did not reduce renal injury markers nor function, but reduced apoptosis and restored tubular dilation 7 days post reperfusion. This suggests that trehalose-dependent autophagy stimulation enhances tissue repair following an IR injury. Our data show that autophagy dynamics are strongly dependent on the severity of IR and that trehalose shows the potential to trigger autophagy-dependent repair processes following renal IR injury.

Keywords: ischemia-reperfusion injury; acute kidney injury; autophagy; apoptosis; trehalose

1. Introduction

Renal ischemia-reperfusion (IR) injury is a major contributor to acute kidney injury (AKI), leading to acute tubular necrosis [1,2]. AKI is a very common condition, affecting 3–18% of hospitalized patients and 33–66% of those admitted to intensive care [3]. AKI is an independent risk factor for death, especially when renal replacement therapy is needed, and is associated with a mortality of 40–70% in critically ill patients [4,5]. Currently, there are no effective treatment strategies for AKI, and measures are supportive while recovery is awaited. Indeed, the kidney's capacity to recover after ischemic injury is remarkable but not perfect [6,7]. In mild injury, this repair process restores renal structure and function; however, when the injury is severe, the repair process can trigger fibrosis, increasing the risk of developing chronic kidney disease [8]. Understanding the link between the severity of injury and the regeneration process could lead to the development of treatments that enhance recovery. A possible link is autophagy, an evolutionary conserved intracellular degradation pathway with homeostatic and damage-mitigating functions.

Macroautophagy, the best studied type of autophagy (and hereafter simply referred to as "autophagy"), manifests as intracellular vesicles (autophagosomes) that envelop cytoplasmic material and subsequently transport and deliver their cargo to the lysosomes for degradation. It involves more than 30 autophagy (Atg) proteins for the initiation, formation, transportation, and fusion of autophagosomes towards lysosomes [9]. Its levels depend on input from various signaling pathways, including nutrient signaling through the mammalian target of rapamycin (mTOR) and energy status monitoring through adenosine monophosphate -activated kinase AMPK. Typically, autophagy is stimulated upon stress as a survival pathway. This way, autophagy recycles damaged and toxic cytoplasmic material into cellular building blocks, which are then used to support anti-stress responses and energy maintenance. Moreover, autophagy is able to degrade damaged mitochondria, preventing the initiation of apoptosis, and therefore might reduce IR injury [10,11]. However, in addition to necrosis and apoptosis [12–14], autophagy has also been positively associated with injury during renal IR [15–19]. Indeed, autophagy can both prevent and assist cell death, depending on the type and duration of the stress, due to the molecular crosstalks between autophagy and cell death mechanisms such as apoptosis and necrosis (reviewed in [20,21]). This autophagy paradox—damaging on the one hand, protecting on the other—implies that the role and dynamics of autophagy during renal IR injury are not well understood [22]. We hypothesized earlier that the role of autophagy in renal IR injury depends on the duration of ischemia, where autophagy can switch from a protective to an injuring mechanism with an increasing ischemia time [23,24].

We now examined this hypothesis by evaluating the dynamics of autophagy, apoptosis, and injury in a rat renal IR model. Subsequently, we assessed the effects of autophagy stimulation on renal IR injury by the administration of trehalose, a naturally occurring disaccharide known to stimulate autophagy [25].

2. Results

2.1. *Transient Renal Injury Following Mild Ischemia*

All Sham and I45 rats (subjected to 45 min of mild ischemia) survived 90 days of reperfusion (R90d). The plasma creatinine was higher after I45 compared to the Sham rats up to R7d (Figure 1A), as were plasmatic aspartate aminotransferase (AST) and heart-fatty acid binding protein (h-FABP), especially early post reperfusion (Figure 1B,C). Terminal deoxynucleotidyl transferase end labeling (TUNEL) staining gradually increased with increasing reperfusion time, with the strongest signal at R6h (Figure S1a). The positive area originated around the blood vessels (R1h) and migrated towards the tubuli at R6h and R24h. Cortical areas were most prominently stained, although some disperse staining was observed in the medulla. It should be noted that besides the expected TUNEL staining of the nuclei, we observed most prominently the staining of the tubular lumen, as previously described [26,27]. TEM revealed swollen and damaged mitochondria at R3h (Figure S1b) in the kidney, confirming the occurrence of intracellular damage. TEM also revealed possible early and late autophagosomes, but clear differences between the Sham and I45 group were not observed. In addition, the mRNA transcription of inflammatory factors intracellular adhesion molecule-1 (ICAM-1) (Figure 1D), interleukins IL-6 and IL-10 (Figure S1c,d) and stress marker heat shock protein 70 (Hsp70) (Figure 1E) significantly increased, with a peak around R3h. These results thus indicate that the kidneys are transiently injured in the I45 model, concomitant with decreased function, enhanced inflammation, and with sustained survival.

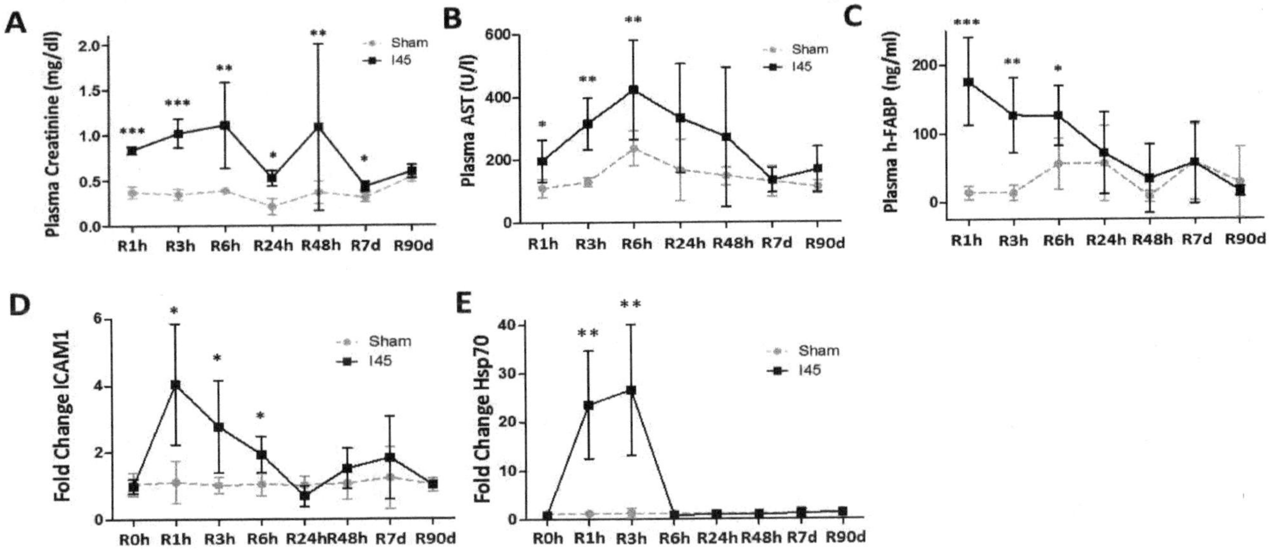

Figure 1. Kidney function is reduced, injury is increased, and tissue inflammatory processes are activated after mild ischemia and reperfusion. Rats, either Sham-operated (Sham) or subjected to 45 min of renal ischemia (I45), were sacrificed at various time points post reperfusion (R0h, R1h, R3h, R6h, R24h, R48h, R7d, and R90d). Plasma was collected to measure the creatinine (**A**), aspartate aminotransferase (AST) (**B**), and heart-fatty acid binding protein (h-FABP) (**C**). Kidneys were collected and analyzed for the mRNA expression of intracellular adhesion molecule-1 (ICAM-1) (**D**) and heat shock protein 70 (Hsp70) (**E**). * $p<0.05$, ** $p<0.01$, *** $p<0.001$. $N=6$.

2.2. *Autophagy Is Suppressed during Ischemia and Reperfusion Following Mild Ischemia*

This rat IR model was now exploited to investigate the autophagic response to mild ischemia. Autophagy markers were assessed by Western blotting on Sham and I45 rat kidney lysates at several time points during reperfusion (R0h, R1h, R3h, R6h, R24h, R48h, R7d, and R90d) (Figure S2). During autophagy, LC3-I is converted into LC3-II, which then recruits to the autophagosomal membrane. As such, the LC3-II levels represent the amount of autophagosomes present at the time of kidney collection. As recommended in the literature, we quantified the ratio of LC3-II over the housekeeping protein Glyceraldehyde 3-phosphate dehydrogenase (GAPDH) [28]. Interestingly, ischemia alone (R0h) led to a reduction in LC3-II (Figure 2A). Since LC3-II eventually is degraded in the lysosomes, a decrease in LC3-II can signify reduced autophagosome formation or enhanced autophagosome clearance [28]. To establish the overall results of IR for the autophagic degradation rate, we also assessed the levels of Sequestosome 1 (Sqstm1/p62), a substrate for autophagic degradation. Ischemia alone (R0h) resulted in an elevation of p62, concomitant with the decrease in LC3-II (Figure 2B), suggesting suppressed autophagy. Since mTOR is the canonical signaling kinase negatively regulating autophagy, we evaluated the phosphorylation of ribosomal protein S6, which is indirectly phosphorylated by mTOR via the activation of p70S6 kinase. Reduced S6 phosphorylation was observed at R0h (Figure 2C), suggesting that the suppression of autophagy during ischemia could be mTOR-independent.

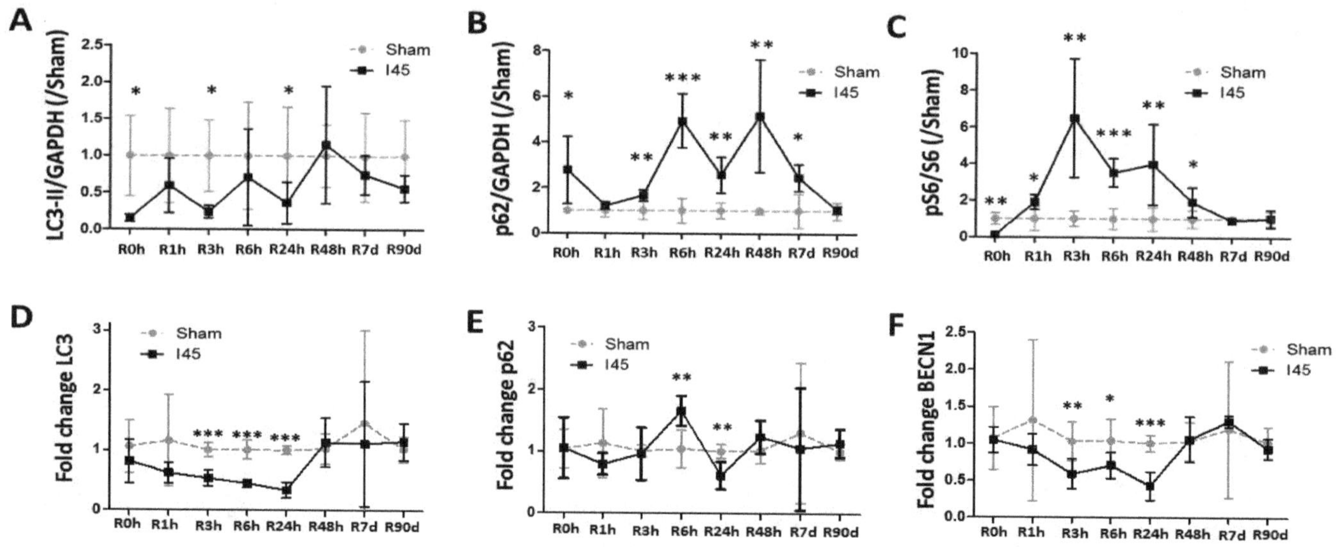

Figure 2. Autophagy is suppressed post reperfusion following mild ischemia. Rats, either Sham-operated (Sham) or subjected to 45 min of renal ischemia (I45), were sacrificed at various time points post reperfusion (R0h, R1h, R3h, R6h, R24h, R48h, R7d, and R90d). Kidney tissue was collected and analyzed by Western blotting for LC3 (**A**), p62 (**B**), S6, and phosphorylated S6 (pS6) (**C**), and by qPCR for the mRNA expression of LC3 (**D**), p62 (**E**), and BECN1 (**F**). * $p < 0.05$, ** $p < 0.01$, *** $p < 0.001$. $N = 6$.

Following mild ischemia, a decrease in LC3-II was generally detected compared to the Sham group, with significant reductions at R0h, R3h, and R24h (Figure 2A). Corresponding with a decrease in LC3-II, the p62 levels were significantly upregulated post reperfusion (Figure 2B), indicating that autophagy is suppressed during reperfusion in this model. Although phosphorylated S6 was decreased during ischemia (R0h), it was strongly increased post reperfusion (Figure 2C), suggesting that the decrease in autophagy could be partially explained by the negative regulation of autophagy by mTOR. It should be noted, however, that S6 can be phosphorylated by other kinases as well [29].

Next, we analyzed whether the results observed on the protein level were also reflected in the mRNA expression of LC3, p62, and BECN1. Interestingly, the LC3 and BECN1 expression were significantly reduced between R3h and R24h (Figure 2D,F). The sqstm1/p62 mRNA levels remained relatively stable, despite an increase at R6h, followed by a decrease at R24h (Figure 2E). As such, it is unlikely that the increase in the p62 levels on a protein level have a transcriptional cause, and most likely reflect the reduction in the autophagic degradation of the p62 protein. In conclusion, these data suggest that autophagy is most prominently suppressed during reperfusion in rats subjected to 45 min of ischemia.

2.3. Apoptosis Is Enhanced during Reperfusion Following Mild Ischemia

We further investigated the apoptotic pathway post reperfusion. Therefore, Western blotting was performed for pro- (Bax, cleaved caspase 3) and anti-apoptotic (Bcl-2) markers on kidney protein lysates from Sham and I45 rats (Figure S3). Despite the reduction in autophagy, apoptosis was not affected following ischemia alone (R0h) (Figure 3A–C). While the Bax protein levels were significantly elevated between R1h and R7d (Figure 3A), the Bcl-2 levels remained stable (Figure 3B). Despite the fast increase in Bax, the levels of cleaved Caspase 3 did not increase before R48h (Figure 3C). Interestingly, a similar trend was observed for the mRNA expression of Bim, a pro-apoptotic BH3-only protein (Figure 3F). Unlike the protein levels, the Bax mRNA expression decreased in I45 rats at R24h and increased at R48h and R90d (Figure 3D). The expression of anti-apoptotic Bcl-2 mRNA was reduced at most time points post reperfusion in I45 rats (Figure 3E). Taken together, these results indicate that the apoptotic machinery is activated late post reperfusion (after 24 h) following mild ischemia in rat kidneys.

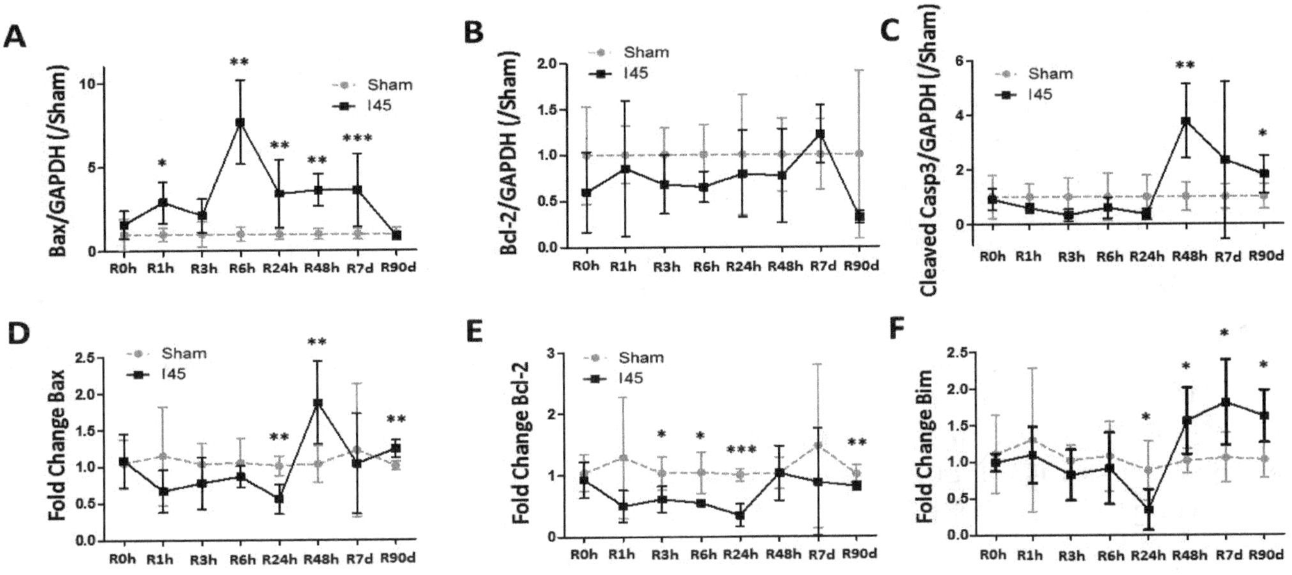

Figure 3. Apoptosis increases post reperfusion following mild ischemia. Rats, either Sham-operated (Sham) or subjected to 45 min of renal ischemia (I45), were sacrificed at various time points post reperfusion (R0h, R1h, R3h, R6h, R24h, R48h, R7d, and R90d). Kidney tissue was collected and analyzed by Western blotting for Bax (**A**), Bcl-2 (**B**), and Cleaved Caspase 3 (**C**), and by qPCR for the mRNA expression of Bax (**D**), Bcl-2 (**E**), and Bim (**F**). * p <0.05, ** p < 0.01, *** p < 0.001. N = 6.

2.4. More Severe Ischemia Increases Kidney Damage

To understand whether autophagy is protective or detrimental for renal IR injury, we first compared the autophagic response in rats subjected to mild (I45) and severe (I60) ischemia. First, in the I60 group, 4/6 rats died within seven days following IR, while in both the I45 and Sham group, all the rats survived. Moreover, the plasma creatinine and AST were also higher in I60 compared to I45 at R3h and R24h (Figure 4A,B), while the plasma h-FABP was only significantly different at R3h (Figure 4C). In addition, the mRNA expression of inflammatory and stress markers ICAM-1 and Hsp70 were higher in I60 versus I45 at R3h (Figure 4D,E). The expressions of IL-6 and -10, however, were lower in I60 compared to I45 (Figure S4a,b). Altogether, the I60 rat model inflicted more kidney damage and inflammation compared to the I45 model.

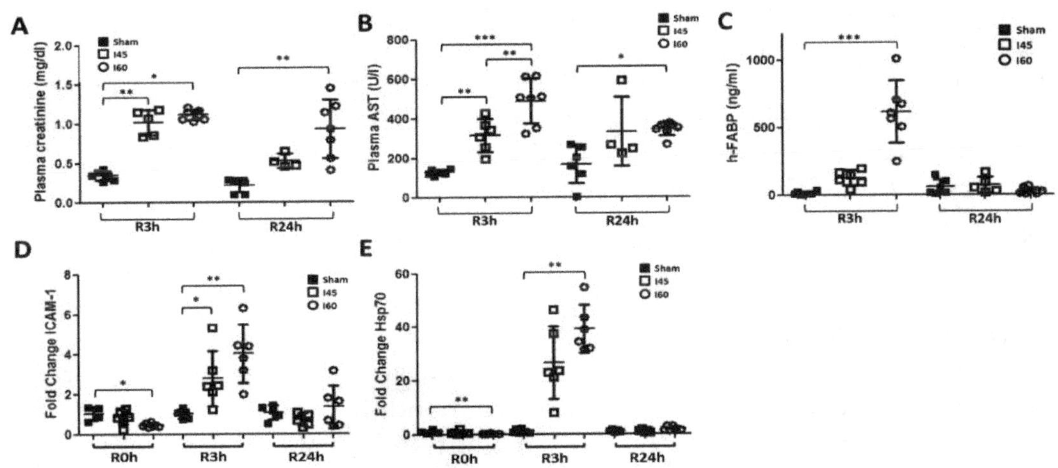

Figure 4. Kidney function is reduced and injury is increased following severe compared to mild or no ischemia. Rats, either Sham-operated (Sham) or subjected to 45 min (I45) or 60 min (I60) of renal ischemia, were sacrificed at various time points post reperfusion (R0h, R3h, and R24h). Plasma was collected to measure the creatinine (**A**), AST (**B**), and h-FABP (**C**). Kidneys were collected and analyzed for the mRNA expression of ICAM-1 (**D**) and Hsp70 (**E**). * p <0.05, ** p < 0.01, *** p < 0.001. N = 6.

2.5. More Autophagy upon Severe Compared to Mild Ischemia

In the I60 model of severe ischemia, we then explored autophagy and apoptosis markers in the kidney. The results observed in the I60 model at the post-reperfusion times R0h, R3h, and R24h (Figure S5a–c) were compared with these time points in the mild ischemia (I45) model. LC3-II decreased in both I45 and I60 in a similar trend, but its levels at R24h were significantly higher in I60 versus I45 (Figure 5A). Interestingly, this was associated with lower p62 levels in the I60 model (Figure 5B and Figure S5b), suggesting a higher autophagic activity in I60 compared to I45. The phosphorylated S6 levels did not significantly differ between I45 and I60 (Figure 5C). On the mRNA level, the LC3 expression was, similarly to the protein levels, increased in I60 versus I45 (Figure 5D), while the p62 levels remained unaltered between the two groups (Figure 5E). The BECN1 expression was significantly lower in I60 versus I45 at R0h, but remained similarly downregulated in both groups afterwards (Figure 5F). Despite these changes in autophagy, no clear trend was observed in the apoptosis markers comparing I60 and I45 (Figure S5d–i). These data thus indicate elevated autophagy upon severe ischemia compared to mild ischemia.

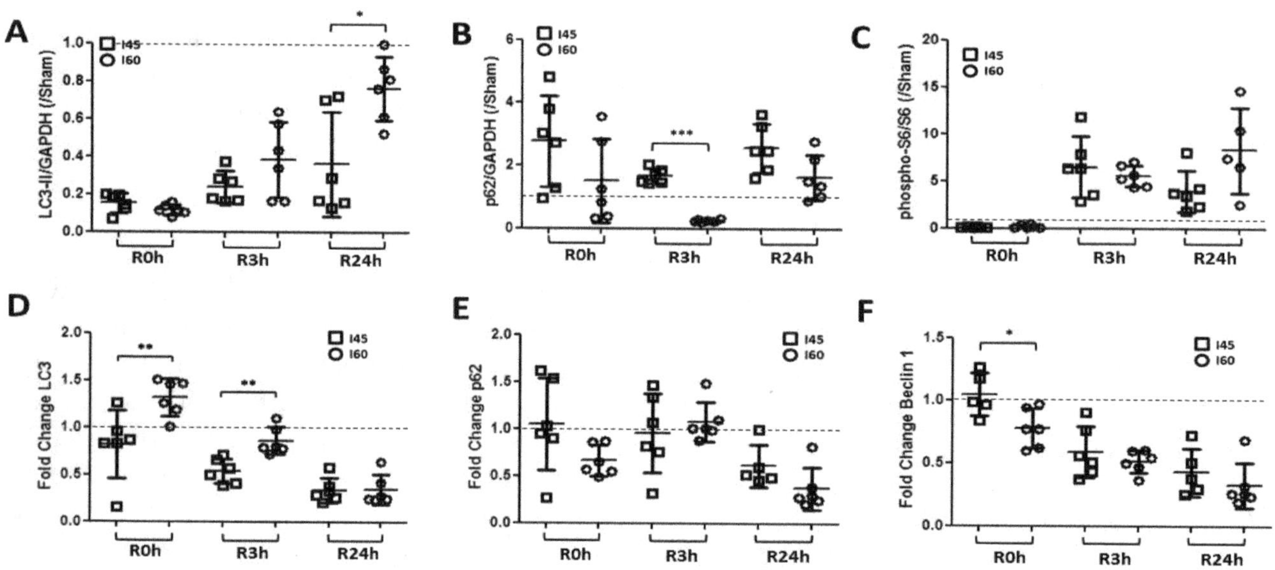

Figure 5. Autophagy is increased during ischemia and after reperfusion following severe ischemia compared to mild ischemia. Rats, either Sham-operated (Sham) or subjected to 45 min (I45) or 60 min (I60) of renal ischemia, were sacrificed at various time points post reperfusion (R0h, R3h, and R24h). Kidneys were collected and analyzed by Western blotting and qPCR for LC3 (**A**), p62 (**B**), S6, and phosphorylated S6 (pS6) (**C**), and by qPCR for the mRNA expression of LC3 (**D**), p62 (**E**), and BECN1 (**F**).The relative change in I45 and I60 compared to the corresponding Sham group (represented by the dashed line at y = 1) was plotted. * $p < 0.05$, ** $p < 0.01$, *** $p < 0.001$. $N = 6$.

2.6. Trehalose Stimulates Autophagy and Reduces IR Injury in the Kidney

To evaluate whether autophagy modulation would alter IR injury, rats were given 2 g/kg body weight trehalose by intraperitoneal injection 48 and 24 h prior to 60 min of ischemia, followed by 24 h or 7 days of reperfusion. Trehalose is a naturally occurring sugar synthesized by bacteria, fungi, and invertebrates, consisting of two glucose molecules connected by a 1-1 α bond. It is an mTOR-independent autophagy inducer that acts partially by inhibiting glucose transport [30]. The kidneys of trehalose-treated rats displayed higher LC3-I and LC3-II levels compared to vehicle-treated rats following 60 min of ischemia and 24 h of reperfusion, without affecting phosphorylated S6, suggesting no change in the mTOR activity and apoptosis (Figure 6A,B). Despite an improvement in survival after R7d (vehicle 50%; trehalose 83%), trehalose did not reduce renal injury at R24h, as evidenced by the similar TUNEL staining (Figure 6C) and plasma AST levels (Figure 6D). The mRNA expression of ICAM-1, Hsp70, and IL-10 even displayed an increasing trend upon trehalose treatment (Figure S6a–d). In addition, the plasma creatinine was increased in the trehalose-treated rats (Figure 6E), suggesting reduced kidney function. However, at R7d, the trehalose-treated rat kidneys showed reduced TUNEL staining (Figure 6F) and an overall improved kidney structure with less dilated tubules (Figure 6G). Together, this suggests that trehalose-induced autophagy does not reduce AKI but improves the repair of the affected tissue.

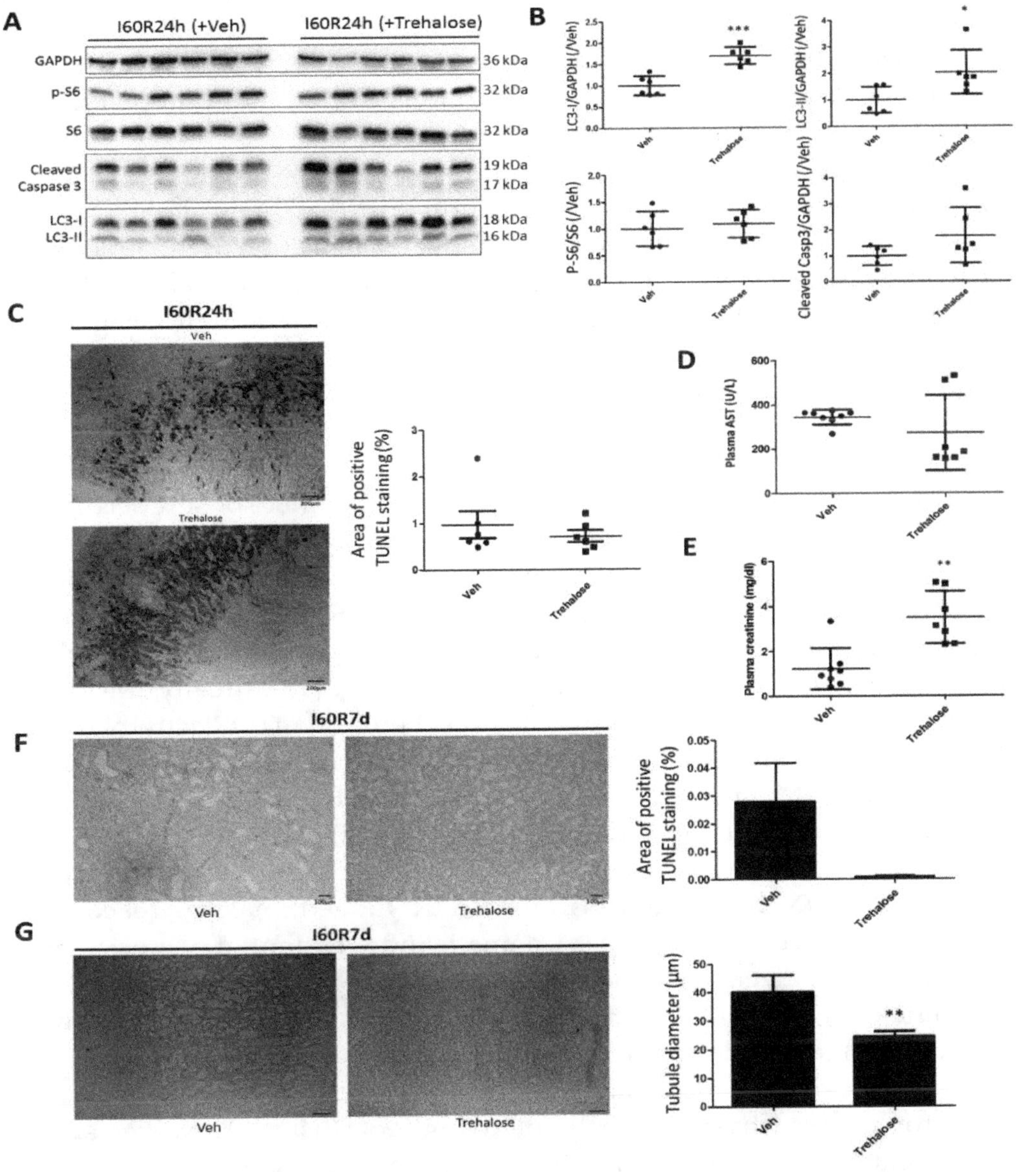

Figure 6. Trehalose induces autophagy and improves the renal structure post reperfusion following severe ischemia. Rats were injected with vehicle (Veh) or trehalose 48 h and 24 h prior to 60 min of renal ischemia (I60), and sacrificed 24 h (I60R24h) or 7 days (I60R7d) post reperfusion. Kidneys of I60R24h were analyzed by Western blotting for the annotated markers (**A**) and compared between Veh- and trehalose-treated for LC3-I, LC3-II, phosphorylated S6 (pS6), and cleaved caspase 3 (**B**). Kidney sections of I60R24h were also stained with TUNEL (**C**) and the plasma levels of AST (**D**) and creatinine (**E**) were determined. In the kidney sections of I60R7d, TUNEL staining was performed (**F**) and the average tubule diameter was assessed (**G**). * $p < 0.05$, ** $p < 0.01$, *** $p < 0.001$. $N = 6$.

3. Discussion

Renal IR injury is a common clinical complication and is the leading cause of AKI. With no effective treatment available to alleviate renal IR injury, it may progress into acute renal failure and increase mortality rates. Therefore, understanding the underlying mechanisms of this injury is crucial to reveal new therapeutic approaches. A central pathway in the progress of renal IR injury is autophagy, an evolutionary conserved intracellular catabolic pathway regulating cellular homeostasis and survival during stress. However, the exact role of autophagy in renal IR injury is still undetermined, as both protective and detrimental effects have been described [23,24]. Indeed, in certain conditions autophagy-dependent cell death can occur. This is suggested to be dependent on the dynamics of autophagy, where excessive or uncontrolled autophagy could trigger the initiation of cell death [19]. The role of autophagy in renal IR injury could therefore be dependent on the ischemic duration of the model, with mild ischemia triggering moderate, protective autophagy and severe ischemia triggering excessive, detrimental autophagy [23,24]. Here, we observed that autophagy dynamics are indeed strongly influenced by these parameters.

First, autophagy was attenuated very rapidly following ischemia (Figure 2). This was not expected, as the lack of oxygen and subsequently energy reduction during ischemia should activate autophagy through AMPK [31]. However, AMPK-dependent autophagy activation occurs upon subtle changes in ATP production, while warm ischemia in rat kidneys leads to a fast and sudden fall in the ATP levels [32]. In view of the ATP dependency of the conjugation reactions leading to the autophagy-specific lipidation of LC3-I into LC3-II [33], this sudden lack of ATP is possibly the cause of the observed decrease in autophagy during ischemia. Similar observations of reduced LC3-II levels have also been observed following renal ischemia in mice [34].

Second, autophagy fluctuated during reperfusion (Figure 2), but overall the attenuation of autophagy during ischemia continues during reperfusion. This effect post reperfusion is most likely due to increased mTOR activity, in which the re-introduction of nutrients during reperfusion likely stimulates mTOR after a suppression caused by nutrient absence during ischemia [35]. This is reflected in the levels of phosphorylated S6, an indirect target of mTOR (Figure 2C). However, it should be noted that the phosphorylation status of S6 is the sum of multiple kinase activities (including mTOR and protein kinase A) and the activity of protein phosphatase-1 [29]. Ideally, the phosphorylation of ULK-1 at Ser757 should be assessed to determine the link between mTOR activity and autophagy [36].

Despite the dynamics of injury and autophagy, apoptosis occurred rather late post reperfusion (R48h). Although TUNEL staining was mostly observed early post reperfusion (R3–6h), this did not correspond with the levels of cleaved caspase 3. In addition, this staining was not typically nucleus-specific, as has been observed previously [26,27]. This suggests that TUNEL staining is indicative of apoptosis-independent DNA damage during renal IR. Indeed, massive reactive oxygen species production has been suggested to induce DNA damage independent of necrosis and apoptosis [37]. These data, therefore, suggest that that the initial (acute) injury post reperfusion is likely more associated with other (inflammatory) types of cell death (e.g., necrosis, caspase3-independent pyrroptosis, ferroptosis, or necroptosis) rather than apoptosis [38,39]. Indeed, in previous work we have shown that necroptosis inhibitor Nec-1 reduces the positive TUNEL staining 3 h post reperfusion in our model [26], suggesting that necroptosis is activated shortly following reperfusion. However, since Nec-1 did not affect the injury markers AST and h-FABP and the plasma creatinine levels, other types of cell death are likely to be activated as well. As such, the observed late apoptosis enhancement 48 h post reperfusion could therefore rather represent a mechanism to remove damaged cells associated with tissue repair.

Third, the autophagy levels are higher when the ischemic duration increases (Figure 5). In general, these data suggest that more severe ischemia is associated with higher autophagy levels and that autophagy dynamics are dependent on the ischemia and reperfusion duration. This could explain the differences in autophagy regulation observed in the literature, as reports often focus on one or few time points post-reperfusion [23]. These differences in the literature are further complicated by the dependency of the IR-induced autophagic response on the gender and age of the model [40], as well as the differences between species. In this context, it is important to note that cell death responses to anoxia-reoxygenation differ between rodent and human cells [41], and that this will likely be reflected in the autophagy dynamics as well. Moreover, in the clinical AKI setting the ischemic time is longer than that in the model presented here. The fact that autophagy dynamics are very dependent on the species and ischemia/reperfusion time, as this study suggests, warrants the need for further evaluation in AKI patients.

As severe ischemia is associated with decreased survival and elevated autophagy, these results bring into question whether autophagy plays an active role in renal damage or is stimulated to prevent renal IR injury. In this respect, trehalose, an autophagy inducer, seemed to have a dual effect following severe ischemia: a (slight) exacerbation of renal injury 24 h post reperfusion on the one hand and an improvement in the kidney tubular structure and reduced apoptosis 7 days following the ischemia on the other (Figure 6 and Figure S6). A similar autophagy-dependent stimulation of tissue remodeling was observed following cardiac injury, in which the beneficial effects of trehalose were blunted by the suppression of autophagy [42]. These observations, together with the lower autophagy levels associated with mild ischemia (Figure 2), suggest that autophagy may be detrimental in the acute phase of IR injury, but protective by promoting tissue repair in the recovery phase. This opens prospects for possible clinical applications of autophagy modulators such as trehalose; for example, as it functions in the repair process following injury, it could be administered peri- or post-operatively during kidney transplantation. In this respect, it is important to note that trehalose is an essential component of the "extracellular type" ET-Kyoto organ preservation solution, which is used in clinical lung transplantation [43], and which was found to be superior in the preservation of rat livers compared to the University of Wisconsin solution [44]. The molecular mechanisms of the beneficial effects of trehalose in renal IR injury, whether this is autophagy-dependent and whether this could be used in the clinical setting, require more investigation.

Due to the limitations of the rat model in this study, autophagy was only analyzed with the Western blotting and qPCR techniques. Nevertheless, it is recommended to analyze autophagy through a series of techniques [28]. Although TEM analysis revealed autophagic vesicles in the kidney tissue (Figure S1b), no clear differences were observed between the Sham and I45 rats. However, TEM is performed on a very small section of the kidney, while the altered autophagy responses are likely restricted to certain renal zones (cf. positive TUNEL staining in the corticomedullary area). Similar experiments in GFP- or RFP-GFP-LC3 mice subjected to various durations of ischemia and reperfusion should gain more insight in the exact dynamics of autophagy. Nonetheless, the combination of the autophagosome marker LC3-II and autophagy degradation marker p62 analyzed in our experiments revealed the expected inverse correlation of LC3-II and p62 dynamics, indicating that these levels indeed reflected autophagy alterations in response to renal ischemia and reperfusion.

In conclusion, the differential dynamics observed in these different IR models thus partially explain the conflicting findings in the literature regarding the role of autophagy in renal IR injury, which is dependent on ischemic duration and the time of reperfusion. As such, it is important to investigate multiple time points post reperfusion and various ischemic lengths. Additionally, modulation with trehalose revealed that autophagy stimulation likely has different outcomes in tissue repair (protective) and in acute IR injury (detrimental). This information is crucial in light of the possible clinical application of (trehalose-dependent) autophagy stimulation in acute kidney injury or kidney transplantation.

4. Materials and Methods

4.1. Ischemia-Reperfusion Injury Model

Female Sprague-Dawley rats (200–250 g; 8–10 weeks old) were housed at the KU Leuven animal facility. After at least 1 week of acclimatization, they were anesthetized by an intraperitoneal injection of 7.5 mg/kg of ketamin (Anesketin®, Eurovet Animal Health BV, Bladel, The Netherlands) and 2.5 mg/kg of xylazin (Xyl-M 2%®, Van Miert & Dams Chemie (VMD), Arendonk, Belgium). Both renal pedicles were dissected free through a midline abdominal incision and clamped "en bloc" with microaneurysm clamps to induce ischemia. Reperfusion was initiated by the removal of the clamps. Sham-operated rats underwent the same surgery without the clamping of the pedicles. Analgesics were administered daily (Vetergesic 0.1 mg/kg, CEVA, Libourne, France) following surgery. At the end of the experiment, pentobarbital (Nembutal 60 mg/kg, CEVA) was injected intraperitoneally and the rats were sacrificed by exsanguination, which allowed plasma sampling directly from the aorta. Plasma was spun down (1000× *g*; 10 min) and snap-frozen. Kidneys were collected and processed immediately, as described below. For the trehalose experiments, sterile PBS (Vehicle) or 2 g/kg bodyweight of trehalose in PBS (in a total volume of ca. 500 μL) was injected intraperitoneally 48 h and 24 h prior to surgery. The rat survival, behavior, and humane endpoints were monitored thrice daily. The animal care and experimental protocols were in accordance with the European guidelines and approved by the Ethical Committee for Animal Experimentation of KU Leuven (P053/2016).

4.2. Experimental Groups

First, to analyze the dynamics of autophagy during reperfusion, Sham-operated rats (Sham) and rats subjected to 45 min of ischemia (I45-mild ischemia) were divided into subgroups with various reperfusion (R) times: R0h, R1h, R3h, R6h, R24h, R48h, R7d, or R90d. Next, to assess the effects of the ischemic time, we compared the I45 mild ischemia group with rats subjected to 60 min of ischemia (severe ischemia-I60), followed by 0 h, 3 h, 24 h, and 7 days of reperfusion. Six rats were included per subgroup.

4.3. Kidney Function and Injury

Kidney function was assessed by plasma creatinine, measured by the kinetic Jaffé method (Hitachi/Roche Modular P, Roche Diagnostics, Diegem, Belgium) by the central laboratory of our University Hospitals. The cellular injury markers aspartate aminotransferase [26,45] (AST, colorimetric method on Hitachi/Roche Modular P) and heart-fatty acid binding protein [26,45,46] (h-FABP, enzyme-linked immunosorbant assay (ELISA)) were assessed according to the manufacturer's instructions (HK414-Hycult Biotech, Uden, The Netherlands).

4.4. Transmission Electron Microscopy

Small samples of the cortex (ca. 1 mm^3) were fixed in 2.5% glutaraldehyde, 0.1 M of sodium cacodylate, and 0.05% $CaCl_2$ (pH 7.4) and further processed for transmission electron microscopy, as described previously [47], with minor modifications (extra staining with 1% tannic acid in veronal acetate for 1h after OsO4 postfixation). A FEI Tecnai microscope was used to examine ultrathin sections at 80–120 kV.

4.5. Western Blotting

Snap-frozen kidney samples were homogenized in a radioimmunoprecipitation assay buffer (RIPA) lysis buffer containing 50 mM of Tris-HCl (pH 7.4); 150 mM of NaCl; 1 mM of EDTA; 1% Ipegal; protease, and phosphatase inhibitors (Roche, Basel, Switzerland). The protein concentration was determined through use of a Bradford protein assay (Sigma-Aldrich, Saint-Louis, MO, USA). Samples were prepared with Laemmli buffer containing β-mercaptoethanol, heated at 95 °C for 3 min and loaded on Any kD Mini-Protean TGX Precast Gel (Bio-Rad Laboratories, Hercules, CA, USA). SDS-PAGE was performed with a constant voltage of 150 V. Next, the proteins were blotted on polyvinylidene difluoride (PVDF) membranes using the semi-dry Trans-Blot Turbo Transfer system (Bio-Rad Laboratories). Membranes were blocked for 1h at room temperature with PBS-Tween (0.1%) containing 5% milk powder (MP), followed by incubation with the primary antibody diluted in PBS-T and 2% MP overnight at 4 °C. Next day, the membranes were washed 3 times with PBS-T and then incubated with the secondary horseradish peroxidase (HRP)-coupled antibody for 45 min with PBS-T + 2% MP. After washing three times with PBS-T, immunoreactive bands were visualized through enhanced chemoluminescence (Pierce ECL Western Blotting Substrate, Thermo Fisher Scientific, Waltham, MA, USA), followed by detection and band intensity quantification using the Chemidoc MP technology and associated Imagelab software (Bio-Rad Laboratories).

4.6. Antibodies

The following antibodies and reagents were used for the Western blotting experiments. Anti-LC3 (5F10, Nanotools), anti-S6 (2217, Cell Signaling Technology, Danvers, MA, USA), anti-phospho-S6 (4858, Cell Signaling Technology), anti-cleaved caspase 3 (9664, Cell Signaling Technology), anti-SQSTM1/p62 (P0067, Sigma-Aldrich, Saint-Louis, MO, USA), anti-Bcl-2 (sc-492, Santa Cruz Biotechnology, Dallas, TX, USA), and anti-Bax (sc-493, Santa Cruz Biotechnology). Anti-GAPDH (G8715, Sigma-Aldrich) served as an internal control. Secondary antibodies are HRP-linked anti-mouse IgG (7076, Cell Signaling Technology) and HRP-linked anti-rabbit IgG (1706515, Bio-Rad Laboratories, Hercules, CA, USA).

4.7. Quantitative Real-Time Polymerase Chain Reaction

RNA was extracted from kidney tissues using Trizol reagent and chloroform, followed by an additional purification step with the RNeasy mini kit (Qiagen, Hilden, Germany), according to the manufacturer's protocol. The mRNA expression levels in kidney tissues were analyzed using quantitative real-time polymerase chain reaction (Q-RT-PCR). Reverse transcription was performed at 37 °C for 1 h with the M-MLV Reverse Transcriptase along with FSBuffer and Rnase out (Life Technologies, Carlsbad, CA, USA). Q-RT-PCR was performed with the PCR mastermix of Applied Biosystems (1.503.193, Foster City, CA, USA). Thermal cycling conditions were composed of cDNA initially denatured at 95 °C for 60 s, and then amplified by PCR for 45 cycles (95 °C for 5 s, 60 °C for 30 s). Experiments were carried out in duplicates. Using the 2-ΔΔCt method [48], the relative quantification in gene expression was determined. Data are expressed as the relative differences (fold change) between the sham and IR samples after correction for GAPDH expression.

4.8. qPCR Taqman Probes

The following reagents from TaqMan Gene Expression Assays (Applied biosystems, Foster Cyti, CA, USA) were used for RT-PCR experiments: GAPDH (Rn01775763_g1), BECN1 (Rn00586976_m1), LC3 (Rn02132764_S1), p62 (Rn00709977_m1), Bcl-2 (Rn99999125_m1), Bax (Rn01480160_g1), Bim (Rn00674175_m1), Hsp70 (Rn00583013_S1), ICAM-1 (Rn00564227_m1), IL-10 (Rn00563409_m1), and IL-6 (Rn01410330_m1).

4.9. Terminal Deoxynucleotidyl Transferase End Labeling

For the detection of oligonucleosomal DNA cleavage via terminal deoxynucleotidyl transferase end labeling (TUNEL), tissue sections were deparaffinized in toluene (2 × 5 min), rehydrated in distilled water (5 min), and pretreated with 3% citric acid (60 min) to remove tissue calcification. Endogenous peroxidase was quenched by incubating sections for 15 min in 0.9% hydrogen peroxide. Thereafter, TUNEL was performed using an ApopTag Plus Peroxidase In Situ Apoptosis Detection Kit (Merck-Millipore, Burlington, MA, USA) according to the instructions of the manufacturer. Slides were observed with an Olympus BX61 microscope at 20× magnification, and pictures were taken with the Olympus Stream Essentials 1.9 software. Quantification of the TUNEL staining was performed with the "color threshold" function of ImageJ, using the color space RGB and the same parameters for each analyzed picture.

4.10. Statistical Analysis

If data were normally distributed, unpaired t-tests were used for the comparison of 2 groups (Sham versus IR group) or a one-way ANOVA for 3 groups (Sham, I45, and I60) with Tukey Multiple Comparison test post-hoc. F-test was performed to compare variances. If the variances were significantly different, Welch's correction was applied. If a group was not normally distributed, non-parametric tests (Mann–Whitney or Kruskal–Wallis test with Dunns post-hoc) were performed. For relative Western blotting and qPCR data, values were normalized to the mean of the control Sham group. Outliers were removed based on the Grubb's test. Normal distribution was analyzed with the Kolmogorov–Smirnov test (for small sample sizes).

Author Contributions: Conceptualization J.-P.D. and I.J.; methodology, J.-P.D. and W.M.; validation, J.-P.D., D.M., J.P., and I.J.; formal analysis, J.-P.D. and S.H.; investigation, J.-P.D., S.H., and I.J.; resources, J.-P.D., D.M., J.P., and I.J.; data curation, J.-P.D.; writing—original draft preparation, J.-P.D.; writing—review and editing, S.H., D.M., W.M., J.P., and I.J.; visualization, J.-P.D.; supervision, J.P. and I.J.; funding acquisition, J.-P.D., D.M., J.P., and I.J. All authors have read and agreed to the published version of the manuscript.

Acknowledgments: We would like to thank Veerle Heedfeld and Tine Wylin (Abdominal Transplantation) for their practical help with the rat and laboratory experiments.

Abbreviations

AKI	Acute kidney injury
AMPK	5′ adenosine monophosphate-activated protein kinase
AST	Aspartate transaminase
Bcl-2	B-Cell lymphoma 2
hFABP	heart-type fatty acid binding protein
Hsp70	Heat shock protein 70
ICAM	Intracellular adhesion molecule
IL	Interleukin
IR	Ischemia-reperfusion
LC3	(microtubule-associated protein 1) Light chain 3
mTOR	mammalian target of rapamycin
Sqstm1	Sequestosome 1
TEM	transmission electron microscopy
TUNEL	Terminal deoxynucleotidyl transferase dUTP nick end labeling
ULK-1	Unc51-like kinase-1

References

1. Bellomo, R.; Kellum, J.A.; Ronco, C. Acute kidney injury. *Lancet* **2012**, *380*, 756–766. [CrossRef]
2. Lameire, N.; Bagga, A.; Cruz, D.; De Maeseneer, J.; Endre, Z.H.; Kellum, J.A.; Liu, K.D.; Mehta, R.L.; Pannu, N.; Van Biesen, W.; et al. Acute kidney injury: An increasing global concern. *Lancet* **2013**, *382*, 170–179. [CrossRef]
3. Hoste, E.; Kellum, J.A.; Selby, N.M.; Zarbock, A.; Palevsky, P.M.; Bagshaw, S.M.; Goldstein, S.L.; Cerdá, J.; Chawla, L.S. Global epidemiology and outcomes of acute kidney injury. *Nat. Rev. Nephrol.* **2018**, *14*, 607–625. [CrossRef] [PubMed]
4. RENAL Replacement Therapy Study Investigators; Bellomo, R.; Cass, A.; Cole, L.; Finfer, S.; Gallagher, M.; Billot, L.; McArthur, C.; McGuinness, S.; Myburgh, J.A.; et al. Intensity of continuous renal-replacement therapy in critically ill patients. *N. Engl. J. Med.* **2009**, *361*, 1627–1638. [PubMed]
5. Palevsky, P.M.; Zhang, J.H.; O'Connor, T.Z.; Chertow, G.M.; Crowley, S.T.; Choudhury, D.; Finkel, K.; Kellum, J.A.; Paganini, E.; Schein, R.M.H.; et al. Intensity of renal support in critically ill patients with acute kidney injury. *N. Engl. J. Med.* **2008**, *359*, 7–20. [PubMed]
6. Bonventre, J.V.; Yang, L. Cellular pathophysiology of ischemic acute kidney injury. *J. Clin. Investig.* **2011**, *121*, 4210–4221. [CrossRef]
7. Sharfuddin, A.A.; Molitoris, B.A. Pathophysiology of ischemic acute kidney injury. *Nat. Rev. Nephrol.* **2011**, *7*, 189–200. [CrossRef]
8. Chawla, L.S.; Kimmel, P.L. Acute kidney injury and chronic kidney disease: An integrated clinical syndrome. *Kidney Int.* **2012**, *82*, 516–524. [CrossRef]

9. Parzych, K.R.; Klionsky, D.J. An Overview of Autophagy: Morphology, Mechanism, and Regulation. *Antioxid Redox Signal.* **2014**, *20*, 460–473. [CrossRef]
10. Pallet, N.; Livingston, M.; Dong, Z. Emerging Functions of Autophagy in Kidney Transplantation. *Am. J. Transplant.* **2013**, *14*, 13–20. [CrossRef]
11. Eltzschig, H.K.; Carmeliet, P. Hypoxia and inflammation. *N. Engl. J. Med.* **2011**, *364*, 656–665. [CrossRef] [PubMed]
12. Daemen, M.A.; Veer, C.v.; Denecker, G.; Heemskerk, V.H.; Wolfs, T.G.A.M.; Clauss, M.; Vandenabeele, P.; Buurman, W.A. Inhibition of apoptosis induced by ischemia-reperfusion prevents inflammation. *J. Clin. Investig.* **1999**, *104*, 541–549. [CrossRef] [PubMed]
13. Daemen, M.A.; de Vries, B.; Buurman, W.A. Apoptosis and inflammation in renal reperfusion injury. *Transplantation* **2002**, *73*, 1693–1700. [CrossRef] [PubMed]
14. Yang, B.; Hosgood, S.A.; Nicholson, M.L. Naked small interfering RNA of caspase-3 in preservation solution and autologous blood perfusate protects isolated ischemic porcine kidneys. *Transplantation* **2011**, *91*, 501–507. [CrossRef] [PubMed]
15. Nakagawa, S.; Nishihara, K.; Inui, K.; Masuda, S. Involvement of autophagy in the pharmacological effects of the mTOR inhibitor everolimus in acute kidney injury. *Eur. J. Pharmacol.* **2012**, *696*, 143–154. [CrossRef] [PubMed]
16. Chien, C.T.; Shyue, S.K.; Lai, M.K. Bcl-xL augmentation potentially reduces ischemia/reperfusion induced proximal and distal tubular apoptosis and autophagy. *Transplantation* **2007**, *84*, 1183–1190. [CrossRef]
17. Isaka, Y.; Suzuki, C.; Abe, T.; Okumi, M.; Ichimaru, N.; Imamura, R.; Kakuta, Y.; Matsui, I.; Takabatake, Y.; Rakugi, H.; et al. Bcl-2 protects tubular epithelial cells from ischemia/reperfusion injury by dual mechanisms. *Transplant. Proc.* **2009**, *41*, 52–54. [CrossRef]
18. Yeh, C.H.; Hsu, S.P.; Yang, C.C.; Chien, C.T.; Wang, N.P. Hypoxic preconditioning reinforces HIF-alpha-dependent HSP70 signaling to reduce ischemic renal failure-induced renal tubular apoptosis and autophagy. *Life Sci.* **2010**, *86*, 115–123. [CrossRef]
19. Wu, H.H.; Hsiao, T.Y.; Chien, C.T.; Lai, M.K. Ischemic conditioning by short periods of reperfusion attenuates renal ischemia/reperfusion induced apoptosis and autophagy in the rat. *J. Biomed. Sci.* **2009**, *16*, 19. [CrossRef]
20. Mariño, G.; Niso-Santano, M.; Baehrecke, E.H.; Kroemer, G. Self-consumption: The interplay of autophagy and apoptosis. *Nat. Rev. Mol. Cell Biol.* **2014**, *15*, 81–94. [CrossRef]
21. Chen, Q.; Kang, J.; Fu, C. The independence of and associations among apoptosis, autophagy, and necrosis. *Signal Transduct. Target. Ther.* **2018**, *3*, 18. [CrossRef]
22. Liu, Y.; Levine, B. Autosis and autophagic cell death: The dark side of autophagy. *Cell Death Differ.* **2015**, *22*, 367–376. [CrossRef] [PubMed]
23. Decuypere, J.P.; Pirenne, J.; Jochmans, I. Autophagy in Renal Ischemia-Reperfusion Injury: Friend or Foe? *Am. J. Transplant.* **2014**, *14*, 1464–1465. [CrossRef] [PubMed]
24. Decuypere, J.P.; Ceulemans, L.J.; Agostinis, P.; Monbaliu, D.; Naesens, M.; Pirenne, J.; Jochmans, I. Autophagy and the kidney: Implications for ischemia-reperfusion injury and therapy. *Am. J. Kidney Dis.* **2015**, *66*, 699–709. [CrossRef] [PubMed]
25. Sarkar, S.; Davies, J.E.; Huang, Z.; Tunnaclliffe, A.; Rubinsztein, D.C. Trehalose, a novel mTOR-independent autophagy enhancer, accelerates the clearance of mutant huntingtin and alpha-synuclein. *J. Biol. Chem.* **2007**, *82*, 5641–5652. [CrossRef]
26. Decuypere, J.P.; Ceulemans, L.J.; Wylin, T.; Martinet, W.; Monbaliu, D.; Pirenne, J.; Jochmans, I. Plasmatic Villin 1 Is a Novel In Vivo Marker of Proximal Tubular Cell Injury During Renal Ischemia-Reperfusion. *Transplantation* **2017**, *101*, e330–e336. [CrossRef] [PubMed]
27. Ikegami, Y.; Goodenough, S.; Inoue, Y.; Dodd, P.R.; Wilce, P.A.; Matsumoto, I. Increased TUNEL positive cells in human alcoholic brains. *Neurosci. Lett.* **2003**, *349*, 201–205. [CrossRef]
28. Klionsky, D.J.; Abdelmohsen, K.; Abe, A.; Abedin, J.; Abeliovich, H.; Arozena, A.A.; Adachi, H.; Adams, C.M.; Adams, P.D.; Adeli, K.; et al. Guidelines for the use and interpretation of assays for monitoring autophagy (3rd edition). *Autophagy* **2016**, *12*, 1–222. [CrossRef]
29. Biever, A.; Valjent, E.; Puighermanal, E. Ribosomal Protein S6 Phosphorylation in the Nervous System: From Regulation to Function. *Front. Mol. Neurosci.* **2015**, *8*, 75. [CrossRef]
30. Mardones, P.; Rubinsztein, D.C.; Hetz, C. Mystery solved: Trehalose kickstarts autophagy by blocking glucose transport. *Sci. Signal.* **2016**, *9*, fs2. [CrossRef]
31. Zhao, M.; Klionsky, D.J. AMPK-dependent phosphorylation of ULK1 induces autophagy. *Cell Metab.* **2011**, *13*, 119–120. [CrossRef] [PubMed]

32. Bore, P.J.; Papatheofanis, I.; Sells, R.A. Adenosine triphosphate regeneration and function in the rat kidney following warm ischaemia. *Transplantation* **1979**, *27*, 235–237. [CrossRef] [PubMed]
33. Glick, D.; Barth, S.; Macleod, K.F. Autophagy: Cellular and molecular mechanisms. *J. Pathol.* **2010**, *221*, 3–12. [CrossRef] [PubMed]
34. Jiang, M.; Liu, K.; Luo, J.; Dong, Z. Autophagy is a renoprotective mechanism during in vitro hypoxia and in vivo ischemia-reperfusion injury. *Am. J. Pathol.* **2010**, *176*, 1181–1192. [CrossRef] [PubMed]
35. Aoyagi, T.; Kusakari, Y.; Xiao, C.-Y.; Inouye, B.T.; Takahashi, M.; Scherrer-Crosbie, M.; Rosenzweig, A.; Hara, K.; Matsui, T. Cardiac mTOR protects the heart against ischemia-reperfusion injury. *Am. J. Heart Physiol. Circ. Physiol.* **2012**, *303*, H75–H85. [CrossRef] [PubMed]
36. Kim, J.; Kundu, M.; Viollet, B.; Guan, K.L. AMPK and mTOR regulate autophagy through direct phosphorylation of Ulk1. *Nat. Cell Biol.* **2011**, *13*, 132–141. [CrossRef]
37. Mulay, S.R.; Thomasova, D.; Ryu, M.; Anders, H.J. MDM2 (murine double minute 2) links inflammation and tubular cell healing during acute kidney injury in mice. *Kidney Int.* **2012**, *81*, 1199–1211. [CrossRef]
38. Linkermann, A.; Chen, G.; Dong, G.; Kunzendorf, U.; Krautwald, S.; Dong, Z. Regulated Cell Death in AKI. *J. Am. Soc. Nephrol.* **2014**, *25*, 2689–2701. [CrossRef]
39. Belavgeni, A.; Meyer, C.; Stumpf, J.; Hugo, C.; Linkermann, A. Ferroptosis and Necroptosis in the Kidney. *Cell Chem. Biol.* **2020**, *27*, 446–462. [CrossRef]
40. Van Erp, A.C.; Hoeksma, D.; Rebolledo, R.A.; Ottens, P.J.; Jochmans, I.; Monbaliu, D.; Pirenne, J.; Leuvenink, H.; Decuypere, J.-P. The Crosstalk between ROS and Autophagy in the Field of Transplantation Medicine. *Oxidative Med. Cell. Longev.* **2017**, *2017*, 7120962. [CrossRef]
41. Eleftheriadis, T.; Pissas, G.; Antoniadi, G.; Liakopoulos, V.; Stefanidis, I. Cell Death Patterns Due to Warm Ischemia or Reperfusion in Renal Tubular Epithelial Cells Originating from Human, Mouse, or the Native Hibernator Hamster. *Biology* **2018**, *7*, 48. [CrossRef] [PubMed]
42. Sciarretta, S.; Yee, D.; Nagarajan, N.; Bianchi, F.; Saito, T.; Valenti, V.; Tong, M.; Del Re, M.P.; Vecchione, C.; Schirone, L.; et al. Trehalose-Induced Activation of Autophagy Improves Cardiac Remodeling After Myocardial Infarction. *J. Am. Coll. Cardiol.* **2018**, *71*, 1999–2010. [CrossRef] [PubMed]
43. Ikeda, M.; Bando, T.; Yamada, T.; Sato, M.; Menjyu, T.; Aoyama, A.; Sato, T.; Chen, F.; Sonobe, M.; Omasa, M.; et al. Clinical application of ET-Kyoto solution for lung transplantation. *Surg. Today* **2015**, *45*, 439–443. [CrossRef]
44. Zhao, X.; Koshiba, T.; Nakamura, T.; Tsuruyama, T.; Li, Y.; Bando, T.; Wada, H.; Tanaka, K. ET-Kyoto solution plus dibutyryl cyclic adenosine monophosphate is superior to University of Wisconsin solution in rat liver preservation. *Cell Transplant.* **2008**, *17*, 99–109. [CrossRef]
45. Jochmans, I.; Lerut, E.; Van Pelt, J.; Monbaliu, D.; Pirenne, J. Circulating AST, H-FABP, and NGAL are early and accurate biomarkers of graft injury and dysfunction in a preclinical model of kidney transplantation. *Ann. Surg.* **2011**, *254*, 784–791. [CrossRef]
46. Shirakabe, A.; Kobayashi, N.; Hata, N.; Shinada, T.; Tomita, K.; Tsurumi, M.; Okazaki, H.; Matsushita, M.; Yamamoto, Y.; Yokoyama, S.; et al. The serum heart-type fatty acid-binding protein (HFABP) levels can be used to detect the presence of acute kidney injury on admission in patients admitted to the non-surgical intensive care unit. *BMC Cardiovasc. Disord.* **2016**, *16*, 174. [CrossRef] [PubMed]
47. Martinet, W.; Timmermans, J.P.; De Meyer, G.R.Y. Methods to assess autophagy in situ—Transmission electron microscopy versus immunohistochemistry. *Methods Enzymol.* **2014**, *543*, 89–114.
48. Livak, K.J.; Schmittgen, T.D. Analysis of relative gene expression data using real-time quantitative PCR and the 2(-Delta Delta C(T)) Method. *Methods* **2001**, *25*, 402–408. [CrossRef]

9

NOX1 Inhibition Attenuates Kidney Ischemia-Reperfusion Injury via Inhibition of ROS-Mediated ERK Signaling

Hee-Yeon Jung †, Se-Hyun Oh †, Ji-Sun Ahn, Eun-Joo Oh, You-Jin Kim, Chan-Duck Kim, Sun-Hee Park, Yong-Lim Kim and Jang-Hee Cho *

Division of Nephrology, Department of Internal Medicine, School of Medicine, Kyungpook National University, Kyungpook National University Hospital, Daegu 41944, Korea; hy-jung@knu.ac.kr (H.-Y.J.); ttily@nate.com (S.-H.O.); ggumsuni@hanmail.net (J.-S.A.); oej1124@naver.com (E.-J.O.); pinkqic1004@naver.com (Y.-J.K.); drcdkim@knu.ac.kr (C.-D.K.); sh-park@knu.ac.kr (S.-H.P.); ylkim@knu.ac.kr (Y.-L.K.)

* Correspondence: jh-cho@knu.ac.kr

† These authors contributed equally to this study.

Abstract: The protective effects of nicotinamide adenine dinucleotide phosphate (NADPH) oxidase (NOX) 1 inhibition against kidney ischemia-reperfusion injury (IRI) remain uncertain. The bilateral kidney pedicles of C57BL/6 mice were clamped for 30 min to induce IRI. Madin–Darby Canine Kidney (MDCK) cells were incubated with H_2O_2 (1.4 mM) for 1 h to induce oxidative stress. ML171, a selective NOX1 inhibitor, and siRNA against NOX1 were treated to inhibit NOX1. NOX expression, oxidative stress, apoptosis assay, and mitogen-activated protein kinase (MAPK) pathway were evaluated. The kidney function deteriorated and the production of reactive oxygen species (ROS), including intracellular H_2O_2 production, increased due to IRI, whereas IRI-mediated kidney dysfunction and ROS generation were significantly attenuated by ML171. H_2O_2 evoked the changes in oxidative stress enzymes such as SOD2 and GPX in MDCK cells, which was mitigated by ML171. Treatment with ML171 and transfection with siRNA against NOX1 decreased the upregulation of NOX1 and NOX4 induced by H_2O_2 in MDCK cells. ML171 decreased caspase-3 activity, the Bcl-2/Bax ratio, and TUNEL-positive tubule cells in IRI mice and H_2O_2-treated MDCK cells. Among the MAPK pathways, ML171 affected ERK signaling by ERK phosphorylation in kidney tissues and tubular cells. NOX1-selective inhibition attenuated kidney IRI via inhibition of ROS-mediated ERK signaling.

Keywords: NOX1; ML171; reactive oxygen species; ERK; ischemia-reperfusion injury; acute kidney injury

---

1. Introduction

Kidney ischemia/reperfusion injury (IRI), which is the interruption and restoration of blood flow, is a basic pathophysiology of acute kidney injury associated with high mortality and morbidity. IRI causes oxygen and nutrition deficiency, inflammatory cell infiltration, oxygen-derived reactive oxygen species (ROS) or nitrogen-derived reactive nitrogen species generation, microvascular damage, and ultimately tissue damage [1–3]. Excessive ROS is among the most important contributors of tissue damage by inducing oxidative damage of deoxyribonucleic acid, proteins, and lipids [4–8].

Nicotinamide adenine dinucleotide 3-phosphate (NADPH) oxidase (NOX) is a major enzyme that uses NADPH to catalyze oxygen conversion to superoxide and produce ROS. Seven NOX isoforms have been identified including NOX1–5, Duox1, and Duox2 [9]. In particular, NOX1-dependent ROS production contributes to cell signaling, cell growth, angiogenesis, motility, and blood pressure regulation [10–12]. Previous studies have reported that NOX1 upregulation was involved in cisplatin-induced kidney injury [13] and NOX1 inhibitor has a protective effect on lung IRI by suppressing inflammatory and autophagy activation [14]. Although several antioxidants and anti-inflammatory agents [15–19] have effects on ROS production and inflammatory reactions, and NOX4 inhibitor [20] has been used in experimental studies to prevent or decrease IRI-induced kidney damage, the protective effect of NOX1 inhibition against kidney IRI is not totally understood.

This study's aim is to identify the effect of NOX1 inhibition on the recovery from IRI through ROS suppression and related mechanisms. We used a pharmacological inhibitor specific for NOX1 (2-acetylphenothiazine, ML171) [21] and siRNA against NOX1.

2. Material and Methods

2.1. Animals

Eight-week-old male C57BL/6 mice that weighed 22–25 g (Samtako, Osan, Korea) were used. They were housed with a free access to standard chow and water and were kept in a 12 h light/dark cycle. They were divided randomly into six groups as follows: control vehicle (Con + Veh, $n = 5$), control with 60 mg/kg ML171 (Con + ML171, $n = 5$), sham operation with vehicle (Sham + Veh, $n = 6$), sham operation with 60 mg/kg of ML171 (Sham + ML171, $n = 6$), ischemia-reperfusion vehicle (IRI + Veh, $n = 8$), and ischemia-reperfusion with 60 mg/kg of ML171 (IRI + ML171, $n = 8$). ML171 (MedChemExpress, Monmouth Junction, NJ 08852, USA) was dissolved in 10% DMSO, 40% PEG300, 5% Tween-80, and 45% normal saline. Animals were injected intraperitoneally with a single daily dose of ML171 (60 mg/kg) or vehicle before 24 h for bilateral IRI and were sacrificed by cardiac puncture under anesthesia at 24 h after reperfusion. Blood and kidneys were harvested for the analyses. Animal experiments were performed according to the guidelines approved by the Animal Care and Use Committee at the Kyungpook National University (KNU-2017-0013).

2.2. Induction of Kidney IRI

For ischemia induction, the mice were anesthetized using isoflurane inhalation and kidney pedicles were completely occluded for 30 min using a microaneurysm clamp. After 30 min of ischemia, the artery clamp was removed to allow reperfusion, and the skin was closed. Identical surgical treatment was performed on sham-operated animals except for the clamping of the kidney pedicles. During the operation, animals were maintained at a temperature of 36.5–37 °C using a temperature-controlled heating device (Harvard Bioscience, Holliston, MA, USA).

2.3. Kidney Function and Histopathological Studies

In mouse serum, blood urea nitrogen (BUN) and creatinine (Cr) levels were evaluated by GCLabs (Yongin, Korea) using the Cobas 8000 modular analyzer system (Roche, Germany). Kidney tissues from each experimental group were immersion-fixed with 4% paraformaldehyde (pH 7.4) and then embedded in paraffin. Two-micrometer tissue sections were prepared and stained with periodic acid-Schiff (PAS) and Masson's trichrome using standard protocols for the determination of histological changes and collagen deposition, respectively. Immunohistochemical analysis of kidney tissues detected the Nox-1 (1:100, ab121009, Abcam) and Nox-4 proteins (1:100, MA5-32090, Invitrogen).

2.4. Cell Culture Treatment

Madin-Darby Canine Kidney (MDCK) cells were obtained from the American Type Culture Collection (CCL-34™, Manassas, VA, USA), which were maintained in Eagle's Minimum Essential Medium (EMEM, ATCC®30-2003™) and supplemented with 10% fetal bovine serum at 37 °C in a humidified atmosphere of 5% CO_2 and 95% air. Cultured MDCK cells were plated on 96-well plates (1.0×10^4 cells/well) for intracellular ROS measurement and on 12-well plates (1.0×10^5 cells/well) for real-time reverse transcriptase-polymerase chain reaction (RT-PCR) and on 6-well plates

(2.0×10^5 cells/well) for measurement of caspase-3 activity and immunoblot analysis. For each experiment, 80–85% confluent cells were incubated with serum-free media for 24 h and were placed into the 0.2% FBS-added medium, which were treated with (1) only medium, (2) ML171 (1 μM), (3) ML171 (2.5 μM), (4) H_2O_2 (1.4 mM), (5) H_2O_2 (1.4 mM) + ML171 (1 μM), or (6) H_2O_2 (1.4 mM) + ML171 (2.5 μM) for an additional 48 h and were pretreated with ML171 (1 μM or 2.5 μM) for 1 h and treated with H_2O_2 (1.4 mM). To further study the effect of Nox-1 inhibition, MDCK cells were transiently transfected with 100 nM siRNA against Nox-1 (AccuTarget™ SMART pool customized siRNA, Bioneer, Daejeon, Korea) or nontargeting siRNA (SignalSilence® Control siRNA, #6568, Cell signaling, Danvers, MA, USA) using Lipofectamine RNAiMax (Thermo Fisher Scientific, Waltham, MA, USA) for 6 h. Subsequently, cells were incubated with H_2O_2 (1.4 mM) for 48 h.

2.5. *Hydrogen Peroxide Assay*

Extracellular H_2O_2 was measured using the Amplex Red Hydrogen Peroxide Assay Kit (Thermo Fisher Scientific) in accordance with the manufacturer's instructions. Briefly, to detect H_2O_2 released from mice kidney and treated MDCK cells, lysis buffer or culture media (50 mL) were reacted with the Amplex Red reagent, along with horseradish peroxidase, to produce resorufin, a red fluorescent oxidation product. Its fluorescence was determined at 530 nm excitation and 590 nm emission using a fluorescence microplate reader (Molecular Devices, Sunnyvale, CA, USA). The concentrations of H_2O_2 were calculated using standard curves.

2.6. *Intracellular ROS Measurement*

Mice kidney and MDCK cells were stained using 10 μM 2′,7′-dichlorodihydrofluorescein diacetate (H_2DCFDA; Molecular Probes, Eugene, OR, USA) for 40 min and visualized using fluorescence microscopy (Nikon, Tokyo, Japan). To quantitatively measure fluorescence signal intensity, the stained kidney tissues and cells in 96-well plates were incubated with lysis buffer (0.1% Triton X-100 plus 0.5M EDTA in PBS), and the intensity was measured at 480 nm excitation and 520 nm emission using a fluorescence microplate reader (Molecular Devices Corp., Silicon Valley, CA, USA). The value of the fluorescence signal was normalized based on the total amount of cellular protein and then expressed as a percentage of the control.

2.7. *Measurement of Caspase-3 Activity*

Caspase-3 activity in the mice kidney and MDCK cells was measured using a colorimetric assay kit (Sigma-Aldrich) in accordance with the manufacturer's protocol. In brief, kidney homogenates were incubated with the fluorometric caspase-3 substrate, Ac-DEVD-pNA, in the assay buffer. To account for nonspecific hydrolysis of the substrate, a control reaction mixture containing the caspase-3 inhibitor, acetyl-DEVD-CHO, in the assay buffer was used. Both mixtures were incubated for 90 min at 37 °C, with the absorbance being read at 405 nm.

2.8. *TUNEL Assay*

Apoptosis was investigated by terminal deoxynucleotidyl transferase-mediated dUTP <nick end labeling (TUNEL) assay using the In Situ Cell Death Detection Kit (Roche, Mannheim, Germany), Fluorescein, for fluorescence and the Click-iT™ TUNEL colorimetric IHC Detection Kit (Life Technologies, Carlsbad, CA, USA) for immunohistochemistry. Briefly, treated cells were fixed with 4% paraformaldehyde for 1 h at room temperature and then permeabilized in the 0.1% Triton X-100/0.1% sodium citrate for 2 min at 4 °C. After washing with PBS, the cells were incubated with 50 uL TUNEL reagent mixture for 1 h at 37 °C and then counterstained with 4′,6-diamidino-2-phenylindole (DAPI; Sigma, St. Louis, MO, USA) to detect cell nucleus for 1 min. Finally, the cells were mounted with the Prolong Gold anti-fade reagent (Invitrogen, Eugene, OR, USA) and then observed under a confocal microscope (Carl Zeiss, Göttingen, Germany). The number of TUNEL-positive cells was randomly counted (three to five sections per experiment). The percentage of apoptotic cells was calculated

as a percentage of the TUNEL-positive cell-to-DAPI ratio. For immunohistochemistry of TUNEL assay, after treating with terminal deoxynucleotidyl transferase (TdT) reaction buffer for 10 min at 37 °C, the TdT reaction mixture was added for 60 min at 37 °C. The streptavidin-peroxidase conjugate solution was incubated for 30 min at room temperature. Then, the sections were washed and mixed with the 3,3′-diaminobenzidine (DAB) reaction to produce a brown color and then counterstained with Mayer's hematoxylin.

2.9. *Quantitative RT-PCRs*

Total RNA was extracted from treated MDCK cells and kidney tissues using Trizol (Invitrogen, Waltham, MA) in accordance to the manufacturer's instructions. One microgram of total RNA was reverse transcribed to cDNA using PrimeScript cDNA Synthesis kit (TaKaRa Shuzo Co., Ltd., Otsu, Japan). Quantitative PCR was performed in the synthesized cDNA using the StepOne Plus Real-time PCR system (Applied Biosystems, Foster City, CA, USA) with SYBER Green PCR master mix (Life Technologies, Carlsbad, CA, USA). The qRT-PCRs were performed in duplicate. The transcript level of target genes was calculated using the $2^{-\Delta\Delta CT}$ method. All primers used for qRT-PCR were designed using the Primer Express 3.0.1 software (Applied Biosystems, Foster City, CA, USA), which are listed in Table 1.

Table 1. Oligonucleotide primer sequences.

Gene	Forward Primer (5′–3′)	Reverse Primer (5′–3′)
Mouse Nox-1	CAG GCC ATG GAT GGA TCT CT	ATG TTT GGA GAC TGG ATG GGA TT
Mouse Nox-2	GCT CTC TCT GAC ATC GGT GAC A	CGA GTC ACG GCC ACA TAC AG
Mouse Nox-4	CAC CAA ACA CAG AAG CAC AAG AC	AAA GCA GGG TAT CAC TCC ATG AA
Mouse GAPDH	TAA AGG GCA TCC TGG GCT ACA CT	TTA CTC CTT GGA GGC CAT GTA GG
Dog Nox-1	CCC CGC TGA GTC TTG GAA	TAA AAT CGG AGA ATC CTT TCA AGA A
Dog Nox-2	GAC ACG CAC GCC TTT GAG T	CCT GCA TCT GGG TCT CTA GCA
Dog Nox-4	CAC TCT TCG GAC TAT ACT GCA TGA TC	TCA TCC CCT GAG CCA AGA AT
Dog p40phox	GGG AAG ACA TCG CCC TGA AT	ACA GCA GCC GCA CCA GAT
Dog SOD2	CGC CGC CTA CGT GAA CA	CTC CAG CGC CTC CAG ATA CT
Dog GPX	GAA TGT GGC GTC GCT CTG A	CGC TGC AGC TCG TTC ATC T
Dog GAPDH	GAT GCC CCC ATG TTT GTG A	TTT GGC TAG AGG AGC CAA GCA

2.10. *Immunoblot Analysis*

Immunoblot analysis detected the marker proteins of apoptosis and mitogen-activated protein kinase (MAPK) pathway, and 20 µg of protein was separated using 10% SDS-polyacrylamide gel electrophoresis and transferred to a nitrocellulose membrane, which was blocked with 10% skimmed milk for 1 h at room temperature and incubated overnight at 4 °C with primary antibodies and then incubated with a horseradish peroxidase-conjugated secondary antibody (Dako, Glostrup, Denmark) for 1 h at room temperature and detected using advanced ECL reagents (Amersham Bioscience, Piscataway, NJ, USA). The intensity of the bands was quantified using the Scion Image software (Scion, Frederick, MD, USA). Primary antibodies that detect proteins are listed in Table 2.

Table 2. List of antibodies used in immunohistochemistry and immunoblotting.

Antibodies	Cat. No.	Company
Dog Bcl-2	ab117115	Abcam
Dog Bax	2772S	Cell signaling
Dog β-actin	A1978	Sigma
Dog p-Erk1 (pT202/pY204) + p-Erk2(pT185/pY187)	ab4819	Abcam
Dog Erk1+Erk2	ab17942	Abcam
Dog p-p38 (phospho T180+Y182)	ab4822	Abcam
Dog p38 (M138)	ab31828	Abcam
Dog p-JNK1 + p-JNK2 (phospho T183+Y185)	ab4821	Abcam
Dog JNK1 + JNK2 + JNK3	ab179461-1	Abcam
Mouse Bcl-2	2876	Cell signaling
Mouse Bax	2772	Cell signaling
Dog, mouse NOX-1	Ab121009	Abcam
Mouse NOX-4	MA5-32090	Invitroten
Mouse a-SMA	Ab5694	Abcam
Mouse fibronectin	Ab2413	Abcam
Mouse GAPDH	2118S	Cell signaling
Mouse p-AKT (Ser473)	9271	Cell signaling
Mouse AKT	9272	Cell signaling
Mouse p-ERK (Thr202/Tyr204)	4370S	Cell signaling
Mouse ERK	9102	Cell signaling
Mouse p-JNK (Thr183/Tyr185)	9251S	Cell signaling
Mouse JNK	9252S	Cell signaling
Mouse p-p38 (Thr180/Tyr182)	9211S	Cell signaling
Mouse p38	9212S	Cell signaling

2.11. *Statistical Analysis*

Data represent mean ± SEM. Statistical analyses were performed using GraphPad Prism 5.01 (GraphPad Software Inc., La Jolla, CA, USA). The difference among the groups was analyzed using a one-way nonparametric ANOVA followed by Tukey's multiple comparison test. Multiple comparison tests were only applied when a significant difference was determined using the ANOVA ($p < 0.05$).

3. Results

3.1. *Effect of ML171 on Attenuation of Kidney Function and Histological Alteration in Kidney IRI*

Figure 1A,B shows the results of kidney function after IRI with treatment of ML171. BUN and Cr levels were significantly increased by IRI compared to the control groups. The levels of serum BUN and Cr were decreased in IRI mouse pretreated with ML171. The PAS and trichrome staining evaluated the histological changes in IRI models (Figure 1C–F). The histological analyses revealed that ML171 attenuated tubular necrosis, loss of the brush border, and cast formation in IRI kidney. Treatment with ML171 decreased collagen deposition in the IRI model.

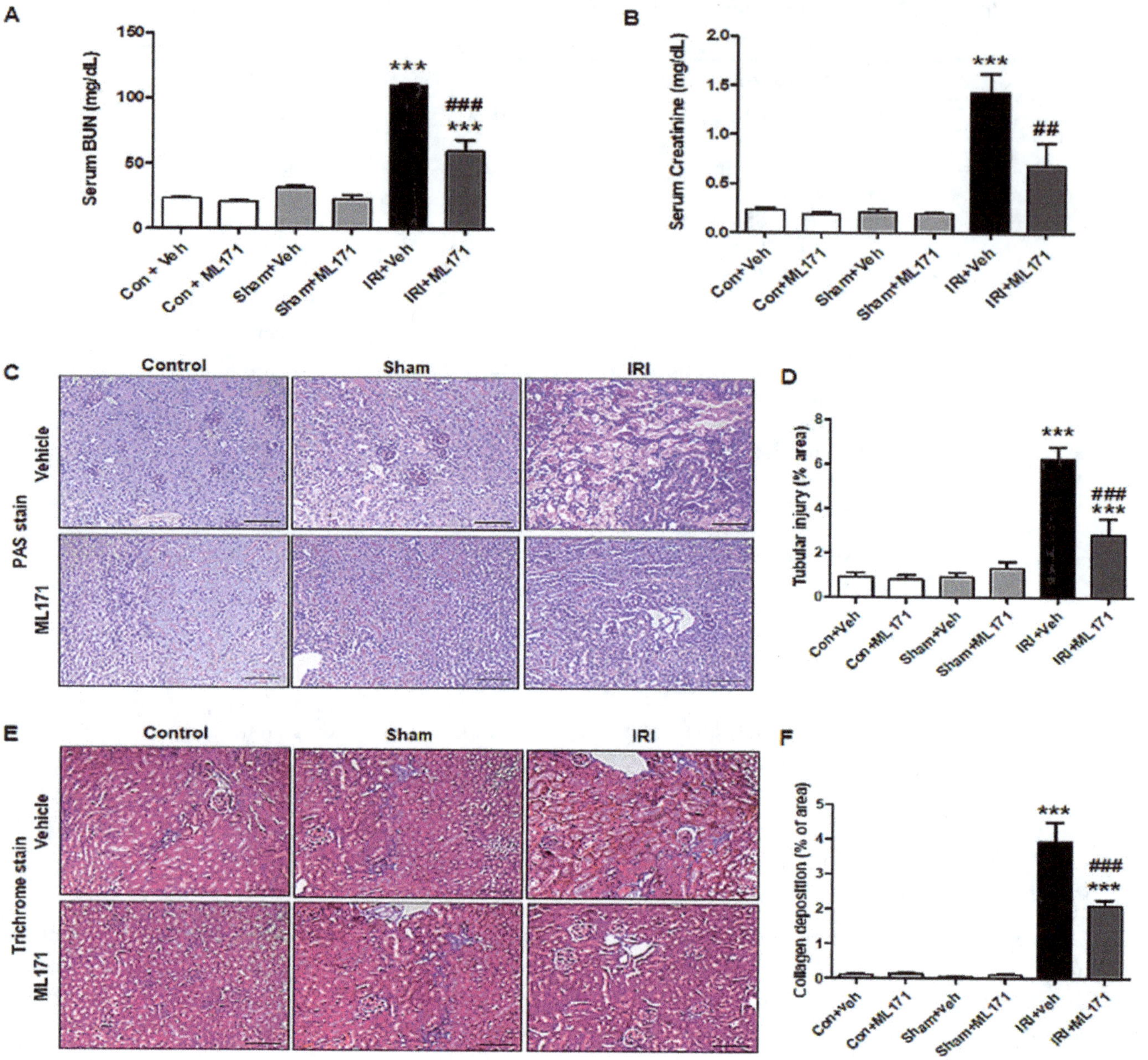

Figure 1. Effect of ML171 on attenuation of kidney function and histological alteration in renal ischemia-reperfusion injury (IRI). The levels of serum blood urea nitrogen (BUN) and creatinine were significantly reduced in ML171-pretreated IRI model (**A**,**B**). The periodic acid-Schiff (PAS)- and trichrome-stained kidney sections in IRI models showed that ML171 decreased tissue damage in renal tubular epithelial cells and collagen deposition (**C**–**F**). Data represent mean ± SEM. *** $p < 0.001$ vs. Con + Veh, ## $p < 0.01$, ### $p < 0.001$ vs. IRI + Veh. The difference among the groups was analyzed using a one-way nonparametric ANOVA followed by Tukey's multiple comparison test.

3.2. *Effect of ML171 on the Expression of NOX Family Subunits and Oxidative Stress Markers in IRI*

To investigate the changes in oxidative stress after IRI, the expression of NOX subunits and generation of ROS were evaluated. Among the NOX subunits, NOX1 and NOX4, but not NOX2 mRNA expression increased after IRI, which was significantly reduced by ML171 (Figure 2A–C). Immunohistochemical staining of NOX1 and NOX4 revealed an increased amount of NOX1 and NOX4 expression in the IRI model and a significant decrease by ML171 treatment (Figure 2D–G). ML171 attenuated the increase of intracellular H_2O_2 in the IRI kidney model (Figure 2H–I).

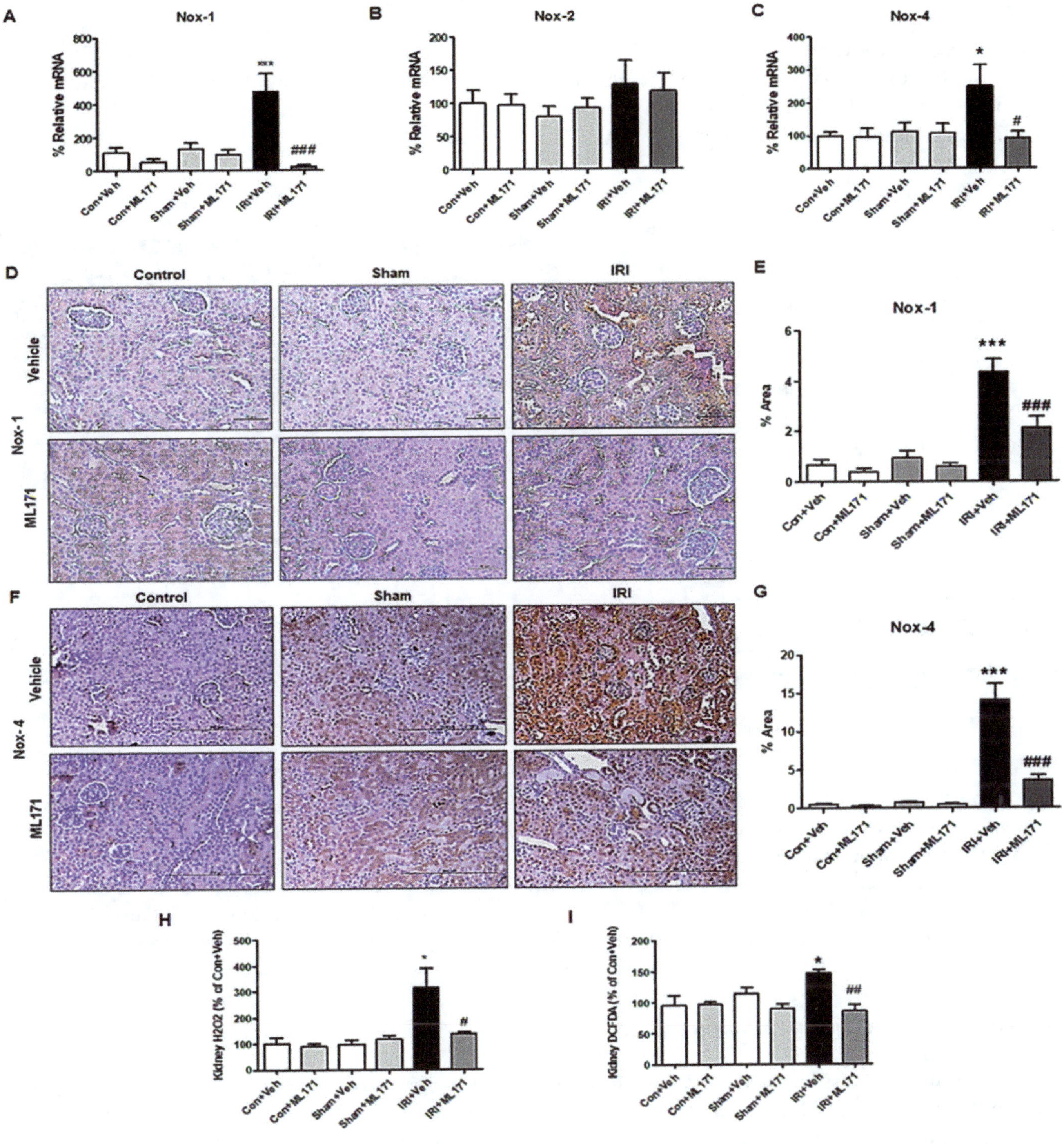

Figure 2. Effect of ML171 on nicotinamide adenine dinucleotide phosphate (NADPH) oxidase (NOX) family subunits and oxidative stress markers in IRI. The increased mRNA expression of NOX1 and NOX4 in IRI were significantly mitigated by ML171 (**A–C**). The immunohistochemical staining of NOX1 and NOX4 showed that the increased expression of NOX1 and NOX4 in IRI was decreased by ML171 (**D–G**). The increased reactive oxygen species (ROS) including H_2O_2 in the IRI model were significantly decreased by ML171 (**H,I**). Data represent mean ± SEM. * $p < 0.05$, *** $p < 0.001$ vs. Con + Veh, # $p < 0.05$, ## $p < 0.01$, ### $p < 0.001$ vs. IRI + Veh. The difference among the groups was analyzed using a one-way nonparametric ANOVA followed by Tukey's multiple comparison test.

3.3. *Effect of ML171 on Apoptosis in Kidney Tubular Cells Following IRI*

Caspase-3 activity decreased in the kidneys after ML171 treatment (Figure 3A), and TUNEL assay showed that apoptosis of kidney tubule cells decreased after MA171 treatment (Figure 3B). Figure 3C also showed that ML171 caused a significantly increased Bcl-2 level and Bcl-2/Bax ratio in the IRI model, suggesting the mitigating effect of ML171 on apoptosis.

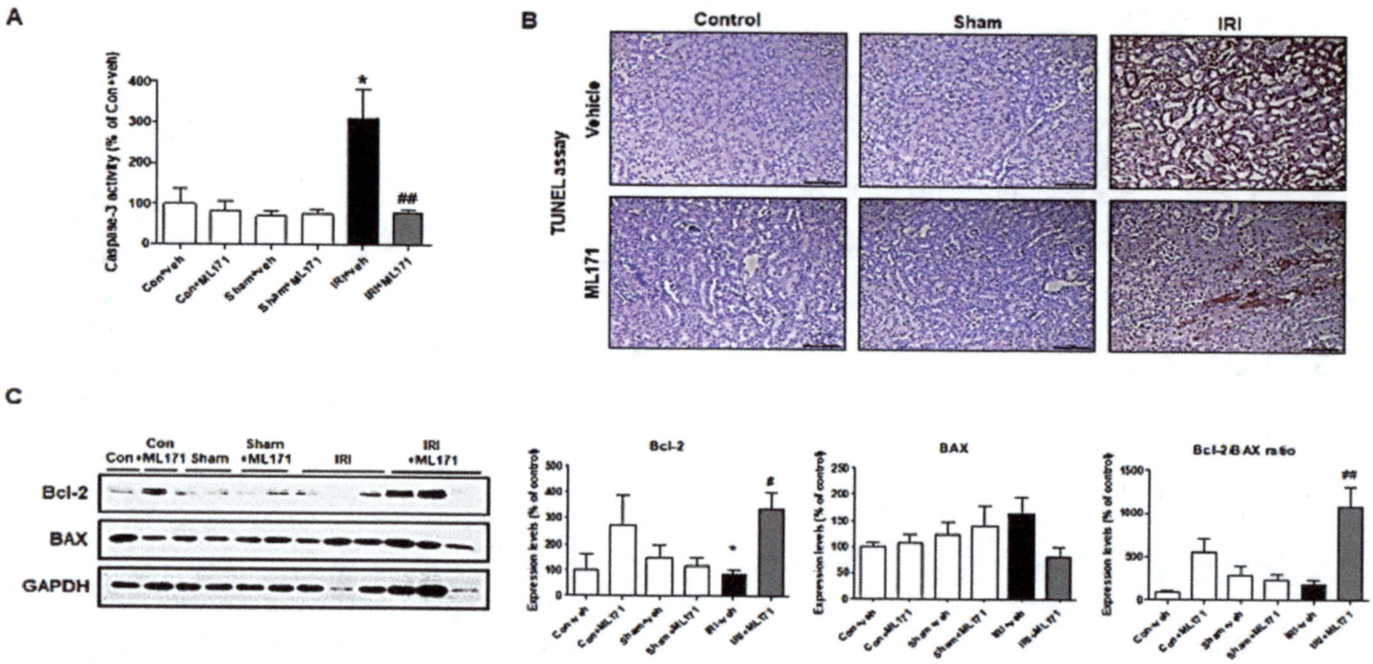

Figure 3. Effect of ML171 on apoptosis in kidney tubular cells following IRI. Caspase-3 activity was significantly decreased in IRI model after ML171 treatment (**A**). TUNEL assay showed that ML171 attenuated the apoptosis of kidney tubule cells (**B**). The Bcl-2 level and Bcl-2/Bax ratio were significantly increased in the IRI model after ML171 treatment (**C**). Data represent mean ± SEM. * $p < 0.05$ vs. Con + Veh, $^{\#}$ $p < 0.05$, $^{\#\#}$ $p < 0.01$ vs. IRI + Veh. The difference among the groups was analyzed using a one-way nonparametric ANOVA followed by Tukey's multiple comparison test.

3.4. *Changes in Phosphorylated Proteins of MAPK Signaling Pathways in Kidney Tissues*

We identified MAPK pathway genes to determine the oxidative stress mechanism induced by IRI. The Western blot of MAPK genes revealed that the phosphorylated extracellular signal-regulated kinase (p-ERK) was significantly increased in the IRI model, which was effectively attenuated by ML171. However, no difference in the expression of phosphorylated p38 and JNK was noted (Figure 4).

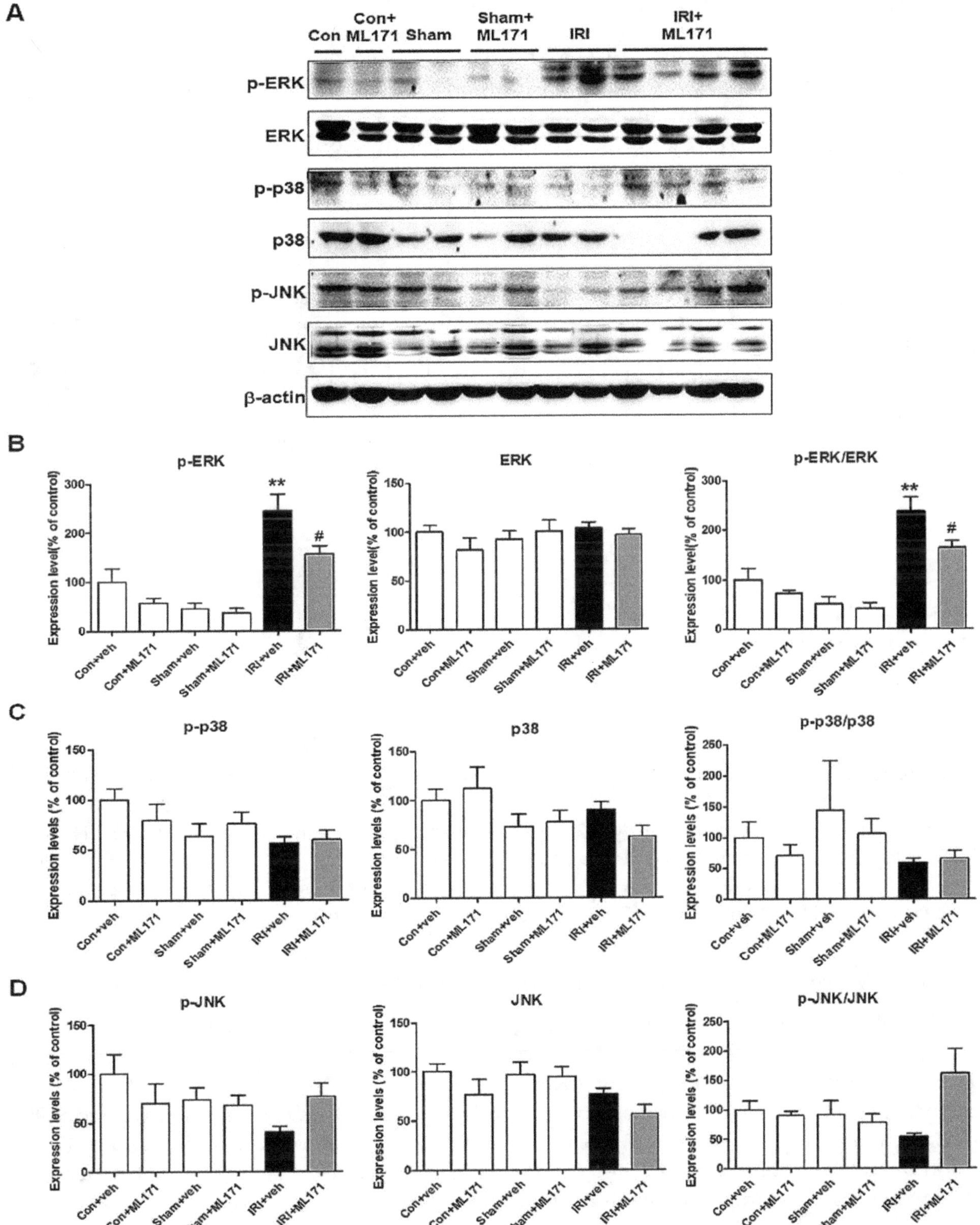

Figure 4. Changes in phosphorylated proteins of mitogen-activated protein kinase (MAPK) signaling pathways in kidney tissues. The genes of MAPK pathway determined the mechanism of oxidative stress-induced IRI. ML171 effectively attenuated increased p-ERK in the IRI model (**A**,**B**). The expression of phosphorylated p38 and JNK was not increased in the IRI model nor affected by ML171 (**C**,**D**). Data represent mean ± SEM. ** $p < 0.01$ vs. Con + Veh, # $p < 0.05$ vs. IRI + Veh. The difference among the groups was analyzed using a one-way nonparametric ANOVA followed by Tukey's multiple comparison test.

3.5. *Effect of ML171 on NOX Subunit Expression and ROS Generation in H_2O_2-Treated MDCK Cells*

MDCK cells were treated with H_2O_2 to induce NOX subunit expression and ROS generation. H_2O_2 increased expression of NOX1, NOX4, and p40^{phox}, but not NOX2. ML171 attenuated the increased expression of NOX subunits induced by H_2O_2 in MDCK cells. H_2O_2 evoked a change in oxidative stress-related enzymes of SOD2 and GPX production, which was mitigated by ML171 treatment (Figure 5).

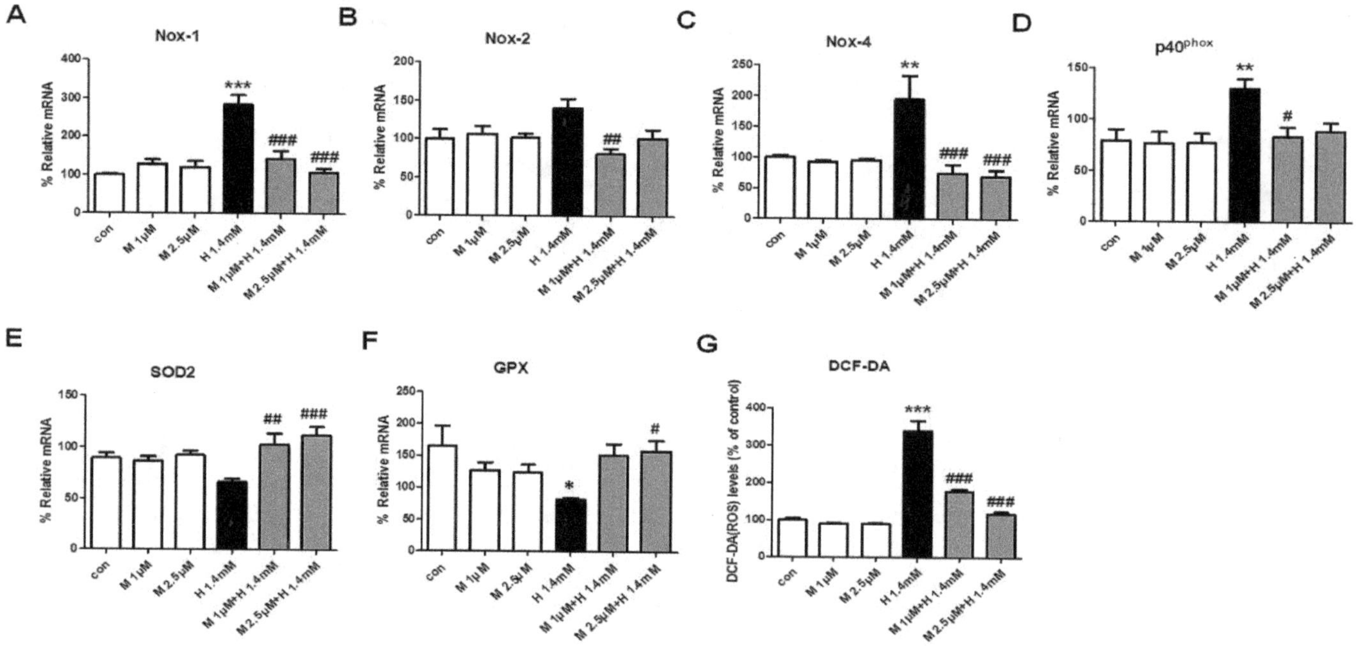

Figure 5. Effect of ML171 on H_2O_2-induced NOX subunit expression and ROS generation in MDCK cells. ML171 decreased NOX1, NOX4, and p40^{phox} expression in H_2O_2-treated MDCK cells (**A–D**). Oxidative stress-related enzymes of SOD2 and GPX production were mitigated by ML171 treatment (**E–G**). Data represent mean ± SEM. * $p < 0.05$, ** $p < 0.01$, *** $p < 0.001$ vs. Con, # $p < 0.05$, ## $p < 0.01$, ### $p < 0.001$ vs. H 1.4 mM. The difference among the groups was analyzed using a one-way nonparametric ANOVA followed by Tukey's multiple comparison test.

3.6. *Effect of siRNA against NOX1 on H_2O_2-Treated MDCK Cells*

MDCK cells were transfected with siRNA against NOX1 to evaluate whether the protective effect of ML171 was mediated with NOX1 and the expression of NOX4 was related with that of NOX1 in MDCK cells. Compared to nontargeting siRNA, siRNA against NOX1 showed a decreased NOX1 expression after H_2O_2 induction. Transfection with siRNA against NOX1 also upregulated SOD2 and GPX mRNA, which is consistent with the effect of ML171 treatment. Surprisingly, H_2O_2-induced expression of NOX4 mRNA was inhibited in MDCK cells with siRNA against NOX1, whereas NOX2 and p40^{phox} expression remained increased (Figure 6).

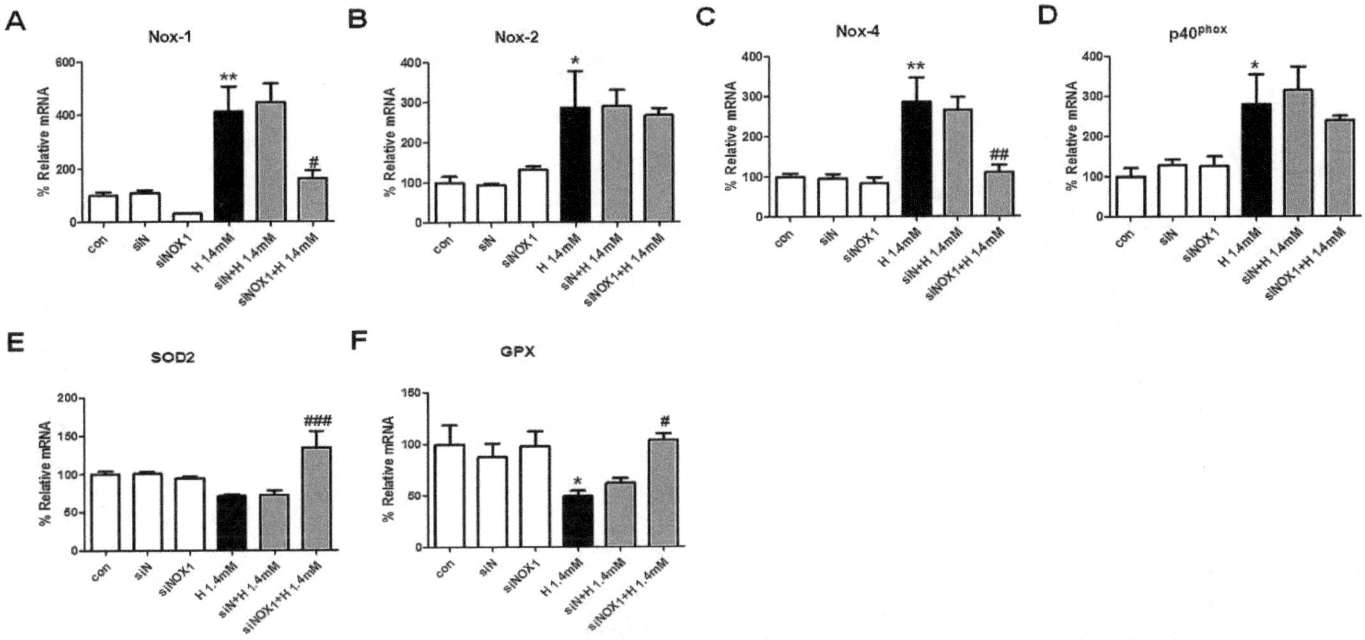

Figure 6. Effect of siRNA against NOX1 on H_2O_2-induced NOX subunit expression and ROS generation in MDCK cells. siRNA against NOX1 reduced NOX1 and NOX4 expression, however, did not affect NOX2 and p40^{phox} expression (**A–D**). Oxidative stress-related enzymes of SOD2 and GPX production were upregulated by siRNA against NOX1 treatment (**E**,**F**). Data represent mean ± SEM. * $p < 0.05$, ** $p < 0.01$ vs. Con, # $p < 0.05$, ## $p < 0.01$, ### $p < 0.001$ vs. H 1.4 mM. The difference among the groups was analyzed using a one-way nonparametric ANOVA followed by Tukey's multiple comparison test.

3.7. Effect of ML171 on the Apoptosis Induced by H_2O_2 in MDCK Cells

The effect of ML171 on the apoptosis induced by oxidative stress was assessed in MDCK cells. Caspase-3 activity increased significantly after H_2O_2 treatment and decreased after ML171 treatment in MDCK cells (Figure 7A). ML171 also attenuated the changes in the expression of Bax and Bcl-2/Bax ratio in H_2O_2-treated MDCK cells (Figure 7B). The TUNEL assay showed that ML171 decreased the H_2O_2-induced apoptosis in tubule cells (Figure 7C,D).

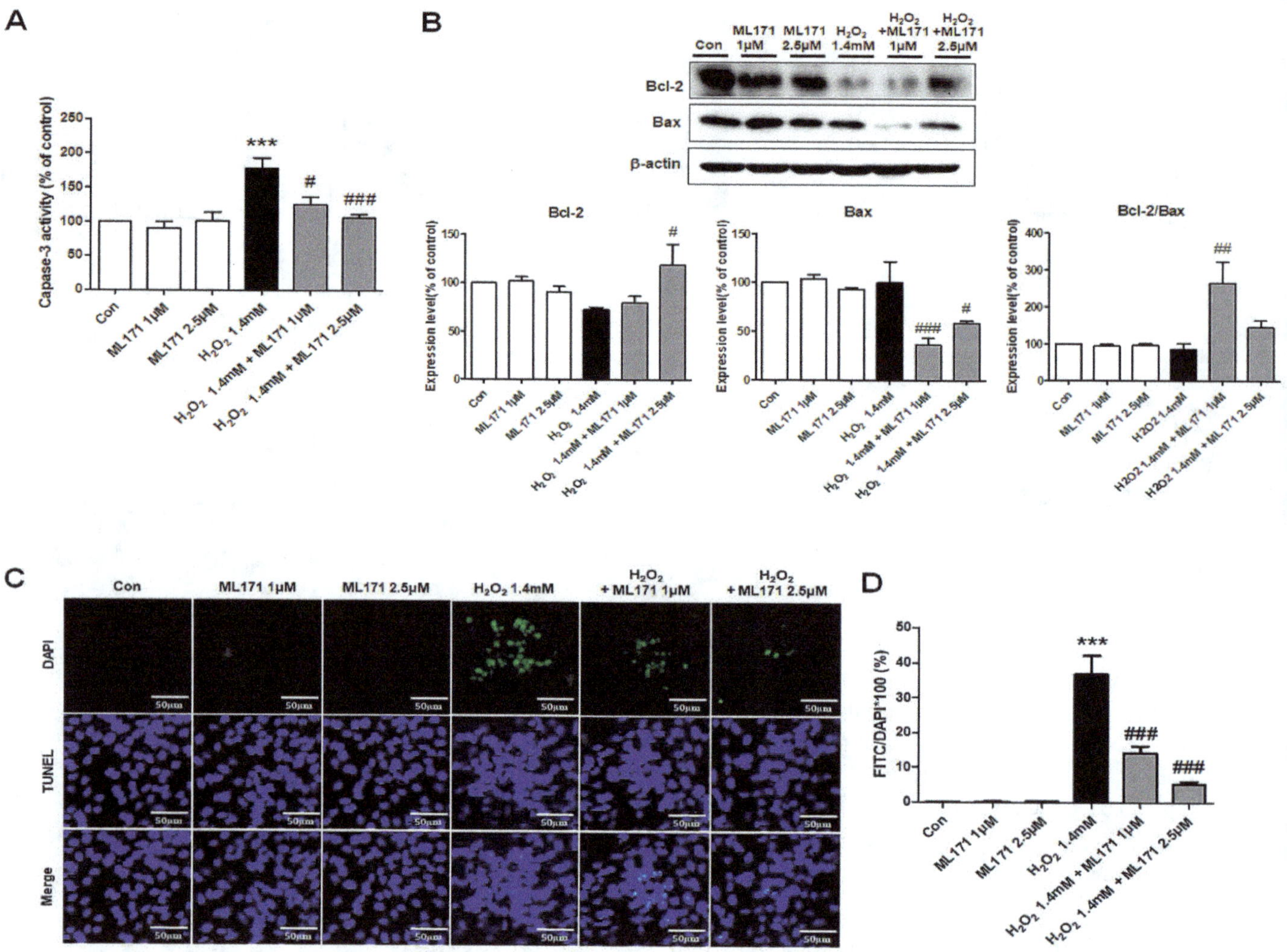

Figure 7. Effect of ML171 on the apoptosis induced by H_2O_2 in MDCK cells. Caspase-3 activity was significantly increased after H_2O_2 induced oxidative stress in MDCK cells and was significantly decreased by ML171 treatment (**A**). ML171 attenuated the changes in the expression of Bax and the Bcl-2/Bax ratio in H_2O_2-treated MDCK cells (**B**). TUNEL assay showed that H_2O_2-induced apoptosis was significantly reduced by ML171 treatment (**C**,**D**). Data represent mean ± SEM. *** $p < 0.001$ vs. Con, # $p < 0.05$, ## $p < 0.01$, ### $p < 0.001$ vs. H 1.4 mM. The difference among the groups was analyzed using a one-way nonparametric ANOVA followed by Tukey's multiple comparison test.

3.8. Changes in Phosphorylated Proteins of MAPK Signaling Pathways in MDCK Cells

We investigated the mechanism with which ML171 blocked oxidative stress and apoptosis in MDCK cells. The p-ERK and p-ERK/ERK ratio significantly increased after H_2O_2 treatment and was significantly reduced by ML171 in MDCK cells. p38 and JNK expressions were not affected by H_2O_2 and ML171, which was consistent with the in vivo experiment results (Figure 8).

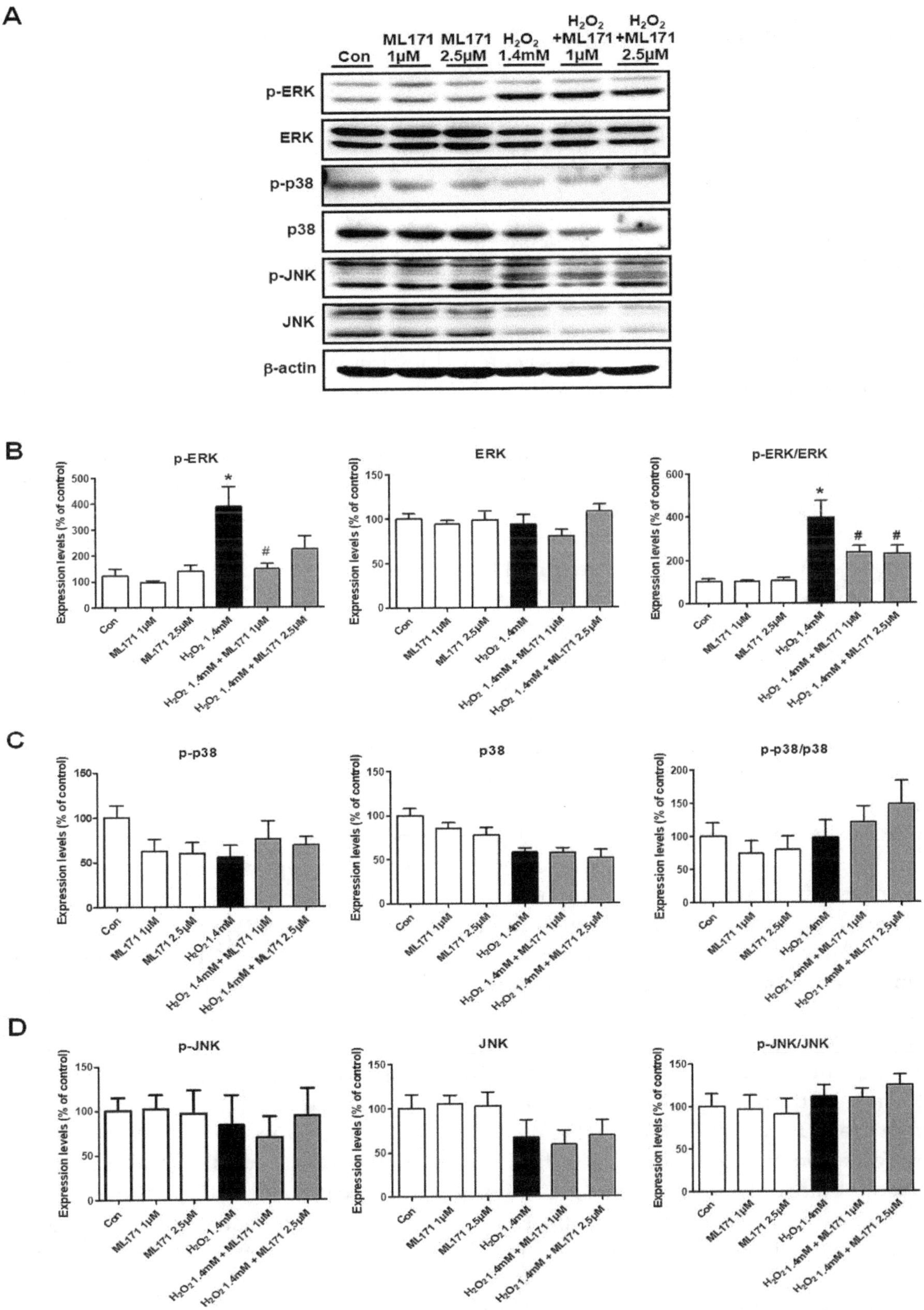

Figure 8. Changes in phosphorylated proteins of MAPK signaling pathways in MDCK cells. Consistent with the results from the in vivo experiment, the increased p-ERK and p-ERK/ERK ratio after H_2O_2 treatment was significantly decreased after ML171 treatment in MDCK cells (**A**,**B**). There were no significant differences in the expression of phosphorylated p38 and JNK after ML171 treatment (**C**,**D**). Data represent mean ± SEM. * $p < 0.05$ vs. Con, # $p < 0.05$ vs. H 1.4 mM. The difference among the groups was analyzed using a one-way nonparametric ANOVA followed by Tukey's multiple comparison test.

4. Discussion

The present study demonstrated that NOX1 inhibition by ML171 attenuated kidney IRI in the mouse model. The ischemic injury decreased significantly in the ML171-treated IRI group compared to that in the IRI group. The tissue injury was associated with the increased ROS production and NOX expression, which was reversed by ML171 treatment. H_2O_2 evoked changes in oxidative stress-related enzymes of SOD2 and GPX production in MDCK cells, which was mitigated by NOX1 inhibition with ML171 and siRNA against NOX1. Treatment with ML171 and transfection with siRNA against NOX1 decreased the expression of NOX1 induced by H_2O_2 exposure in MDCK cells. ML171 caused a significant increase in the Bcl-2 level and decrease in caspase-3 activity in IRI mice and H_2O_2-treated MDCK cells. ML171 affected ERK signaling by the phosphorylation of ERK in kidney tissues and tubular cells. The present study was the first to suggest that NOX1 inhibition could protect kidney IRI by inhibition of ROS-mediated ERK signaling.

Ischemic damage of the kidney causes acute kidney injury, which is responsible for the hypoxic damage induced by the production of ROS as well as the decrease in kidney blood flow [22,23]. ROS acts as signaling molecules including regulation of vascular tone, monitoring of oxygen tension, and signal transduction from membrane receptors in physiological situations, but in excess, it causes tissue damage [24–26]. NOX, one of the main sources of ROS, catalyzes the transfer of electrons from NADPH to molecular oxygen to produce ROS [27].

NOX4 is the most distributed NOX isoform in the kidney and has been studied in various kidney diseases. NOX4 expression in proximal tubular cells increased after exposure to high glucose, and NOX4 inhibition with GKT136901 decreased albuminuria in diabetic mice [28,29]. NOX4 deficiency was associated with the increased tubular injury after IRI [30], and hypoxia to kidney tubule cell upregulated NOX4 expression via a TGF-β1/Smad signaling pathway [31]. NOX2 also plays a role especially in the development of diabetic nephropathy, and its expression was upregulated in the kidneys of diabetic mice [32–34]. NOX2 is the classic phagocytic NOX and its main role is free radical generation [35,36]. It has been reported that NOX2 inhibition could prevent kidney damage and delayed graft function after IRI by the inhibition fibrosis and oxidative stress [37].

NOX1 is also expressed in the kidney cortex [38–40], and the associations with ischemic injury have been reported in other organs. NOX1 was a therapeutic target in ischemic retinopathy and IRI in the heart [41,42]. The role of NOX1 in kidney injury has been reported in cisplatin nephrotoxicity. Cardamonin, a flavone with anti-inflammatory activity, inhibited NOX1 expression in the cisplatin nephrotoxicity model, decreasing inflammation and apoptosis in the injured kidney [13]. The study on a NOX inhibitor has also revealed its protective effect in the kidney IRI. Apocynin, a nonspecific NOX inhibitor, ameliorated the histological damages after IRI by reducing oxidative stress markers, demonstrating that NOX1 was associated with kidney injury and downregulation of NOX could prevent kidney damage. However, it was difficult to attribute the action specifically to NOX1 inhibition, since two drugs did not selectively inhibit NOX1. In contrast, ML171 is a known potent NOX1 inhibitor with isoform selectivity only for NOX1 [21]. In the present study, NOX1 expression significantly increased in the kidney after IRI and MDCK cells treated with H_2O_2. ML171 effectively suppressed NOX1 upregulation induced by IRI, and the suppression of NOX1 by ML171 was also observed in H_2O_2-treated tubular cells, which are the main site of IRI. The treatment of ML171 showed improvement of serum BUN and Cr levels in the IRI group, suggesting significant amelioration of the ischemic injury. Therefore, this is the first study to demonstrate the renoprotective effect of NOX1 selective inhibition through the IRI animal model.

The expression of NOX1, NOX2, and NOX4 is closely related to each other [43]. Angiotensin II increases oxidative stress by upregulating the kidney cortical gene product for NOX1 and $p22^{phox}$, a catalytic core of the NOX [38]. Rats with the silenced $p22^{phox}$ gene reduced NOX1, NOX2, and NOX4 expression in the kidney cortex during infusion of angiotensin II [40]. Aoyama et al. showed that angiotensin II-induced NOX4 expression was inhibited by NOX1 knock-out hepatocytes, suggesting that NOX1 could induce NOX4 upregulation [44]. Our results are consistent with the previous study in that NOX4 expression was downregulated after transfection with siRNA against NOX1 into H_2O_2-treated MDCK cells. The reduced expression of NOX4 by ML171 treatment might be associated with the causal interaction between NOX1 and NOX4, which could also be explained by the downregulation after reduced oxidative stress by NOX1 inhibition or a partial inhibitory effect of ML171 on NOX4 [45].

H_2O_2 is a major marker of oxidative stress, giving rise to tissue injury after IRI [46,47]. In the present study, H_2O_2 increased significantly in the kidney after IRI. DCFDA, a compound used to measure generalized oxidative stress including intracellular H_2O_2 production, also significantly increased in the tubular cells treated with H_2O_2. Therefore, the injury with H_2O_2 in the MDCK cells is comparable to the injury induced by IRI in the kidney. SOD2 and GPX are two important components of the defensive mechanisms against oxidative stress by preventing the reactive free radical formation [48–51]. ML171 reduced H_2O_2 in the IRI mouse, and the effect was manifested as a subsequent increase in SOD2 and GPX in MDCK cells, suggesting the prevention of kidney damage with oxidative stress by selective NOX1 inhibition.

MAPK is associated with the activation of NOX1 [52]. ERK and p38 as well as JNK are members of MAPK that have proline-directed kinase activity. However, a certain stimulus selectively activates a specific member of the MAPK pathway [53]. Among them, ERK signaling pathway was involved in the present study. Only phosphorylation of ERK increased after ischemia and H_2O_2 exposure. ERK phosphorylates $p47^{phox}$ and contributes to NOX1 complex assembly [53]. Our results are consistent with the previous report that suggested the association of ERK with the cellular survival of the kidney with IRI [54].

We also investigated the possible mechanisms by which NOX1 inhibition prevented tubular injury. ROS generated by ischemia or oxidative stress are well-known inducers of apoptosis by activating caspase-3 in kidney tubular cells [6]. It was supported by TUNEL-positive kidney tubular epithelial cells and decreased Bcl-2/Bax ratios [55,56]. ML171 treatment before IRI significantly decreased caspase-3 activity, decreased the number of TUNEL-positive cells, and increased Bcl-2/Bax ratios compared with the IRI group. This suggests that the renoprotective effects of NOX1 inhibition are mediated via modulating kidney tubular cell apoptosis after IRI.

Our study has several limitations. First, our results were not validated with the other oxidative stress injury models such as cisplatin nephrotoxicity or contrast-induced nephropathy. However, the IRI model is a prototype of oxidative stress injury to kidney, and, although other models may show slight differences, we tried to determine NOX1's role in the basic injury model. Second, further experiments with a more specific way to inhibit NOX1 expression are needed to find NOX1's effect in IRI. GKT771, a highly selective NOX1 inhibitor [57] or NOXA1ds, a peptide NOX1 inhibitor with greater specificity and isoform selectivity [58], might reveal the specific effect of NOX1-selective inhibition. Third, our experiment was not performed on murine or human kidney epithelial cell lines. An animal toxicity test and further experiment with human kidney epithelial cells must be accompanied to apply the present results to human medicine. Nevertheless, this is the first study to investigate the renoprotective effect of NOX1 inhibition on the kidneys and kidney tubule cells, which makes it a candidate for treatment of acute kidney injury.

5. Conclusions

NOX1-selective inhibition by ML171 attenuated kidney IRI via inhibition of ROS-mediated ERK signaling. NOX1 inhibition by ML171 and siRNA against NOX1 reduced the oxidative stress-induced apoptosis in MDCK cells, indicating NOX1 selective inhibition's potential as a therapeutic target for acute kidney injury associated with ROS generation and subsequent apoptosis.

6. Patent

The results of this paper were patented under the name "Composition for preventing or treating ischemia-reperfusion injury comprising NADPH oxidase 1" on 20 April 2020 (Number: 10-2020-0047663).

Author Contributions: Conceptualization, H.-Y.J., S.-H.O., and J.-H.C.; Methodology, H.-Y.J., S.-H.O., J.-S.A., E.-J.O., Y.-J.K, and J.-H.C.; Formal Analysis, H.-Y.J., S.-H.O., J.-S.A., E.-J.O., Y.-J.K., and J.-H.C.; Investigation, H.-Y.J., S.-H.O., C.-D.K., S.-H.P., Y.-L.K., and J.-H.C.; Data Curation, H.-Y.J., S.-H.O., J.-S.A., E.-J.O., Y.-J.K., and J.-H.C.; Writing—Original Draft Preparation, H.-Y.J., S.-H.O., and J.-H.C.; Writing—Review and Editing, H.-Y.J. and J.-H.C. All authors have read and agreed to the published version of the manuscript.

Abbreviations

BUN	Blood urea nitrogen
Cr	Creatinine
IRI	Ischemia-reperfusion injury
KHIDI	Korea Health Industry Development Institute
MAPK	Mitogen-activated protein kinase
MDCK	Madin–Darby Canine Kidney
NADPH	Nicotinamide adenine dinucleotide phosphate
PAS	Periodic acid-Schiff
ROS	Reactive oxygen species
TdT	Terminal deoxynucleotidyl transferase

References

1. Kalogeris, T.; Baines, C.P.; Krenz, M.; Korthuis, R.J. Cell biology of ischemia/reperfusion injury. *Int. Rev. Cell Mol. Biol.* **2012**, *298*, 229–317. [CrossRef] [PubMed]
2. Noiri, E.; Nakao, A.; Uchida, K.; Tsukahara, H.; Ohno, M.; Fujita, T.; Brodsky, S.; Goligorsky, M.S. Oxidative and nitrosative stress in acute renal ischemia. *Am. J. Physiol. Renal Physiol.* **2001**, *281*, F948–F957. [CrossRef] [PubMed]
3. Han, S.J.; Lee, H.T. Mechanisms and therapeutic targets of ischemic acute kidney injury. *Kidney Res. Clin. Pract.* **2019**, *38*, 427–440. [CrossRef] [PubMed]
4. Kennedy, S.E.; Erlich, J.H. Murine renal ischaemia-reperfusion injury. *Nephrology (Carlton)* **2008**, *13*, 390–396. [CrossRef]
5. Lien, Y.H.; Lai, L.W.; Silva, A.L. Pathogenesis of renal ischemia/reperfusion injury: Lessons from knockout mice. *Life Sci.* **2003**, *74*, 543–552. [CrossRef]
6. Dobashi, K.; Ghosh, B.; Orak, J.K.; Singh, I.; Singh, A.K. Kidney ischemia-reperfusion: Modulation of antioxidant defenses. *Mol. Cell. Biochem.* **2000**, *205*, 1–11. [CrossRef]
7. Kim, J.; Seok, Y.M.; Jung, K.J.; Park, K.M. Reactive oxygen species/oxidative stress contributes to progression of kidney fibrosis following transient ischemic injury in mice. *Am. J. Physiol. Renal Physiol.* **2009**, *297*, F461–F470. [CrossRef]
8. Kim, J.; Jang, H.S.; Park, K.M. Reactive oxygen species generated by renal ischemia and reperfusion trigger protection against subsequent renal ischemia and reperfusion injury in mice. *Am. J. Physiol. Renal Physiol.* **2010**, *298*, F158–F166. [CrossRef]
9. Sedeek, M.; Nasrallah, R.; Touyz, R.M.; Hebert, R.L. NADPH oxidases, reactive oxygen species, and the kidney: Friend and foe. *J. Am. Soc. Nephrol.* **2013**, *24*, 1512–1518. [CrossRef]

10. Arbiser, J.L.; Petros, J.; Klafter, R.; Govindajaran, B.; McLaughlin, E.R.; Brown, L.F.; Cohen, C.; Moses, M.; Kilroy, S.; Arnold, R.S.; et al. Reactive oxygen generated by Nox1 triggers the angiogenic switch. *Proc. Natl. Acad. Sci. USA* **2002**, *99*, 715–720. [CrossRef]
11. Gavazzi, G.; Banfi, B.; Deffert, C.; Fiette, L.; Schappi, M.; Herrmann, F.; Krause, K.H. Decreased blood pressure in NOX1-deficient mice. *FEBS Lett.* **2006**, *580*, 497–504. [CrossRef] [PubMed]
12. Sadok, A.; Bourgarel-Rey, V.; Gattacceca, F.; Penel, C.; Lehmann, M.; Kovacic, H. Nox1-dependent superoxide production controls colon adenocarcinoma cell migration. *Biochim. Biophys. Acta* **2008**, *1783*, 23–33. [CrossRef] [PubMed]
13. El-Naga, R.N. Pre-treatment with cardamonin protects against cisplatin-induced nephrotoxicity in rats: Impact on NOX-1, inflammation and apoptosis. *Toxicol. Appl. Pharmacol.* **2014**, *274*, 87–95. [CrossRef] [PubMed]
14. Cui, Y.; Wang, Y.; Li, G.; Ma, W.; Zhou, X.S.; Wang, J.; Liu, B. The Nox1/Nox4 inhibitor attenuates acute lung injury induced by ischemia-reperfusion in mice. *PLoS ONE* **2018**, *13*, e0209444. [CrossRef] [PubMed]
15. Hosseini, F.; Naseri, M.K.; Badavi, M.; Ghaffari, M.A.; Shahbazian, H.; Rashidi, I. Effect of beta carotene on lipid peroxidation and antioxidant status following renal ischemia/reperfusion injury in rat. *Scand. J. Clin. Lab. Investig.* **2010**, *70*, 259–263. [CrossRef] [PubMed]
16. Beytur, A.; Binbay, M.; Sarihan, M.E.; Parlakpinar, H.; Polat, A.; Gunaydin, M.O.; Acet, A. Dose-dependent protective effect of ivabradine against ischemia-reperfusion-induced renal injury in rats. *Kidney Blood Press. Res.* **2012**, *35*, 114–119. [CrossRef]
17. Alan, C.; Kocoglu, H.; Altintas, R.; Alici, B.; Resit Ersay, A. Protective effect of decorin on acute ischaemia-reperfusion injury in the rat kidney. *Arch. Med. Sci.* **2011**, *7*, 211–216. [CrossRef]
18. Xu, Y.F.; Liu, M.; Peng, B.; Che, J.P.; Zhang, H.M.; Yan, Y.; Wang, G.C.; Wu, Y.C.; Zheng, J.H. Protective effects of SP600125 on renal ischemia-reperfusion injury in rats. *J. Surg. Res.* **2011**, *169*, e77–e84. [CrossRef]
19. Talab, S.S.; Elmi, A.; Emami, H.; Nezami, B.G.; Assa, S.; Ghasemi, M.; Tavangar, S.M.; Dehpour, A.R. Protective effects of acute lithium preconditioning against renal ischemia/reperfusion injury in rat: Role of nitric oxide and cyclooxygenase systems. *Eur. J. Pharmacol.* **2012**, *681*, 94–99. [CrossRef]
20. Jeong, B.Y.; Lee, H.Y.; Park, C.G.; Kang, J.; Yu, S.L.; Choi, D.R.; Han, S.Y.; Park, M.H.; Cho, S.; Lee, S.Y.; et al. Oxidative stress caused by activation of NADPH oxidase 4 promotes contrast-induced acute kidney injury. *PLoS ONE* **2018**, *13*, e0191034. [CrossRef]
21. Gianni, D.; Taulet, N.; Zhang, H.; DerMardirossian, C.; Kister, J.; Martinez, L.; Roush, W.R.; Brown, S.J.; Bokoch, G.M.; Rosen, H. A novel and specific NADPH oxidase-1 (Nox1) small-molecule inhibitor blocks the formation of functional invadopodia in human colon cancer cells. *ACS Chem. Biol.* **2010**, *5*, 981–993. [CrossRef] [PubMed]
22. Bonventre, J.V. Mechanisms of ischemic acute renal failure. *Kidney Int.* **1993**, *43*, 1160–1178. [CrossRef] [PubMed]
23. Sheridan, A.M.; Bonventre, J.V. Cell biology and molecular mechanisms of injury in ischemic acute renal failure. *Curr. Opin. Nephrol. Hypertens.* **2000**, *9*, 427–434. [CrossRef] [PubMed]
24. Droge, W. Free radicals in the physiological control of cell function. *Physiol. Rev.* **2002**, *82*, 47–95. [CrossRef] [PubMed]
25. Nordberg, J.; Arner, E.S. Reactive oxygen species, antioxidants, and the mammalian thioredoxin system. *Free Radic. Biol. Med.* **2001**, *31*, 1287–1312. [CrossRef]
26. Sen, C.K.; Packer, L. Antioxidant and redox regulation of gene transcription. *FASEB J.* **1996**, *10*, 709–720. [CrossRef]
27. Wang, D.; Chen, Y.; Chabrashvili, T.; Aslam, S.; Borrego Conde, L.J.; Umans, J.G.; Wilcox, C.S. Role of oxidative stress in endothelial dysfunction and enhanced responses to angiotensin II of afferent arterioles from rabbits infused with angiotensin II. *J. Am. Soc. Nephrol.* **2003**, *14*, 2783–2789. [CrossRef]
28. Sedeek, M.; Callera, G.; Montezano, A.; Gutsol, A.; Heitz, F.; Szyndralewiez, C.; Page, P.; Kennedy, C.R.; Burns, K.D.; Touyz, R.M.; et al. Critical role of Nox4-based NADPH oxidase in glucose-induced oxidative stress in the kidney: Implications in type 2 diabetic nephropathy. *Am. J. Physiol. Renal Physiol.* **2010**, *299*, F1348–F1358. [CrossRef]
29. Sedeek, M.; Gutsol, A.; Montezano, A.C.; Burger, D.; Nguyen Dinh Cat, A.; Kennedy, C.R.; Burns, K.D.; Cooper, M.E.; Jandeleit-Dahm, K.; Page, P.; et al. Renoprotective effects of a novel Nox1/4 inhibitor in a mouse model of Type 2 diabetes. *Clin. Sci.* **2013**, *124*, 191–202. [CrossRef]

30. Nlandu-Khodo, S.; Dissard, R.; Hasler, U.; Schafer, M.; Pircher, H.; Jansen-Durr, P.; Krause, K.H.; Martin, P.Y.; de Seigneux, S. NADPH oxidase 4 deficiency increases tubular cell death during acute ischemic reperfusion injury. *Sci. Rep.* **2016**, *6*, 38598. [CrossRef]
31. Cho, S.; Yu, S.L.; Kang, J.; Jeong, B.Y.; Lee, H.Y.; Park, C.G.; Yu, Y.B.; Jin, D.C.; Hwang, W.M.; Yun, S.R.; et al. NADPH oxidase 4 mediates TGF-beta1/Smad signaling pathway induced acute kidney injury in hypoxia. *PLoS ONE* **2019**, *14*, e0219483. [CrossRef]
32. Fukuda, M.; Nakamura, T.; Kataoka, K.; Nako, H.; Tokutomi, Y.; Dong, Y.F.; Ogawa, H.; Kim-Mitsuyama, S. Potentiation by candesartan of protective effects of pioglitazone against type 2 diabetic cardiovascular and renal complications in obese mice. *J. Hypertens.* **2010**, *28*, 340–352. [CrossRef] [PubMed]
33. Ohshiro, Y.; Ma, R.C.; Yasuda, Y.; Hiraoka-Yamamoto, J.; Clermont, A.C.; Isshiki, K.; Yagi, K.; Arikawa, E.; Kern, T.S.; King, G.L. Reduction of diabetes-induced oxidative stress, fibrotic cytokine expression, and renal dysfunction in protein kinase Cbeta-null mice. *Diabetes* **2006**, *55*, 3112–3120. [CrossRef] [PubMed]
34. Chew, P.; Yuen, D.Y.; Stefanovic, N.; Pete, J.; Coughlan, M.T.; Jandeleit-Dahm, K.A.; Thomas, M.C.; Rosenfeldt, F.; Cooper, M.E.; de Haan, J.B. Antiatherosclerotic and renoprotective effects of ebselen in the diabetic apolipoprotein E/GPx1-double knockout mouse. *Diabetes* **2010**, *59*, 3198–3207. [CrossRef]
35. Djamali, A.; Vidyasagar, A.; Adulla, M.; Hullett, D.; Reese, S. Nox-2 Is a Modulator of fibrogenesis in kidney allografts. *Am. J. Transplant.* **2009**, *9*, 74–82. [CrossRef]
36. Djamali, A.; Reese, S.; Hafez, O.; Vidyasagar, A.; Jacobson, L.; Swain, W.; Kolehmainen, C.; Huang, L.; Wilson, N.A.; Torrealba, J.R. Nox2 is a mediator of chronic CsA nephrotoxicity. *Am. J. Transplant.* **2012**, *12*, 1997–2007. [CrossRef]
37. Karim, A.S.; Reese, S.R.; Wilson, N.A.; Jacobson, L.M.; Zhong, W.; Djamali, A. Nox2 Is a mediator of ischemia reperfusion injury. *Am. J. Transplant.* **2015**, *15*, 2888–2899. [CrossRef]
38. Chabrashvili, T.; Kitiyakara, C.; Blau, J.; Karber, A.; Aslam, S.; Welch, W.J.; Wilcox, C.S. Effects of ANG II type 1 and 2 receptors on oxidative stress, renal NADPH oxidase, and SOD expression. *Am. J. Physiol. Regul. Integr. Comp. Physiol.* **2003**, *285*, R117–R124. [CrossRef]
39. Kitiyakara, C.; Chabrashvili, T.; Chen, Y.; Blau, J.; Karber, A.; Aslam, S.; Welch, W.J.; Wilcox, C.S. Salt intake, oxidative stress, and renal expression of NADPH oxidase and superoxide dismutase. *J. Am. Soc. Nephrol.* **2003**, *14*, 2775–2782. [CrossRef]
40. Modlinger, P.; Chabrashvili, T.; Gill, P.S.; Mendonca, M.; Harrison, D.G.; Griendling, K.K.; Li, M.; Raggio, J.; Wellstein, A.; Chen, Y.; et al. RNA silencing in vivo reveals role of p22phox in rat angiotensin slow pressor response. *Hypertension* **2006**, *47*, 238–244. [CrossRef]
41. Wilkinson-Berka, J.L.; Deliyanti, D.; Rana, I.; Miller, A.G.; Agrotis, A.; Armani, R.; Szyndralewiez, C.; Wingler, K.; Touyz, R.M.; Cooper, M.E.; et al. NADPH oxidase, NOX1, mediates vascular injury in ischemic retinopathy. *Antioxid. Redox Sign.* **2014**, *20*, 2726–2740. [CrossRef] [PubMed]
42. Braunersreuther, V.; Montecucco, F.; Asrih, M.; Pelli, G.; Galan, K.; Frias, M.; Burger, F.; Quindere, A.L.; Montessuit, C.; Krause, K.H.; et al. Role of NADPH oxidase isoforms NOX1, NOX2 and NOX4 in myocardial ischemia/reperfusion injury. *J. Mol. Cell. Cardiol.* **2013**, *64*, 99–107. [CrossRef] [PubMed]
43. Gill, P.S.; Wilcox, C.S. NADPH oxidases in the kidney. *Antioxid. Redox Sign.* **2006**, *8*, 1597–1607. [CrossRef] [PubMed]
44. Aoyama, T.; Paik, Y.H.; Watanabe, S.; Laleu, B.; Gaggini, F.; Fioraso-Cartier, L.; Molango, S.; Heitz, F.; Merlot, C.; Szyndralewiez, C.; et al. Nicotinamide adenine dinucleotide phosphate oxidase in experimental liver fibrosis: GKT137831 as a novel potential therapeutic agent. *Hepatology* **2012**, *56*, 2316–2327. [CrossRef]
45. Dao, V.T.; Elbatreek, M.H.; Altenhofer, S.; Casas, A.I.; Pachado, M.P.; Neullens, C.T.; Knaus, U.G.; Schmidt, H. Isoform-selective NADPH oxidase inhibitor panel for pharmacological target validation. *Free Radic. Biol. Med.* **2020**, *148*, 60–69. [CrossRef]
46. Choi, H.I.; Kim, H.J.; Park, J.S.; Kim, I.J.; Bae, E.H.; Ma, S.K.; Kim, S.W. PGC-1alpha attenuates hydrogen peroxide-induced apoptotic cell death by upregulating Nrf-2 via GSK3beta inactivation mediated by activated p38 in HK-2 cells. *Sci. Rep.* **2017**, *7*, 4319. [CrossRef]
47. Park, J.S.; Choi, H.I.; Bae, E.H.; Ma, S.K.; Kim, S.W. Small heterodimer partner attenuates hydrogen peroxide-induced expression of cyclooxygenase-2 and inducible nitric oxide synthase by suppression of activator protein-1 and nuclear factor-kappaB in renal proximal tubule epithelial cells. *Int. J. Mol. Med.* **2017**, *39*, 701–710. [CrossRef]

48. Slyshenkov, V.S.; Rakowska, M.; Moiseenok, A.G.; Wojtczak, L. Pantothenic acid and its derivatives protect Ehrlich ascites tumor cells against lipid peroxidation. *Free Radic. Biol. Med.* **1995**, *19*, 767–772. [CrossRef]
49. van Haaften, R.I.; Haenen, G.R.; Evelo, C.T.; Bast, A. Effect of vitamin E on glutathione-dependent enzymes. *Drug Metab. Rev.* **2003**, *35*, 215–253. [CrossRef]
50. Parlakpinar, H.; Olmez, E.; Acet, A.; Ozturk, F.; Tasdemir, S.; Ates, B.; Gul, M.; Otlu, A. Beneficial effects of apricot-feeding on myocardial ischemia-reperfusion injury in rats. *Food Chem. Toxicol.* **2009**, *47*, 802–808. [CrossRef]
51. Walker, E.M., Jr.; Gale, G.R. Methods of reduction of cisplatin nephrotoxicity. *Ann. Clin. Lab. Sci.* **1981**, *11*, 397–410. [PubMed]
52. El Benna, J.; Faust, L.P.; Babior, B.M. The phosphorylation of the respiratory burst oxidase component p47phox during neutrophil activation. Phosphorylation of sites recognized by protein kinase C and by proline-directed kinases. *J. Biol. Chem.* **1994**, *269*, 23431–23436. [PubMed]
53. El Benna, J.; Han, J.; Park, J.W.; Schmid, E.; Ulevitch, R.J.; Babior, B.M. Activation of p38 in stimulated human neutrophils: Phosphorylation of the oxidase component p47phox by p38 and ERK but not by JNK. *Arch. Biochem. Biophys.* **1996**, *334*, 395–400. [CrossRef] [PubMed]
54. Luo, F.; Shi, J.; Shi, Q.; Xu, X.; Xia, Y.; He, X. Mitogen-Activated protein kinases and hypoxic/ischemic nephropathy. *Cell. Physiol. Biochem.* **2016**, *39*, 1051–1067. [CrossRef] [PubMed]
55. Chien, C.T.; Chang, T.C.; Tsai, C.Y.; Shyue, S.K.; Lai, M.K. Adenovirus-mediated bcl-2 gene transfer inhibits renal ischemia/reperfusion induced tubular oxidative stress and apoptosis. *Am. J. Transplant.* **2005**, *5*, 1194–1203. [CrossRef]
56. Havasi, A.; Li, Z.; Wang, Z.; Martin, J.L.; Botla, V.; Ruchalski, K.; Schwartz, J.H.; Borkan, S.C. Hsp27 inhibits Bax activation and apoptosis via a phosphatidylinositol 3-kinase-dependent mechanism. *J. Biol. Chem.* **2008**, *283*, 12305–12313. [CrossRef]
57. Stalin, J.; Garrido-Urbani, S.; Heitz, F.; Szyndralewiez, C.; Jemelin, S.; Coquoz, O.; Ruegg, C.; Imhof, B.A. Inhibition of host NOX1 blocks tumor growth and enhances checkpoint inhibitor-based immunotherapy. *Life Sci. Alliance* **2019**, *2*. [CrossRef]
58. Ranayhossaini, D.J.; Rodriguez, A.I.; Sahoo, S.; Chen, B.B.; Mallampalli, R.K.; Kelley, E.E.; Csanyi, G.; Gladwin, M.T.; Romero, G.; Pagano, P.J. Selective recapitulation of conserved and nonconserved regions of putative NOXA1 protein activation domain confers isoform-specific inhibition of Nox1 oxidase and attenuation of endothelial cell migration. *J. Biol. Chem.* **2013**, *288*, 36437–36450. [CrossRef]

Cilastatin Preconditioning Attenuates Renal Ischemia-Reperfusion Injury via Hypoxia Inducible Factor-1α Activation

Yu Ah Hong [1], So Young Jung [2], Keum Jin Yang [2], Dai Sig Im [3,4], Kyung Hwan Jeong [5], Cheol Whee Park [1] and Hyeon Seok Hwang [5,*]

1 Division of Nephrology, Department of Internal Medicine, The Catholic University of Korea, Seoul 06591, Korea; amorfati@catholic.ac.kr (Y.A.H.); cheolwhee@catholic.ac.kr (C.W.P.)
2 Clinical Research Institute, Daejeon St. Mary's Hospital, Daejeon 34943, Korea; syzzim84@gmail.com (S.Y.J.); nadia@cnu.ac.kr (K.J.Y.)
3 Department of Chemistry, College of Natural Sciences, Soonchunhyang University, Asan 31538, Korea; dsim@sch.ac.kr
4 SH Company, 507, SCH BIT Business Incubator B/D, 22 Soonchunhyang-ro, Shinchang, Asan, Chungnam 31538, Korea 5 Division of Nephrology, Department of Internal Medicine, College of Medicine, Kyung Hee University, Seoul 02447, Korea; khjeong@khu.ac.kr
* Correspondence: hwanghsne@gmail.com

Abstract: Cilastatin is a specific inhibitor of renal dehydrodipeptidase-1. We investigated whether cilastatin preconditioning attenuates renal ischemia-reperfusion (IR) injury via hypoxia inducible factor-1α (HIF-1α) activation. Human proximal tubular cell line (HK-2) was exposed to ischemia, and male C57BL/6 mice were subjected to bilateral kidney ischemia and reperfusion. The effects of cilastatin preconditioning were investigated both in vitro and in vivo. In HK-2 cells, cilastatin upregulated HIF-1α expression in a time- and dose-dependent manner. Cilastatin enhanced HIF-1α translation via the phosphorylation of Akt and mTOR was followed by the upregulation of erythropoietin (EPO) and vascular endothelial growth factor (VEGF). Cilastatin did not affect the expressions of PHD and VHL. However, HIF-1α ubiquitination was significantly decreased after cilastatin treatment. Cilastatin prevented the IR-induced cell death. These cilastatin effects were reversed by co-treatment of HIF-1α inhibitor or HIF-1α small interfering RNA. Similarly, HIF-1α expression and its upstream and downstream signaling were significantly enhanced in cilastatin-treated kidney. In mouse kidney with IR injury, cilastatin treatment decreased HIF-1α ubiquitination independent of PHD and VHL expression. Serum creatinine level and tubular necrosis, and apoptosis were reduced in cilastatin-treated kidney with IR injury, and co-treatment of cilastatin with an HIF-1α inhibitor reversed these effects. Thus, cilastatin preconditioning attenuated renal IR injury via HIF-1α activation.

Keywords: cilastatin; hypoxia inducible factor-1-α; ischemia-reperfusion injury

---

1. Introduction

Renal ischemia-reperfusion (IR) injury is a major cause of acute kidney injury [1]. Acute ischemic injury produces excessive apoptotic cell death, and several studies have explored various stimuli to reduce injury processes [2,3]. Hypoxia-inducible factor-1α (HIF-1α) is the master regulator of cell response to hypoxia [4]. It increases the expression of several genes, including angiogenic growth factors, erythropoietin, and nitric oxide synthases [5–7]. Activation of these genes enhances adaptation to hypoxia and improves cell survival. Therefore, it is reasonable that HIF-1α activation before IR injury might exhibit protective effects.

Cilastatin is a molecule designed to inhibit brush border–sorted dehydrogenase peptide-1 (DHP-1). In current clinical settings, cilastatin is used to prevent the hydrolysis of antibiotics and decrease antibiotic-induced nephrotoxicity [8]. Previous in vitro and in vivo experimental studies have demonstrated that cilastatin has antioxidant and anti-apoptotic effects in drug-induced nephropathy, such as cisplatin, calcineurin inhibitor, and vancomycin [9–12]. These effects of cilastatin were associated with reduced accumulation of drug within the kidney and renal proximal tubular epithelial cells. However, the cilastatin effect is rarely investigated in the non-pharmacological renal injury. Moreover, it is unclear that cilastatin exhibits protective effects on kidney injuries.

Cilastatin binds to lipid raft in which DHP-1 is embedded. The lipid raft acts as a major platform for signaling regulation and controls Akt signaling pathways [13,14]. The Akt/mammalian target of rapamycin (mTOR) pathway is potent regulator of HIF-1α expression at translational or transcriptional level [15,16]. Therefore, cilastatin treatment can modulate the HIF-1α activity via lipid raft-related signaling pathway. However, it is less known that the cilastatin as a preconditioning stimulus activates HIF-1α pathway and the underlying mechanism of cilastatin treatment is not evaluated in the renal IR injury.

Therefore, we investigated whether preconditioning with cilastatin exhibits renoprotective effects in a mouse model of IR injury, and whether cilastatin is effective in preventing proximal tubular cell death after IR injury. We hypothesized that cilastatin treatment activates HIF-1α signaling pathway, which leads to protective effects against renal IR injury.

2. Results

2.1. *Cilastatin Upregulates HIF-1α and Its Downstream Effector in HK-2 Cells*

Figure 1 shows the effects of cilastatin on HIF-1α expression in HK-2 cells. The expression of HIF-1α was significantly increased after cilastatin treatment in a dose- and time-dependent manner (Figure 1A,B). However, the HIF-1α mRNA level was not affected in cilastatin-treated HK-2 cells (Figure S1). Downstream effectors of HIF-1α, such as erythropoietin (EPO) and vascular endothelial growth factor (VEGF), were significantly upregulated after cilastatin treatment, respectively (Figure 1C).

2.2. *Cilastatin Upregulates HIF-1α and Its Downstream Effector in HK-2 Cells*

We studied the involved phase of protein synthesis for HIF-1α in HK-2 cells. The Akt/mTOR pathway was evaluated to assess the upstream signaling of HIF-1α, which translated the HIF-1α protein. The phosphorylation of Akt was significantly increased with maximal expression occurring at 6 h after cilastatin treatment. The phosphorylation of mTOR was also enhanced in a time-dependent manner (Figure 2A). To confirm whether HIF-1α upregulation was dependent on Akt/mTOR pathway, we exposed the cells to cilastatin in the presence of rapamycin, an mTOR inhibitor. Cilastatin increased HIF-1α expression, and co-treatment of rapamycin with cilastatin significantly reversed the HIF-1α upregulation (Figure 2B).

We conducted further experiments to investigate whether HIF-1α upregulation is dependent on lipid raft, because lipid raft modulates p-Akt/Akt signaling pathways [13,14]. The disruption of lipid raft with methyl-β-cyclodextrin (MβCD) significantly suppressed the HIF-1α expression when cilastatin increased HIF-1α expression (Figure 2C).

2.3. *PHD/VHL-Independent Ubiquitination Pathway is Involved in Cilastatin-Mediated HIF-1α Upregulation in HK-2 cells*

To identify whether cilastatin preconditioning activates HIF-1α by impairing its degradation pathway, the expression levels of prolyl hydroxylase domain (PHD) and von Hippel-Lindau (VHL) protein were evaluated. Cilastatin did not significantly alter the expression of PHD and VHL (Figure 3) compared to control. Therefore, cilastatin did not activate HIF-1α through the canonical HIF-1α degradation pathway. We further evaluated the interaction between HIF-1α and ubiquitin. In contrast to previous results, HIF-1α/ubiquitin complex formation was decreased after cilastatin preconditioning compared to control cells. These results suggested that cilastatin-induced HIF-1α activation was closely associated with decreased ubiquitination independent of PHD and VHL expression.

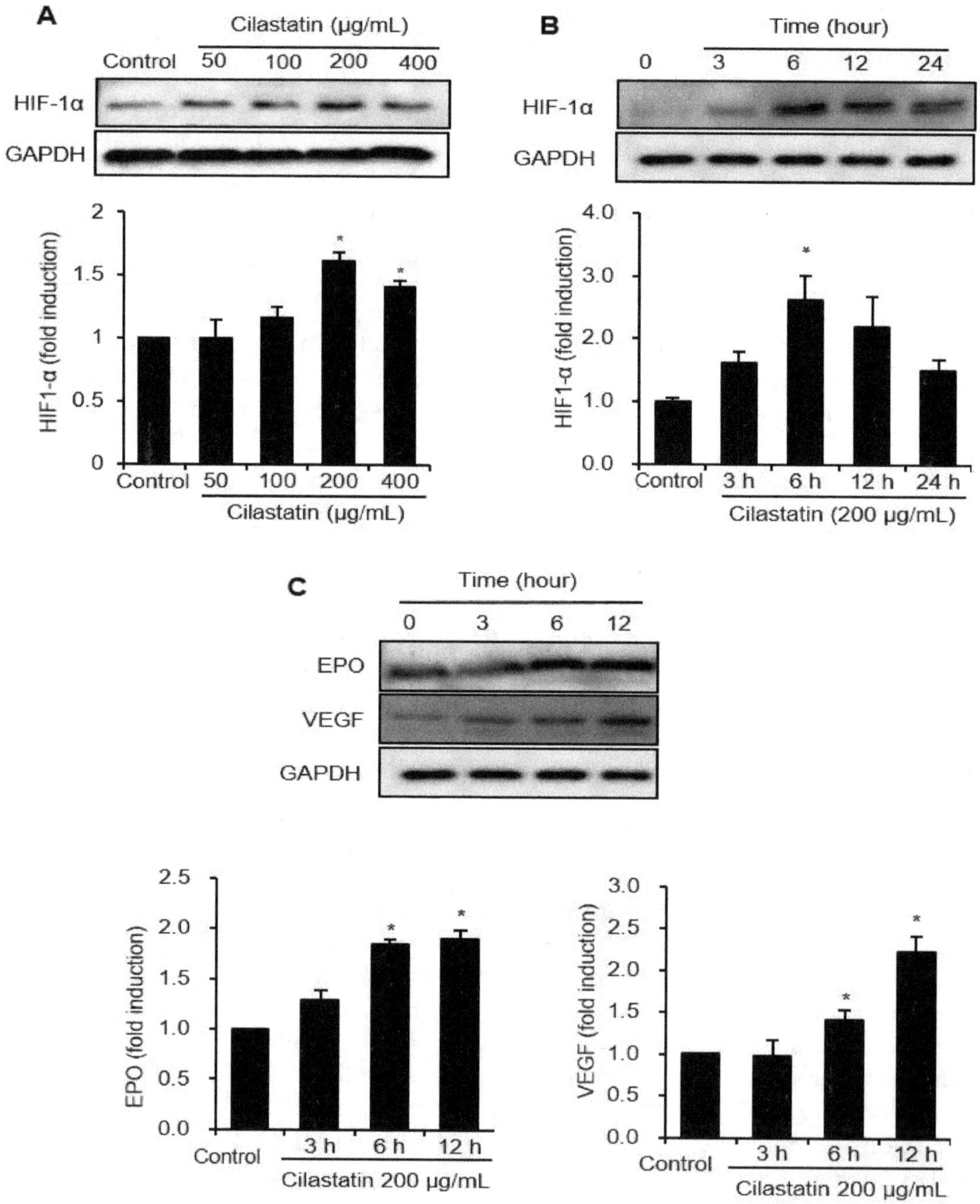

Figure 1. Cilastatin treatment upregulated the expressions of HIF-1α and its downstream pathway in HK-2 cells. (**A**) Semiquantitative immunoblotting revealed upregulation of HIF-1α expression by cilastatin treatment in a dose-dependent manner. (**B**) Semiquantitative immunoblotting revealed upregulation of HIF-1α expression by treatment with 200 μg/mL cilastatin in a time-dependent manner. (**C**) The expressions of VEGF and EPO proteins, determined by semiquantitative immunoblotting, were significantly elevated by treatment with 200 μg/mL cilastatin in a time-dependent manner as compared to untreated control. The data are presented as means ± SEM. * $p < 0.05$ vs. control.

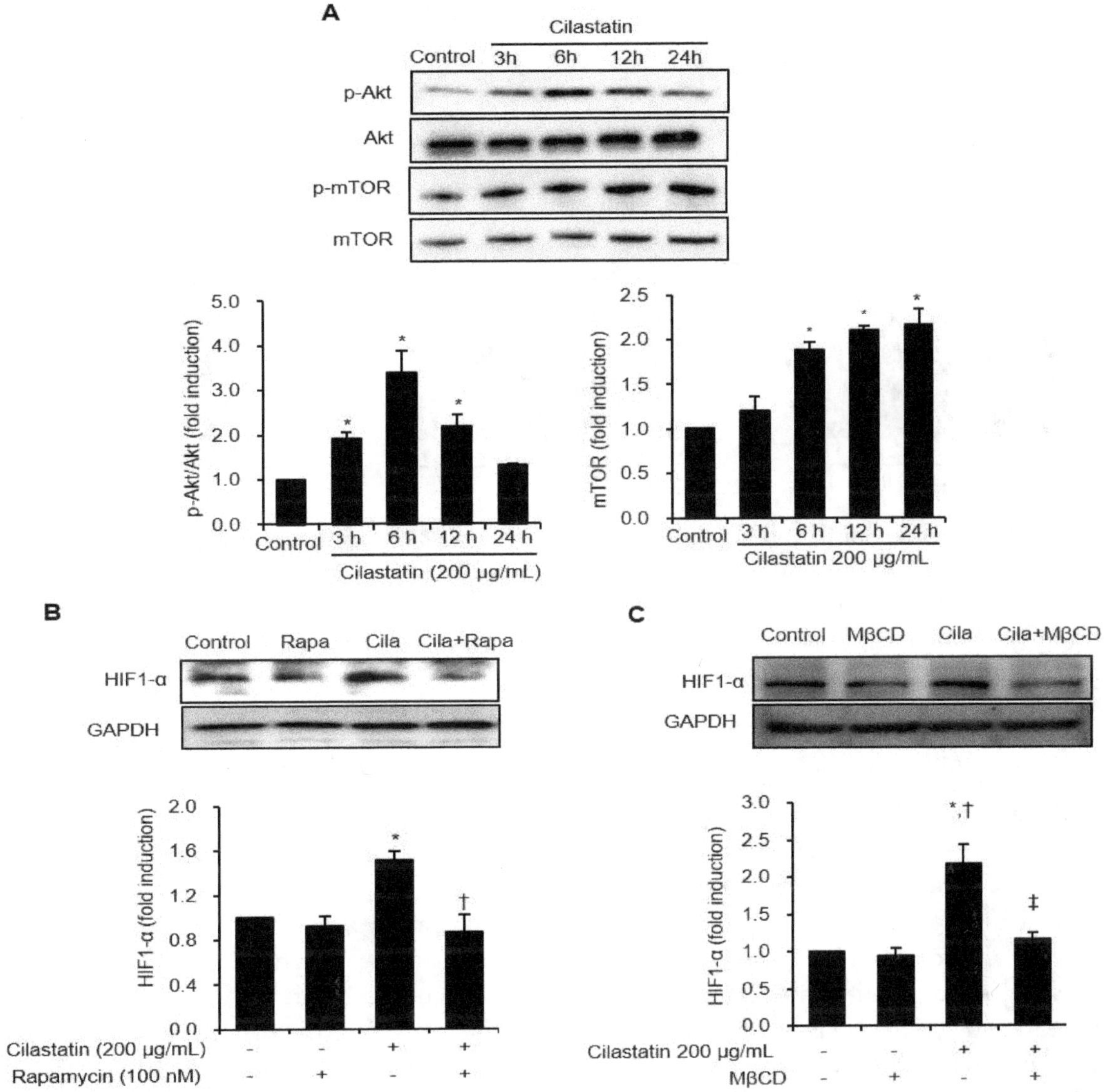

Figure 2. Cilastatin treatment induced HIF-1α expression via Akt/mTOR dependent pathway in HK-2 cells. (**A**) Semiquantitative immunoblotting revealed increase in Akt and mTOR expression by treatment with 200 μg/mL cilastatin in a time-dependent manner. The data are presented as means ± SEM. $^*p < 0.05$ vs. control. (**B**) Cilastatin pretreatment increased HIF-1α expression and the treatment of rapamycin, an mTOR inhibitor, significantly decreased HIF-1α expression despite cilastatin pretreatment. The data are presented as means ± SEM. * $p < 0.05$ vs. control, † $p < 0.05$ vs. rapamycin, and ‡$p < 0.05$ vs. cilastatin. (**C**) Cilastatin treatment increased HIF-1α expression and the destruction of lipid raft by MβCD significantly decreased HIF-1α expression despite cilastatin treatment. The data are presented as means ± SEM. * $p < 0.05$ vs. control, † $p < 0.05$ vs. MβCD, and ‡ $p < 0.05$ vs. cilastatin.

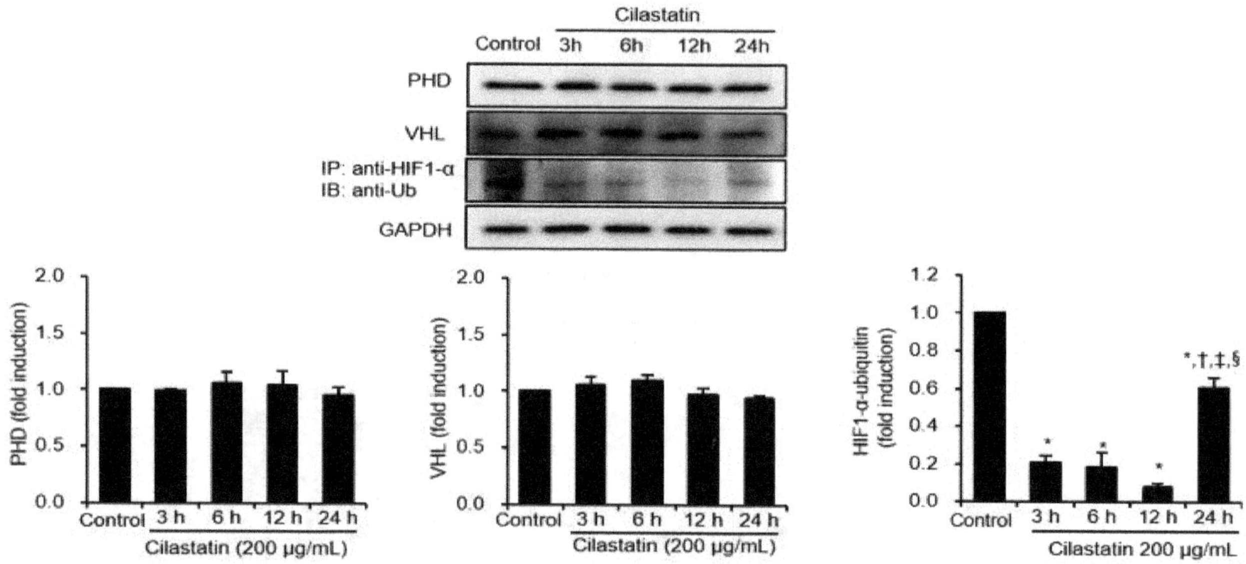

Figure 3. Cilastatin preconditioning upregulated HIF-1α expression via the inhibition of ubiquitination in HK-2 cells. Semiquantitative immunoblotting showed that cilastatin pretreatment did not affect the levels of VHL and PHD expressions. Immunoprecipitation showed that HIF-1α/ubiquitin complex formation was significantly suppressed in cilastatin-treated HK-2 cells compared to control in a time-dependent manner, but it was significantly increased at 24 h after cilastatin pretreatment. The data are presented as means ± SEM. **p* < 0.05 vs. control, †,‡,§ *p* < 0.05 vs. 3 h, 6 h, and 12 h after cilastatin treatment.

2.4. Cilastatin Preconditioning Enhances HIF-1α-Mediated Cell Survival in IR-Exposed HK-2 Cells

We evaluated whether cilastatin preconditioning provided protection against IR injury in HK-2 cells and whether HIF-1α mediated its protective effects. Cilastatin preconditioning and IR exposure increased HIF-1α level compared with control group (Figure 4A). Cilastatin preconditioning further enhanced the HIF-1α expression in IR-exposed cells than in non-exposed cells. IR exposure significantly reduced cell viability compared to the control group and cilastatin prevented this IR-induced cell death. The protective effect of cilastatin in IR-exposed cells was reversed by the co-treatment of YC-1, which downregulated HIF-1α at the post-translational level (Figure 4B). To evaluate whether the enhanced cell survival was associated with the specific activation of HIF-1α, we performed further experiments using HIF-1α small interfering (si) RNA. The viability of cells treated with HIF-1α siRNA was similar to that of control cells and HIF-1α siRNA treatment blocked the protective effects of cilastatin (Figure 4C).

2.5. Cilastatin Upregulates HIF-1α Expression Via Akt/mTOR Pathway in Mouse Kidney

Next, we investigated the effect of cilastatin treatment in mouse kidney. The expression of HIF-1α was significantly increased after cilastatin treatment in a time-dependent pattern (Figure 5A). The effect of cilastatin treatment on the ubiquitination pathway was evaluated in mouse kidney, and it was found that cilastatin did not affect the expressions of PHD and VHL. The expression of VEGF, which is downstream of HIF-1α, was also increased in mouse kidney. Similar to in vitro study, cilastatin treatment significantly increased the phosphorylation of both Akt and mTOR (Figure 5B).

2.6. Cilastatin Preconditioning Activates HIF-1α Signaling Pathway in Renal IR Injury

As shown in Figure 6, HIF-1α/ubiquitin complex formation was significantly suppressed in mice with IR injury, and cilastatin preconditioning further inhibited this complex formation. HIF-1α expression in immunoblot was significantly increased in mice with IR injury, and it was further increased after cilastatin preconditioning. The expression of EPO, a downstream effector of HIF-1α, was significantly increased in sham-operated mice with cilastatin preconditioning. IR injury reduced the EPO expression in mouse kidney, which recovered in cilastatin-treated mice with IR injury.

2.7. *Cilastatin Preconditioning Protects Against Renal IR Injury*

Serum creatinine levels were significantly increased at 24 h after IR injury compared with those in sham-operated mice (Figure 7A). Cilastatin preconditioning improved serum creatinine levels compared with the mice without cilastatin preconditioning. Histologic examination of tissue sections indicated extensive tubular necrosis in the kidneys of ischemic mice compared with those of sham-operated mice (Figure 7B). Tubular necrosis was improved in the cilastatin-treated mice with IR injury compared with those not treated with cilastatin.

2.8. *Cilastatin Preconditioning Attenuates Apoptosis in Renal IR Injury*

The number of terminal deoxynucleotidyl transferase-mediated dUTP nick end-labeling (TUNEL)-positive cells was increased in mice with IR injury compared to those of sham-operated mice, and it was decreased in cilastatin-treated mice with IR injury (Figure 8A). IR injury increased the expression of the proapoptotic protein Bcl-2-associated X (Bax) and decreased the expression of the antiapoptotic protein B-cell lymphoma 2 (Bcl-2). Cilastatin preconditioning significantly attenuated Bax levels and increased Bcl-2 expression in ischemic mouse kidney (Figure 8B).

2.9. *Cilastatin Protects Against Renal IR Injury Via HIF-1α Pathway*

Cilastatin attenuates renal dysfunction in mouse kidney with IR injury, and co-treatment with YC-1 restored IR injury to a great extent (Figure 9A). The quantitative tubular necrosis score of YC-1 co-treated ischemic mouse kidney was significantly higher than that of the mouse kidney treated with only cilastatin (Figure 9B).

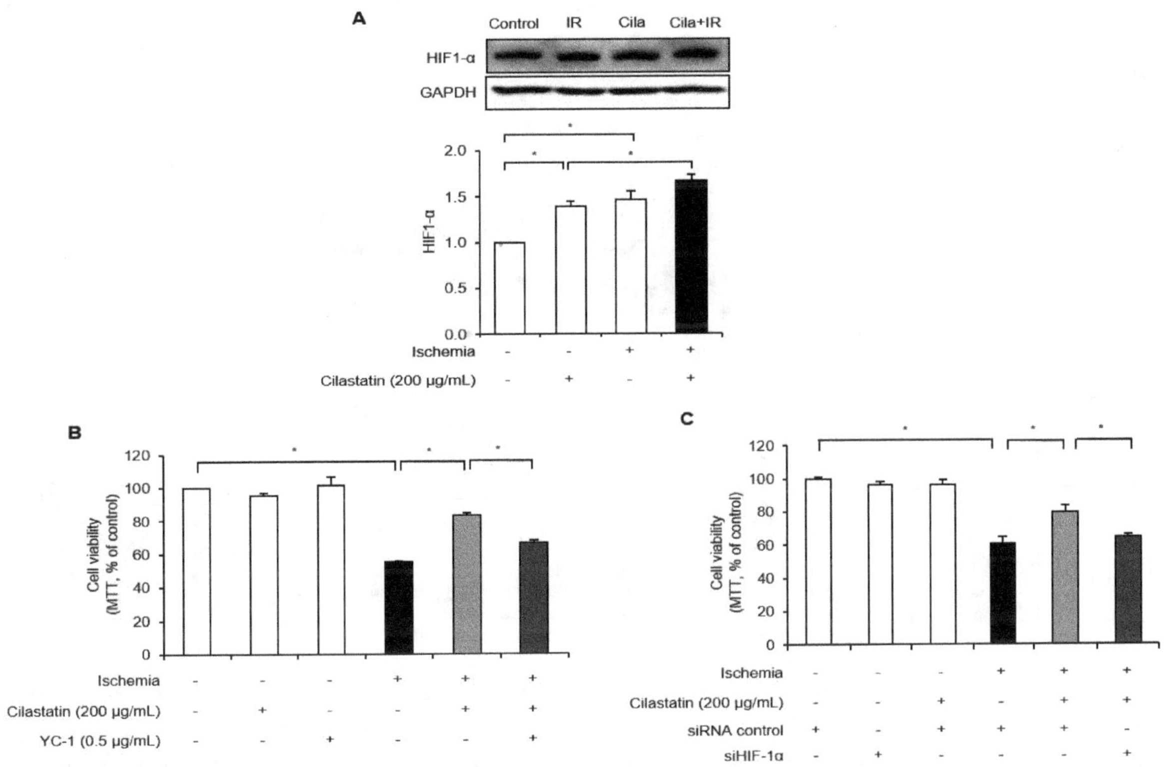

Figure 4. Cilastatin preconditioning protected IR-induced cell death via the activation of HIF-1α in HK-2 cells. (**A**) Semiquantitative immunoblotting of HIF-1α expression revealed that IR injury upregulated HIF-1α expression and cilastatin pretreatment further enhanced HIF-1α expression in IR-exposed cells. Cilastatin treatment also prevented IR-induced cell death. Co-treatment with cilastatin and (**B**) HIF-1α inhibitor, YC-1, or (**C**) HIF-1α siRNA restored cell death similar to those of IR-exposed cells without cilastatin treatment. The data are presented as means ± SEM. * $p < 0.05$.

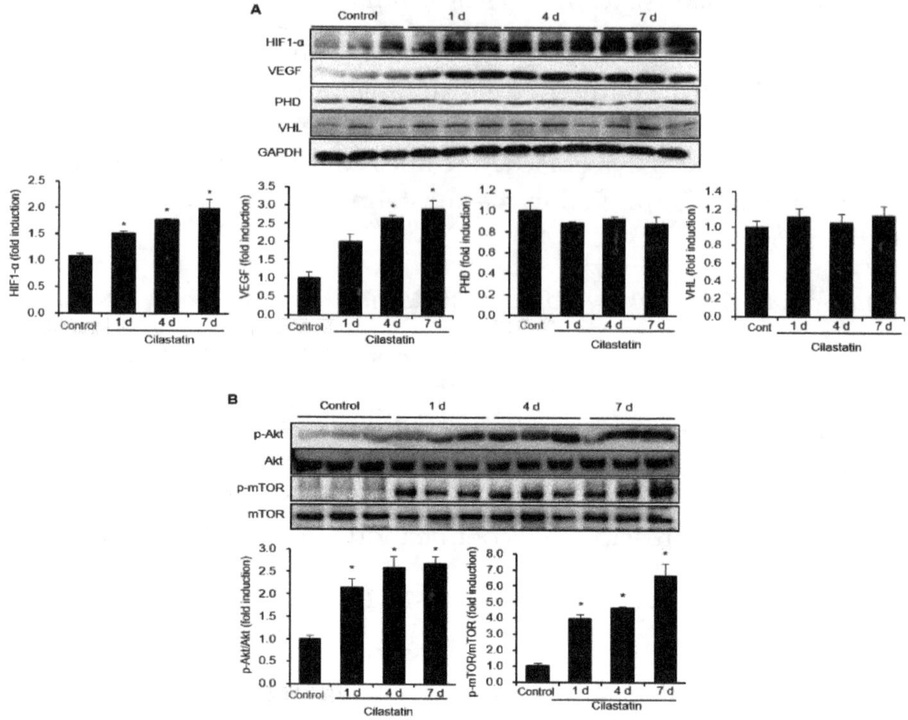

Figure 5. Cilastatin treatment upregulated HIF-1α expression and its upstream and downstream signaling pathways in mouse kidney. (**A**) Cilastatin treatment enhanced HIF-1α and VEGF expression in a time-dependent manner in mouse kidney, but it did not affect VHL and PHD expression. (**B**) Cilastatin treatment enhanced Akt and mt Or phosphorylation in a time-dependent manner in mouse kidney. The data are presented as means ± SEM. * $p < 0.05$.

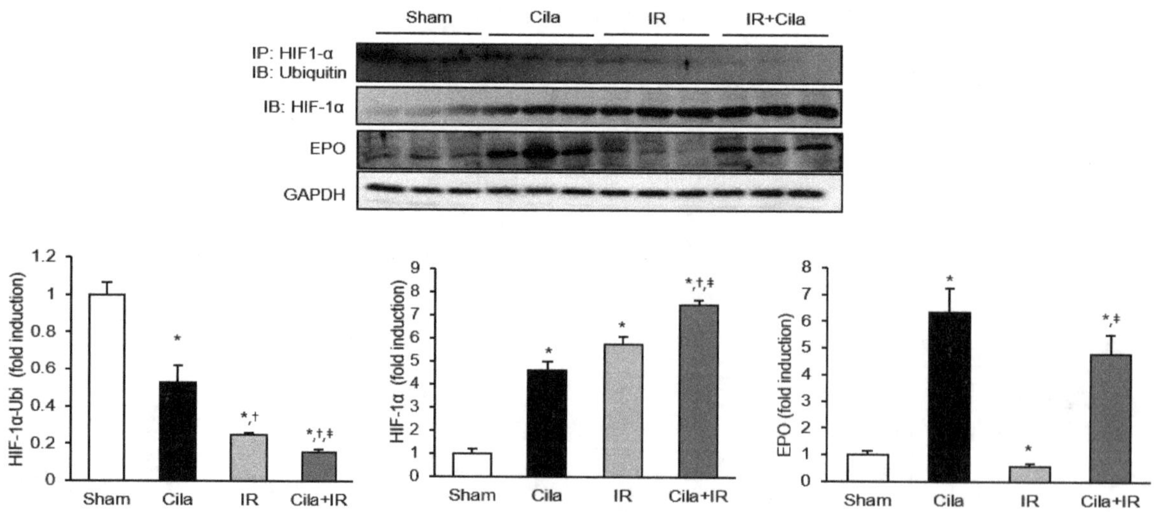

Figure 6. Cilastatin preconditioning upregulated HIF-1α expression and its downstream signaling pathway and decreased the ubiquitination of HIF-1α in mouse kidney with IR injury. Immunoprecipitation showed that HIF-1α/ubiquitin complex formation was significantly decreased in mouse kidney with IR injury compared to sham-operated mice; however, it more significantly decreased in cilastatin-treated mouse kidney with IR injury. Therefore, semiquantitative immunoblotting revealed that HIF-1α expression markedly increased in cilastatin-treated mouse kidney with IR injury compared to other groups. EPO expression was significantly increased in cilastatin-treated mouse kidney and was decreased in mouse kidney with IR injury; however, it increased in cilastatin-treated mouse kidney with IR injury. The data are presented as means ± SEM.* $p < 0.05$ vs. sham group; † $p < 0.05$ vs. Cila group; ‡ $p < 0.05$ vs. IR group.

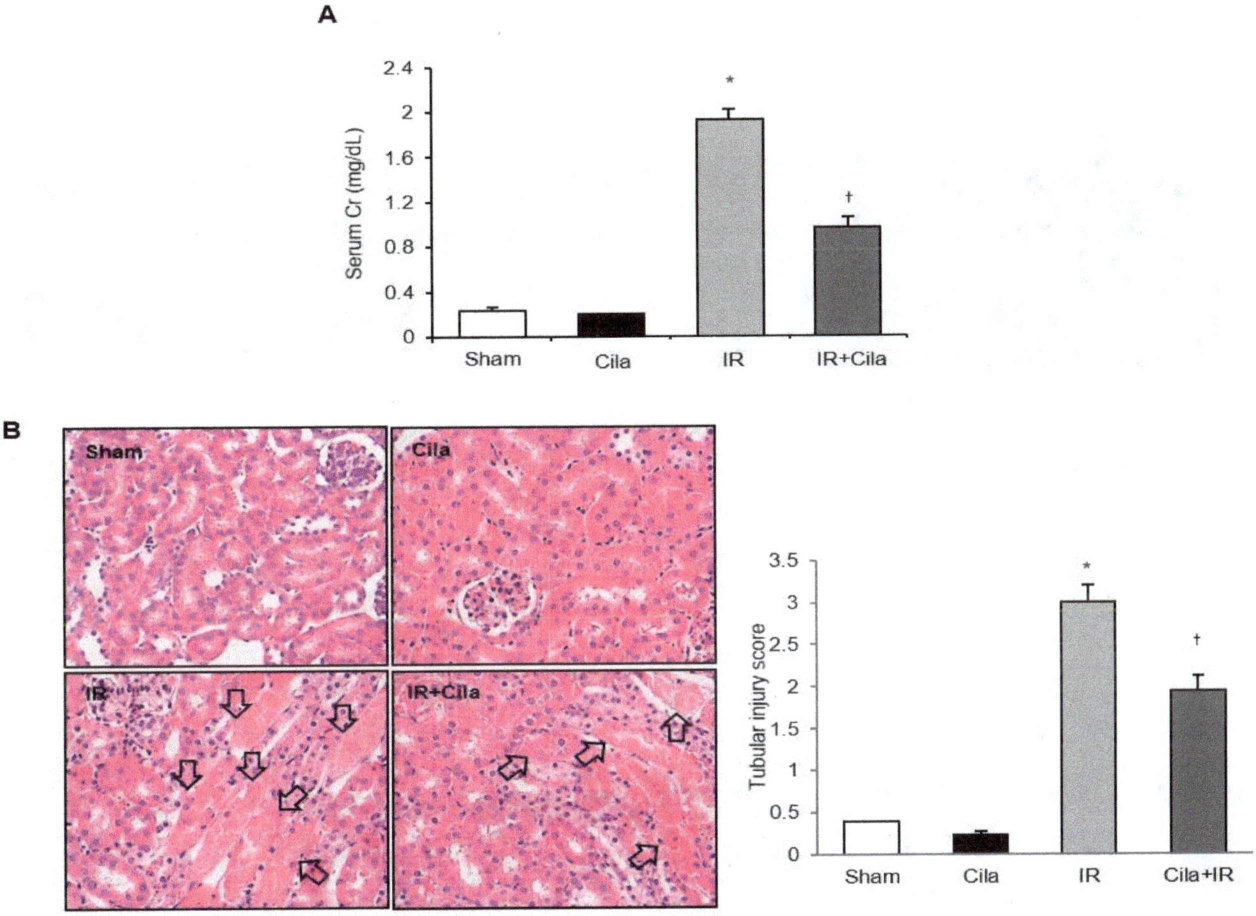

Figure 7. Cilastatin preconditioning improved renal function and tubular necrosis in mouse kidney with IR injury. (**A**) Serum creatinine levels were significantly increased at 24 h after IR injury compared with serum creatinine levels in sham-operated mice. Cilastatin pretreatment improved serum creatinine level in mouse kidney with IR injury. (**B**) The representative staining with hematoxylin and eosin showed a decreased tubular necrosis (arrows) in the cilastatin-treated mouse kidney with IR injury compared with mouse kidney with IR injury not treated with cilastatin (original magnification, × 200). The data are presented as means ± SEM. * $p < 0.05$ vs. sham and Cila group; † $p < 0.05$ vs. IR group.

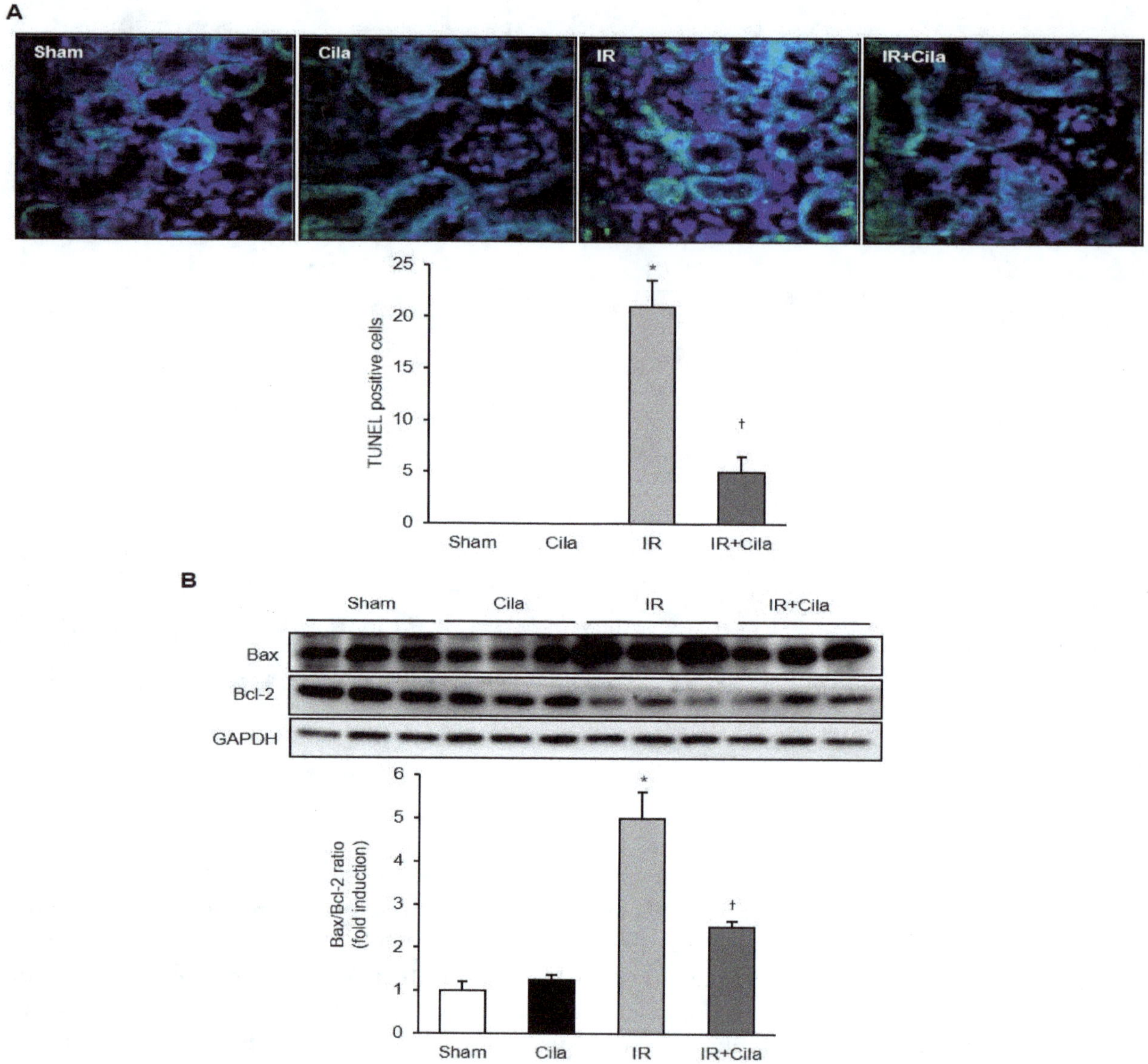

Figure 8. Cilastatin preconditioning attenuates apoptosis in mouse kidney with IR injury. (**A**) TUNEL assay revealed that cilastatin pretreatment significantly attenuated number of TUNEL-positive cells in mouse kidney with IR injury (original magnification, ×400). (**B**) Semiquantitative immunoblotting indicated that the level of pro-apoptotic marker, Bax, decreased in cilastatin-treated mouse kidney with IR injury, compared with mouse kidney with IR injury alone. Significant increase in levels of anti-apoptotic marker protein, Bcl-2, was noted after cilastatin pretreatment in mouse kidney with IR injury. The data are presented as means ± SEM. * $p < 0.05$ vs. sham and cila group; † $p < 0.05$ vs. IR group.

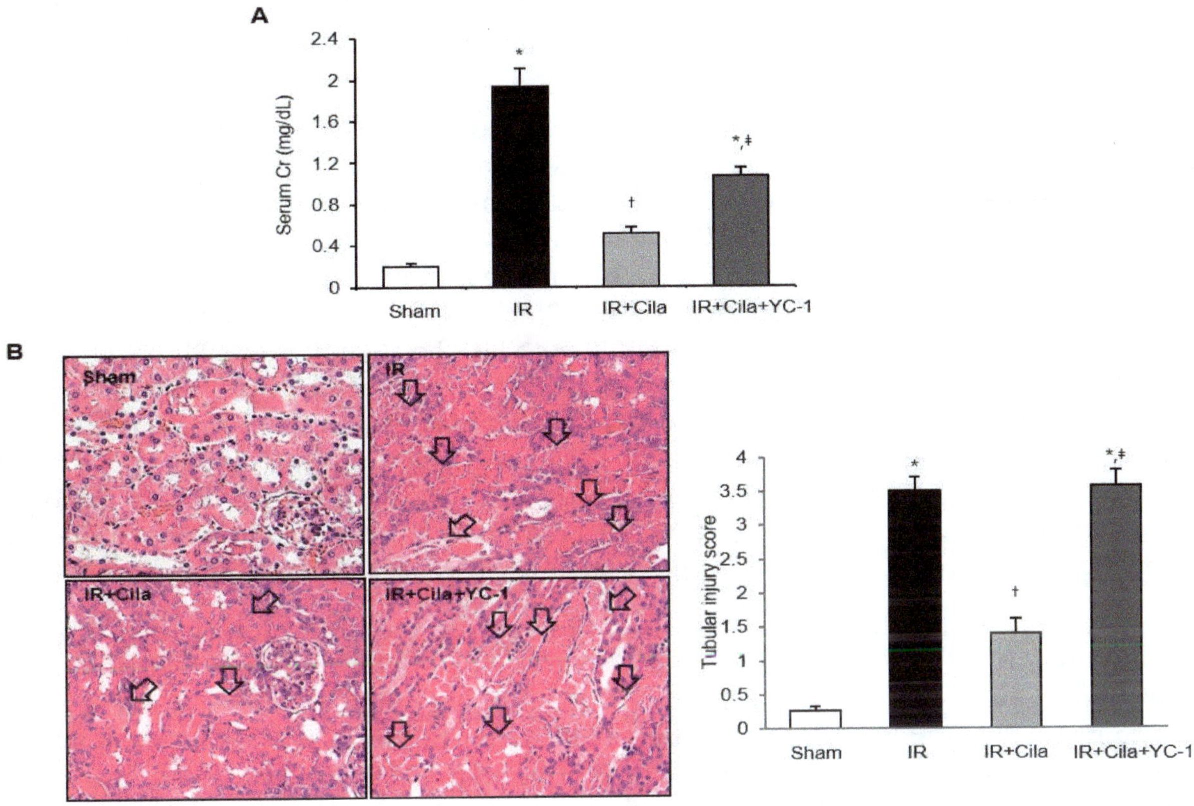

Figure 9. The co-treatment of YC-1, an HIF-1α inhibitor, with cilastatin worsened renal function and tubular necrosis in mouse kidney with IR injury. (**A**) Serum creatinine levels were significantly increased at 24 h after IR injury and decreased in mouse kidney with IR injury with cilastatin pretreatment. Co-treatment with cilastatin and YC-1 exacerbated renal function in mouse kidney with IR injury. (**B**) The representative staining with hematoxylin and eosin showed a decreased tubular necrosis (arrows) in the cilastatin-treated mouse kidney with IR injury, and aggravated tubular necrosis in mouse kidney with IR injury co-treated with cilastatin and YC-1 (original magnification, × 200). The data are presented as means ± SEM. * $p < 0.05$ vs. sham; † $p < 0.05$ vs. IR group; ‡ $p < 0.05$ vs. IR + Cila group.

3. Discussion

Our study demonstrated that cilastatin preconditioning induced the upregulation of HIF-1α via activation of Akt/mTOR pathway and inhibition of PHD/VHL-independent ubiquitination pathway. The cilastatin-induced HIF-1α upregulation prevented proximal tubular cell death during IR injury. In mouse kidney, cilastatin preconditioning again upregulated HIF-1α expression in the same fashion and the activated HIF-1α pathway suppressed renal dysfunction, tubular damage, and apoptotic cell death after IR injury. These findings suggested that cilastatin preconditioning exhibits protective effects against renal IR injury via HIF-1α activation.

Preconditioning refers to exposure to a stimulus to protect organs or tissues before subjection to ischemic injury, and HIF-1α has been implicated as an attractive target pathway for ischemic preconditioning for prevention against acute kidney injury [17,18]. Our study demonstrated that cilastatin preconditioning increased the expression of HIF-1α protein and enhanced its downstream pathway. In addition, the destruction of lipid raft blocked cilastatin-induced HIF-1α expression. These findings suggested that cilastatin effectively activates HIF-1α signaling pathway and that cell membrane structure having an affinity with cilastatin is important to activate a preconditioning target.

HIF-1α is mainly located in proximal tubular cells and can be upregulated at transcriptional or translational level [17,19]. Therefore, we investigated the mRNA level of HIF-1α and Akt/mTOR pathway. We found that phosphorylated Akt/mTOR level was abundant after cilastatin preconditioning and the inhibition of mTOR pathway reduced the HIF-1α expression in cilastatin-treated HK-2 cells.

However, cilastatin preconditioning did not increase the HIF-1α mRNA level in HK-2 cells. These findings demonstrated that cilastatin induces the expression of HIF-1α at the translational level, not at the transcriptional level.

HIF-1α expression can be enhanced via the enhanced Akt/mTOR pathway or by impairment of ubiquitin-proteasome degradation pathway [20,21]. Under normoxic conditions, PHD enzymes hydroxylated a subunit of HIF-1α and VHL captured them to undergo ubiquitin-protease pathway resulting in HIF-1α degradation [21,22]. However, ubiquitination of HIF-1α is also modulated via an oxygen/PHD/VHL-independent pathway involving the p53, glycogen synthase kinase 3, and the molecular chaperone 90 kDa heat-shock proteins [23–25]. In the present study, we demonstrated that the expressions of PHD and VHL were not altered in both HK-2 cells and mouse kidney after cilastatin preconditioning. On the other hand, immunoprecipitation analysis showed that the interactive binding between HIF-1α and ubiquitin was significantly decreased in cilastatin-treated cells under normoxic condition. Furthermore, the interaction between HIF-1α and ubiquitin was significantly decreased in mouse kidney with IR injury, and was further suppressed in cilastatin-treated mouse kidney with IR injury. These findings suggested that cilastatin may suppress HIF-1α degradation via the PHD and VHL-independent ubiquitin pathway in both normoxic and hypoxic condition.

Upregulation of renal HIF-1α plays an important role in the protection against IR injury and several studies reported HIF-1α as a potential therapeutic target [26,27]. Our study demonstrated that IR injury increased the expression of HIF-1α in proximal tubular cells and mouse kidney, and cilastatin preconditioning further increased the expression of HIF-1α. In addition, HIF-1α siRNA transfection or co-treatment with an YC-1 significantly reversed the protective effects of cilastatin in terms of proximal tubular cell death, renal dysfunction, and tubular necrosis. These data suggested that activation of HIF-1α signaling pathway plays a pivotal role in the renoprotective effect of cilastatin in IR injury.

HIF-1α regulates the adaptive response to hypoxia and other stresses by orchestrating the transcription of protective genes [17]. EPO, a representative downstream effector of HIF-1α, prevents apoptotic cell death, and promotes tubular cell regeneration during renal IR injury [28,29]. HIF-1α activation also activates the anti-apoptotic protein, bcl-2 in renal IR injury [30,31]. Our study showed that cilastatin preconditioning upregulated the expression of EPO and decreased apoptosis in mouse kidney with IR injury. These findings suggested that cilastatin-induced HIF-1α upregulation activates downstream effectors to reduce apoptosis during renal IR injury.

There are some interesting points and limitation in this study. Nuclear factor-erythroid-2-related factor 2 (Nrf2) is a transcription factor that regulates genes encoding antioxidant and detoxifying molecules [32,33]. It is known that Nrf2 has preventive effects against drug nephrotoxicity and ischemia reperfusion injury [34,35]. Therefore, cilastatin effects on Nrf2 is the attractive target as potential protective mechanism. Furthermore, we found Akt phosphorylation was decreased at 12 and 24 hours in cilastatin preconditioning. The reduced Akt activity was simply associated with limited working time of cilastatin. Otherwise, feedback from mTOR activation might negatively regulate the Akt activity [36,37]. The phosphorylation of mTOR at 12 h and 24 h in this experiment also supports this hypothesis. Finally, preconditioning effect of cilastatin has limitation in the clinical setting, because renal damage is already underway without preconditioning patients. Therefore, further experiments on the rescue effect of cilastatin after IR injury are required to increase the clinical usefulness.

In conclusion, cilastatin preconditioning protects against renal IR injury via the HIF-1α dependent pathway. Cilastatin preconditioning upregulated the HIF-1α expression by enhancing translational efficiency involving the Akt/mTOR pathway and by suppressing PHD/VHL-independent ubiquitination pathway. Our study provided evidence of the protective effects of cilastatin in non-pharmacological renal injury and demonstrated that the wide clinical application of cilastatin could be expected to prevent acute kidney injury.

4. Materials and Methods

4.1. Human Proximal Tubular Cell Culturing

HK-2 cells were purchased from American Type Culture Collection (Manassas, VA, USA). The cells were grown and passaged in Dulbecco's modified Eagle's medium (DMEM) supplemented with 10% fetal bovine serum, 50 U/mL penicillin, and 50 µg/mL streptomycin. The cells were cultivated in a humidified 5% CO2 environment at 37 °C. HK-2 cells were plated and cultured to 80% confluence.

HK-2 cells were treated with different doses of cilastatin for different times. The control cells were treated with distilled water. We also harvested the cells 24 h after co-treatment of cilastatin and MβCD (Sigma-Aldrich, St Louis, MO, USA), or mTOR inhibitor (rapamycin, Sigma-Aldrich, St Louis, MO, USA).

HK-2 cells were placed in serum-free media for 16 h at 80% confluence and were pretreated with cilastatin, HIF-1α inhibitor, YC-1 [38], or HIF-1α siRNA (Bioneer, Daejeon, Korea) for 1 h. Scrambled siRNA were complexed with a transfection reagent (Invitrogen, Carlsbad, CA, USA). After washing with phosphate-buffered saline (PBS), they were exposed to ischemia by immersing the cellular monolayer in mineral oil (Sigma-Aldrich, St Louis, MO, USA) for 90 min [39]. Then, the cells were washed twice and then received the same treatment.

4.2. Cell Viability

A commercially available MTT assay kit (EZ-Cytox; Daeil Lab Service, Seoul, Korea) determined cell viability. After exposure to ischemia and 24 h reperfusion, 10 µL of cell viability assay reagent was added. The optical densities of the samples were determined at 450 nm in a microplate reader (Bio-Rad Laboratories, Hercules, CA, USA).

4.3. Animal Model of Renal IR Injury

Seven- to eight-week-old male C57BL/6J mice were housed under a 12 h light–dark cycle, and food and water were freely available. Crystalline cilastatin was kindly provided by Im DS (Department of Chemistry, Soonchunhyang University, Cheonan, Korea). The experimental protocol was approved by the animal experiments' ethics committee of Daejeon St. Mary's Hospital (1st February 2016, CMCDJ-AP-2016-009).

Mice were divided into five groups (sham, sham + cilastatin, IR, IR + cilastatin, and IR + cilastatin + YC-1) and each group consisted of six mice. Cilastatin was diluted in saline, and 300 mg/kg of cilastatin, with or without YC-1 (5 mg/kg/day), was intraperitoneally injected daily for seven consecutive days before ischemia induction. The sham and IR groups of mice received the same volume of saline. Renal IR injury was performed under tiletamine–zolazepam (30 mg/kg) and xylazine (10 mg/kg) anesthesia. The mice were subjected to renal IR injury using previously described methods [40–42]. The bilateral renal pedicles were occluded for 23 min using microvascular clamps. A homoeothermic pad maintained the core body temperature of mice. The mice were sacrificed 24 h after ischemia and tissue and blood samples were collected.

4.4. Functional and Morphological Changes due to Kidney Injury

Serum creatinine level was measured by an IDEXX VetTest® Chemistry Analyzer (IDEXX Laboratories, Inc., Westbrook, ME, USA). The kidney tissues were fixed in 10% formalin buffer, embedded in paraffin, and then, cut into 3.5 mm-thick sections. Hematoxylin and eosin staining was performed to evaluate the degree of tubular damage. Markers of tubular damage were scored by calculating the percentage of tubules in the corticomedullary junction that displayed cell necrosis, loss of brush border, cast formation, and tubular dilation, as follows: 0, none; 1, ≤10%; 2, 11–25%; 3, 26–50%; 4, 51–75% and 5, ≥76%. The tubular necrosis score was quantified per high power field of each kidney and at least 20 fields were reviewed from each slide.

4.5. Immunofluorescence Staining

The number of apoptotic HK-2 cells was counted by TUNEL using a TUNEL Apoptosis Detection kit (Intergen, Purchase, NY, USA). The immunofluorescence images for TUNEL assay were captured by confocal microscopy (LSM5 Live Configuration Variotwo VRGB; Zeiss, Oberkochen, Germany). The number of positive cells was quantified per high-power field (HPF) of each kidney, and at least 20 fields were reviewed for each slide.

4.6. Immunoblotting Analyses of HK-2 Cells And Kidney Tissue

We performed the immunoblotting analyses for mouse kidneys and HK-2 cell lysates as described previously [42]. Kidney tissues were homogenized and resolved by SDS-polyacrylamide gel electrophoresis (SDS-PAGE) after centrifugation. HK-2 cells were harvested, washed with cold PBS, and resuspended in lysis buffer. Equal amounts of protein were electroblotted onto a nitrocellulose membrane. The membrane was blocked and incubated with primary antibodies directed against HIF-1α (Abcam, Cambridge, UK), Akt (Cell Signaling Technology, Beverly, MA, USA), pS473 Akt (Cell Signaling Technology), mTOR (Cell Signaling Technology), pSer2448 mTOR (Cell Signaling Technology), PHD (Cell Signaling Technology), VHL (von Hippel-Lindau, Santa Cruz Biotechnology), EPO (Abcam), VEGF (Abcam, Cambridge, UK), Bax (Cell Signaling Technology), Bcl-2 (Cell Signaling Technology), and glyceraldehyde-3-phosphate dehydrogenase (GAPDH, Cell Signaling Technology). They were then incubated with horseradish peroxidase-conjugated anti-rabbit IgG or anti-mouse IgG antibody (Invitrogen, Carlsbad, CA, USA). Positive bands were detected and analyzed using the ChemiDoc XRS Image system (Bio-Rad Laboratories, Hercules, CA, USA).

4.7. Real-Time Reverse Transcription PCR

Total RNA was isolated from kidney tissues and HK-2 cells using a NucleoSpin® RNA II kit (Macherey-Nagel, Düren, Germany). cDNA was synthesized using Reverse Transcriptase Premix (Elpis Biotech, Daejeon, Korea) and amplified in a Power SYBR®Green polymerase chain reaction (PCR) Master Mix (Applied Biosystems, Warrington, UK) with gene-specific primer pairs (HIF-1α: F; 5′-TGCCCCAGATTCAAGATCAGC-3′, R; 5′-GGCTGGGAAAAGT TAGGAGTGT-3′) Quantitative real-time PCR was performed on an ABI 7500 FAST instrument (Applied Biosystems, Warrington, UK). The expression levels of mRNAs were normalized to the expression of GAPDH.

4.8. Immunoprecipitation

Cultured HK-2 cells and kidney tissues were lysed with kinase buffer and then 1 mg of lysate was immunoprecipitated using 1 µg of anti-ubiquitin antibody (Santa Cruz Biotechnology) and protein G Sepharose 4 Fast Flow (GE Healthcare, Danderyd, Sweden). After washing with KB without 1% NO40, immunoblotting was performed using HIF-1α antibody (Biorbyt Ltd., Cambridge, UK).

4.9. Statistical Analysis

Data are expressed as the mean ± standard error of the mean (SEM) of ≥3 independent experiments. Differences between the two groups were determined using Student's t test or the Mann–Whitney U test. Multiple comparisons were performed using one-way analysis of variance and Tukey's post hoc test. Statistical analysis was performed using SPSS software (version 22.0; IBM, Armonk, NY). Results were considered significant when $p < 0.05$.

Author Contributions: Conceptualization, Y.A.H., C.W.P. and H.S.H.; methodology, S.Y.J. and K.J.Y.; software, H.S.H.; validation, K.H.J. and C.W.P.; formal analysis, Y.A.H.; investigation, S.Y.J. and K.J.Y.; resources, D.S.I. and H.S.H.; data curation, S.Y.J.; writing—original draft preparation, Y.A.H.; writing—review and editing, H.S.H.; visualization, K.H.J.; supervision, K.H.J. and C.W.P.; project administration, D.S.I.; funding acquisition, Y.A.H., D.S.I. and H.S.H. All authors have read and agreed to the published version of the manuscript.

Abbreviations

IR	Ischemia–reperfusion
HIF-1α	Hypoxia-inducible factor-1α
DHP-1	Dehydrogenase peptide-1
mTOR	Mammalian target of rapamycin
EPO	Erythropoietin
VEGF	Vascular endothelial growth factor
MβCD	Methyl-β-cyclodextrin
PHD	Prolyl hydroxylase
VHL	Von Hippel-Lindau
si	Small interfering
TUNEL	terminal deoxynucleotidyl transferase-mediated dUTP nick end-labeling
Nrf2	nuclear factor-erythroid-2-related factor 2
Bax	Bcl-2-associated X protein
Bcl-2	B-cell lymphoma 2
GAPDH	glyceraldehyde-3-phosphate dehydrogenase
PCR	polymerase chain reaction

References

1. Liano, F.; Pascual, J. Epidemiology of acute renal failure: A prospective, multicenter, community-based study. Madrid Acute Renal Failure Study Group. *Kidney Int.* **1996**, *50*, 811–818. [CrossRef] [PubMed]
2. Smith, S.F.; Hosgood, S.A.; Nicholson, M.L. Ischemia-reperfusion injury in renal transplantation: 3 key signaling pathways in tubular epithelial cells. *Kidney Int.* **2019**, *95*, 50–56. [CrossRef] [PubMed]
3. Baer, P.C.; Koch, B.; Geiger, H. Kidney Inflammation, Injury and Regeneration. *Int. J. Mol. Sci.* **2020**, *21*, 1164. [CrossRef] [PubMed]
4. Semenza, G.L. Hypoxia-inducible factor 1: Oxygen homeostasis and disease pathophysiology. *Trends Mol. Med.* **2001**, *7*, 345–350. [CrossRef]
5. Haase, V.H. Hypoxic regulation of erythropoiesis and iron metabolism. *Am. J. Physiol. Renal Physiol.* **2010**, *299*, F1–F13. [CrossRef]
6. Sethi, K.; Rao, K.; Bolton, D.; Patel, O.; Ischia, J. Targeting HIF-1α to Prevent Renal Ischemia-Reperfusion Injury: Does It Work? *Int. J. Cell Biol.* **2018**, *2018*, 9852791. [CrossRef]
7. Kaelin, W.G.; Ratcliffe, P.J., Jr. Oxygen sensing by metazoans: The central role of the HIF hydroxylase pathway. *Mol. Cell* **2008**, *30*, 393–402. [CrossRef]
8. Buckley, M.M.; Brogden, R.N.; Barradell, L.B.; Goa, K.L. Imipenem/Cilastatin: A Reappraisal of its Antibacterial Activity, Pharmacokinetic Properties and Therapeutic Efficacy. *Drugs* **1992**, *44*, 408–444. [CrossRef]
9. Perez, M.; Castilla, M.; Torres, A.M.; Lázaro, J.A.; Sarmiento, E.; Tejedor, A. Inhibition of brush border dipeptidase with cilastatin reduces toxic accumulation of cyclosporin A in kidney proximal tubule epithelial cells. *Nephrol. Dial. Transplant.* **2004**, *19*, 2445–2455. [CrossRef]
10. Camano, S.; Lazaro, A.; Moreno-Gordaliza, E.; Torres, A.M.; de Lucas, C.; Humanes, B.; Lazaro, J.A.; Milagros Gomez-Gomez, M.; Bosca, L.; Tejedor, A. Cilastatin attenuates cisplatin-induced proximal tubular cell damage. *J. Pharmacol. Exp. Ther.* **2010**, *334*, 419–429. [CrossRef]
11. Luo, K.; Lim, S.W.; Jin, J.; Jin, L.; Gil, H.W.; Im, D.S.; Hwang, H.S.; Yang, C.W. Cilastatin protects against tacrolimus-induced nephrotoxicity via anti-oxidative and anti-apoptotic properties. *BMC Nephrol.* **2019**, *20*, 221. [CrossRef] [PubMed]

12. Im, D.S.; Shin, H.J.; Yang, K.J.; Jung, S.Y.; Song, H.Y.; Hwang, H.S.; Gil, H.W. Cilastatin attenuates vancomycin-induced nephrotoxicity via P-glycoprotein. *Toxicol. Lett.* **2017**, *277*, 9–17. [CrossRef] [PubMed]
13. Reis-Sobreiro, M.; Roué, G.; Moros, A.; Gajate, C.; de la Iglesia-Vicente, J.; Colomer, D.; Mollinedo, F. Lipid raft-mediated Akt signaling as a therapeutic target in mantle cell lymphoma. *Blood Cancer J.* **2013**, *3*, e118. [CrossRef] [PubMed]
14. Parkin, E.T.; Turner, A.J.; Hooper, N.M. Differential effects of glycosphingolipids on the detergent-insolubility of the glycosylphosphatidylinositol-anchored membrane dipeptidase. *Biochem. J.* **2001**, *358*, 209–216. [CrossRef]
15. Harada, H.; Itasaka, S.; Kizaka-Kondoh, S.; Shibuya, K.; Morinibu, A.; Shinomiya, K.; Hiraoka, M. The Akt/mTOR pathway assures the synthesis of HIF-1alpha protein in a glucose- and reoxygenation-dependent manner in irradiated tumors. *J. Biol. Chem.* **2009**, *284*, 5332–5342. [CrossRef]
16. Pore, N.; Jiang, Z.; Shu, H.K.; Bernhard, E.; Kao, G.D.; Maity, A. Akt1 activation can augment hypoxia-inducible factor-1alpha expression by increasing protein translation through a mammalian target of rapamycin-independent pathway. *Mol. Cancer Res.* **2006**, *4*, 471–479. [CrossRef]
17. Bernhardt, W.M.; Campean, V.; Kany, S.; Jürgensen, J.S.; Weidemann, A.; Warnecke, C.; Arend, M.; Klaus, S.; Günzler, V.; Amann, K.; et al. Preconditional activation of hypoxia-inducible factors ameliorates ischemic acute renal failure. *J. Am. Soc. Nephrol.* **2006**, *17*, 1970–1978. [CrossRef]
18. Kapitsinou, P.P.; Haase, V.H. Molecular mechanisms of ischemic preconditioning in the kidney. *Am. J. Physiol. Renal Physiol.* **2015**, *309*, F821–F834. [CrossRef]
19. Rosenberger, C.; Mandriota, S.; Jürgensen, J.S.; Wiesener, M.S.; Hörstrup, J.H.; Frei, U.; Ratcliffe, P.J.; Maxwell, P.H.; Bachmann, S.; Eckardt, K.U. Expression of hypoxia-inducible factor-1alpha and -2alpha in hypoxic and ischemic rat kidneys. *J. Am. Soc. Nephrol.* **2002**, *13*, 1721–1732. [CrossRef]
20. Lee, J.W.; Bae, S.H.; Jeong, J.W.; Kim, S.H.; Kim, K.W. Hypoxia-inducible factor (HIF-1)alpha: Its protein stability and biological functions. *Exp. Mol. Med.* **2004**, *36*, 1–12. [CrossRef]
21. Salceda, S.; Caro, J. Hypoxia-inducible factor 1alpha (HIF-1alpha) protein is rapidly degraded by the ubiquitin-proteasome system under normoxic conditions. Its stabilization by hypoxia depends on redox-induced changes. *J. Biol. Chem.* **1997**, *272*, 22642–22647. [CrossRef] [PubMed]
22. Schofield, C.J.; Ratcliffe, P.J. Oxygen sensing by HIF hydroxylases. *Nat. Rev. Mol. Cell Biol.* **2004**, *5*, 343–354. [CrossRef] [PubMed]
23. Chen, D.; Li, M.; Luo, J.; Gu, W. Direct interactions between HIF-1 alpha and Mdm2 modulate p53 function. *J. Biol. Chem.* **2003**, *278*, 13595–13598. [CrossRef] [PubMed]
24. Flugel, D.; Gorlach, A.; Michiels, C.; Kietzmann, T. Glycogen synthase kinase 3 phosphorylates hypoxia-inducible factor 1alpha and mediates its destabilization in a VHL-independent manner. *Mol. Cell Biol.* **2007**, *27*, 3253–3265. [CrossRef] [PubMed]
25. Van de Sluis, B.; Groot, A.J.; Vermeulen, J.; van der Wall, E.; van Diest, P.J.; Wijmenga, C.; Klomp, L.W.; Vooijs, M. COMMD1 Promotes pVHL and O2-Independent Proteolysis of HIF-1alpha via HSP90/70. *PLoS ONE* **2009**, *4*, e7332. [CrossRef] [PubMed]
26. Hill, P.; Shukla, D.; Tran, M.G.; Aragones, J.; Cook, H.T.; Carmeliet, P.; Maxwell, P.H. Inhibition of hypoxia inducible factor hydroxylases protects against renal ischemia-reperfusion injury. *J. Am. Soc. Nephrol.* **2008**, *19*, 39–46. [CrossRef]
27. Ong, S.G.; Hausenloy, D.J. Hypoxia-inducible factor as a therapeutic target for cardioprotection. *Pharmacol. Ther.* **2012**, *136*, 69–81. [CrossRef]
28. Zhang, Y.B.; Wang, X.; Meister, E.A.; Gong, K.R.; Yan, S.C.; Lu, G.W.; Ji, X.M.; Shao, G. The effects of CoCl2 on HIF-1α protein under experimental conditions of autoprogressive hypoxia using mouse models. *Int. J. Mol. Sci.* **2014**, *18*, 10999–11012. [CrossRef]
29. Imamura, R.; Moriyama, T.; Isaka, Y.; Namba, Y.; Ichimaru, N.; Takahara, S.; Okuyama, A. Erythropoietin protects the kidneys against ischemia reperfusion injury by activating hypoxia inducible factor-1alpha. *Transplantation* **2007**, *83*, 1371–1379. [CrossRef]
30. Yang, C.C.; Lin, L.C.; Wu, M.S.; Chien, C.T.; Lai, M.K. Repetitive hypoxic preconditioning attenuates renal ischemia/reperfusion induced oxidative injury via upregulating HIF-1 alpha-dependent bcl-2 signaling. *Transplantation* **2009**, *88*, 1251–1260. [CrossRef]

31. Jamadarkhana, P.; Chaudhary, A.; Chhipa, L.; Dubey, A.; Mohanan, A.; Gupta, R.; Deshpande, S. Treatment with a novel hypoxia-inducible factor hydroxylase inhibitor (TRC160334) ameliorates ischemic acute kidney injury. *Am. J. Nephrol.* **2012**, *36*, 208–218. [CrossRef] [PubMed]
32. Ruiz, S.; Pergola, P.E.; Zager, R.A.; Vaziri, N.D. Targeting the transcription factor Nrf2 to ameliorate oxidative stress and inflammation in chronic kidney disease. *Kidney Int.* **2013**, *83*, 1029–1041. [CrossRef] [PubMed]
33. Nezu, M.; Suzuki, N. Roles of Nrf2 in Protecting the Kidney from Oxidative Damage. *Int. J. Mol. Sci.* **2020**, *21*, 2951. [CrossRef] [PubMed]
34. Jakobs, P.; Serbulea, V.; Leitinger, N.; Eckers, A.; Haendeler, J. Nuclear Factor (Erythroid-Derived 2)-Like 2 and Thioredoxin-1 in Atherosclerosis and Ischemia/Reperfusion Injury in the Heart. *Antioxid. Redox Signal.* **2017**, *26*, 630–644. [CrossRef]
35. Limonciel, A.; Jennings, P. A review of the evidence that ochratoxin A is an Nrf2 inhibitor: Implications for nephrotoxicity and renal carcinogenicity. *Toxins* **2014**, *6*, 371–379. [CrossRef]
36. Manning, B.D.; Toker, A. AKT/PKB Signaling: Navigating the Network. *Cell* **2017**, *169*, 381–405. [CrossRef]
37. Hsu, P.P.; Kang, S.A.; Rameseder, J.; Zhang, Y.; Ottina, K.A.; Lim, D.; Peterson, T.R.; Choi, Y.; Gray, N.S.; Yaffe, M.B.; et al. The mTOR-regulated phosphoproteome reveals a mechanism of mTORC1-mediated inhibition of growth factor signaling. *Science* **2011**, *332*, 1317–1322. [CrossRef]
38. Yeo, E.J.; Chun, Y.S.; Cho, Y.S.; Kim, J.; Lee, J.C.; Kim, M.S.; Park, J.W. YC-1: A potential anticancer drug targeting hypoxia-inducible factor 1. *J. Natl. Cancer Inst.* **2003**, *95*, 516–525. [CrossRef]
39. Meldrum, K.K.; Meldrum, D.R.; Hile, K.L.; Burnett, A.L.; Harken, A.H. A novel model of ischemia in renal tubular cells which closely parallels in vivo injury. *J. Surg. Res.* **2001**, *99*, 288–293. [CrossRef]
40. Hwang, H.S.; Yang, K.J.; Park, K.C.; Choi, H.S.; Kim, S.H.; Hong, S.Y.; Jeon, B.H.; Chang, Y.K.; Park, C.W.; Kim, S.Y.; et al. Pretreatment with paricalcitol attenuates inflammation in ischemia-reperfusion injury via the up-regulation of cyclooxygenase-2 and prostaglandin E2. *Nephrol. Dial. Transplant.* **2013**, *28*, 1156–1166. [CrossRef]
41. Imtiazul, I.M.; Asma, R.; Lee, J.H.; Cho, N.J.; Park, S.; Song, H.Y.; Gil, H.W. Change of surfactant protein D and A after renal ischemia reperfusion injury. *PLoS ONE* **2019**, *14*, e0227097. [CrossRef] [PubMed]
42. Hong, Y.A.; Yang, K.J.; Jung, S.Y.; Park, K.C.; Choi, H.; Oh, J.M.; Lee, S.J.; Chang, Y.K.; Park, C.W.; Yang, C.W.; et al. Paricalcitol Pretreatment Attenuates Renal Ischemia-Reperfusion Injury via Prostaglandin E2 Receptor EP4 Pathway. *Oxid. Med. Cell. Longev.* **2017**, *2017*, 5031926. [PubMed]

B Cell Activating Factor (BAFF) is Required for the Development of Intra-Renal Tertiary Lymphoid Organs in Experimental Kidney Transplantation in Rats

Louisa Steines *, Helen Poth, Marlene Herrmann, Antonia Schuster, Bernhard Banas and Tobias Bergler

Department of Nephrology, University Hospital Regensburg, 93042 Regensburg, Germany; helen_reinfrank@web.de (H.P.); marlene-herrmann@gmx.net (M.H.); antonia-margarete.schuster@ukr.de (A.S.); bernhard.banas@ukr.de (B.B.); tobias.bergler@ukr.de (T.B.)

* Correspondence: Louisa.Steines@ukr.de

Abstract: Intra-renal tertiary lymphoid organs (TLOs) are associated with worsened outcome in kidney transplantation (Ktx). We used an anti-BAFF (B cell activating factor) intervention to investigate whether BAFF is required for TLO formation in a full MHC-mismatch Ktx model in rats. Rats received either therapeutic immunosuppression (no rejection, NR) or subtherapeutic immunosuppression (chronic rejection, CR) and were sacrificed on d56. One group additionally received an anti-BAFF antibody (CR + AB). Intra-renal T ($CD3^+$) and B ($CD20^+$) cells, their proliferation ($Ki67^+$), and IgG^+ plasma cells were analyzed by immunofluorescence microscopy. Formation of T and B cell zones and TLOs was assessed. Intra-renal expression of TLO-promoting factors, molecules of T:B crosstalk, and B cell differentiation was analyzed by qPCR. Intra-renal B and T cell zones and TLOs were detected in CR and were associated with elevated intra-renal mRNA expression of TLO-promoting factors, including CXCL13, CCL19, lymphotoxin-β, and BAFF. Intra-renal plasma cells were also elevated in CR. Anti-BAFF treatment significantly decreased intra-renal B cell zones and TLO, as well as intra-renal B cell-derived TLO-promoting factors and B cell differentiation markers. We conclude that BAFF-dependent intra-renal B cells promote TLO formation and advance local adaptive alloimmune responses in chronic rejection.

Keywords: tertiary lymphoid organs; kidney transplantation; B cells; BAFF

1. Introduction

Kidney transplantation is the best available treatment for many patients with end-stage kidney failure; however, kidney allograft survival is limited, with a 10-year graft survival rate of only 56% [1]. A shortage of organs for donation is therefore exacerbated by premature allograft failure. On top of this, patients with multiple consecutive transplants have a higher risk of graft failure due to rejection [2]. Improving allograft survival is therefore an important aim in renal and transplantation medicine.

Apart from antibody-mediated rejection (ABMR), which is a major cause of allograft failure [3], kidney allograft inflammation is an important predictor of reduced allograft survival [4]. Subclinical inflammation is associated with poorer outcomes [4,5] and may precede irreversible interstitial fibrosis [6]. Due to its prognostic relevance, inflammation in areas of fibrosis has recently been incorporated into Banff rejection grading as an independent score ("iIFTA", inflammation with interstitial fibrosis and tubular atrophy). The role of B cells in allograft inflammation has not been fully clarified. Intra-graft B cell clusters have been observed in animal and human transplant studies, and have been related to poorer outcomes [7,8]. Furthermore, overproportional amounts of B cells were found in allografts with subclinical rejection and fibrotic changes compared to grafts with subclinical rejection without fibrosis [9], suggesting a role of B cells in chronic rejection.

B cells can form organized follicular structures together with T cells and other immune cells [10,11]. Within these structures, termed tertiary lymphoid organs (TLOs), B cells can affect local immune activation [12]. TLOs resemble lymphoid follicles within secondary lymphoid organs and occur at sites of chronic inflammation. They have been detected in systemic lupus erythematodes (SLE), rheumatoid arthritis, multiple sclerosis, atherosclerosis, as well as heart and kidney transplantation, as reviewed by Pitzalis [13]. The formation of TLO is driven by local expression of factors required for formation of secondary lymphoid tissue, such as CCL19, CCL21, CXCL13, and lymphotoxin-α/β [14,15]. Furthermore, TLOs are sites of local activation of adaptive immunity, where locally antigen-activated B cells receive additional signals, clonally proliferate [16], and become a local source of donor-specific antibodies (DSAs) [12].

B cells are important mediators of TLO development due to their expression of lymphotoxin-α/β [17]. They can remain within allografts even after peripheral depletion of B cells using Rituximab [18]. B cell activating factor (BAFF) is an important survival factor for B cells and plasma cells [19]. In Ktx patients, elevated serum BAFF levels have also been associated with pre-sensitization, anti-HLA antibody formation, ABMR, and reduced graft survival [20,21]. We have previously demonstrated expression of BAFF in experimental rat kidney allografts [22], and also showed that anti-BAFF treatment interfered with humoral responses in Ktx using the same model [23]. However, a necessity of BAFF for TLO development has not previously been shown. Here, we tested the effects of an anti-BAFF antibody on intra-renal infiltrates of T and B cells, their microanatomical organization into TLOs, intra-renal expression of TLO-promoting factors and B cell differentiation factors, as part of local adaptive alloresponses in chronic rejection.

2. Results

2.1. *Anti-BAFF Treatment Alters the T and B Cell Composition of Intra-Renal Infiltrates*

We first examined the overall area of intra-renal infiltrates in the different experimental groups using immunohistochemistry. Infiltrates were significantly more expansive in CR and CR + AB compared to NR (CR vs. NR: 0.16 ± 0.05 vs. 0.01 ± 0.01 mm^2, $p = 0.0012$; CR + AB vs. NR: 0.10 ± 0.08 vs. 0.01 ± 0.01 mm^2, $p = 0.030$) (Figure 1A). The expansion of intra-renal infiltrates appeared to be reduced in CR + AB compared to CR, but the difference was not significant. Analysis of the microanatomical localization of infiltrates showed that the majority of infiltrates were localized in the vicinity of arterioles (perivascular), followed by localization surrounding glomeruli (periglomerular) and few were located interstitially without apparent contact to arterioles or glomeruli (Figure 1B). We then assessed the number of T (CD3$^+$) and B (CD20$^+$) cells within kidney sections, and found that there were significantly more T cells in CR and CR + AB compared to NR (CR vs. NR: 610 ± 204 vs. 30 ± 40 cells/mm^2, $p = 0.0032$; CR + AB vs. NR: 479 ± 338 vs. 30 ± 40 cells/mm^2, $p = 0.019$), but CR and CR + AB did not differ significantly in intra-renal T cell content (Figure 1C). The number of B cells was also significantly elevated in CR compared to NR (CR vs. NR: 431 ± 232 vs. 6 ± 13 cells/mm^2, $p = 0.0006$). Anti-BAFF treatment substantially reduced the number of intra-renal B cells (CR vs. CR + AB: 431 ± 232 vs. 60 ± 51 cells/mm^2, $p = 0.0013$) (Figure 1C). Since T cells were non-significantly reduced in CR + AB compared to CR, we also assessed the ratio of B:T cells and found that this was elevated in CR compared to NR (0.67 ± 0.29 vs. 0.12 ± 0.16, $p = 0.0067$), and significantly reduced after anti-BAFF treatment (CR vs. CR + AB: 0.67 ± 0.29 vs. 0.12 ± 0.05, $p = 0.0016$) (Figure 1D).

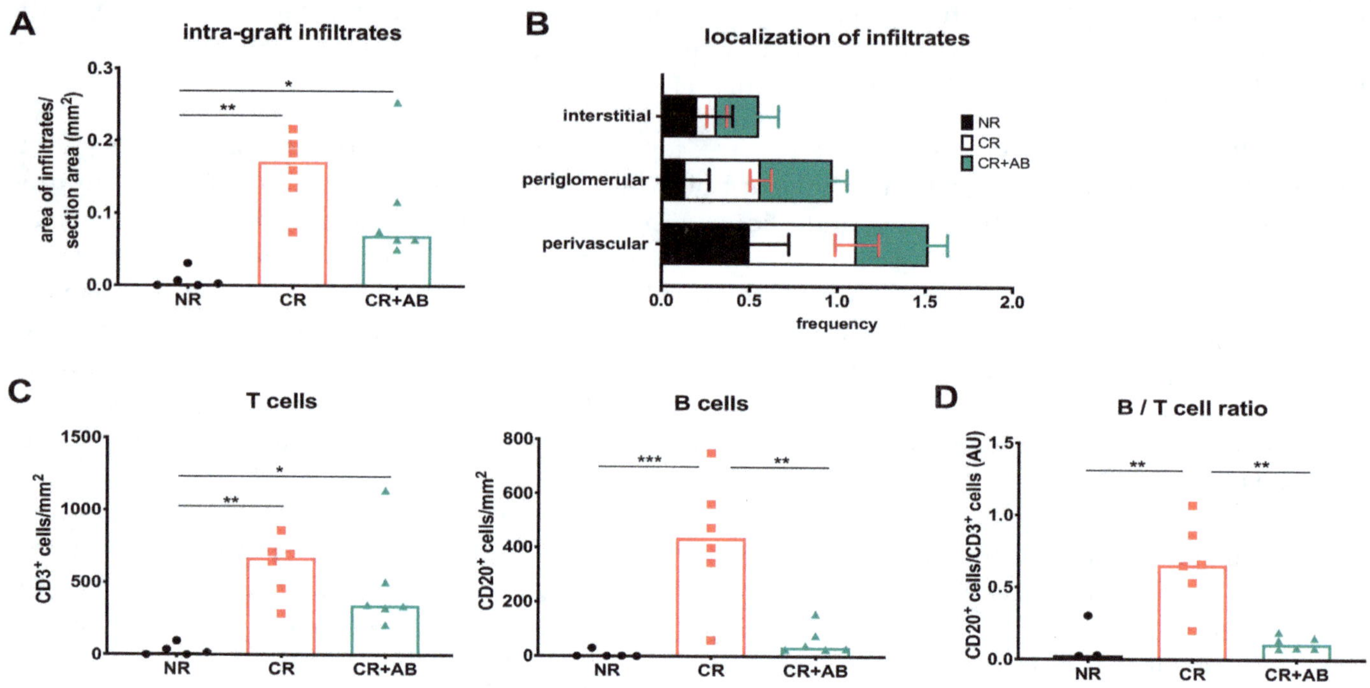

Figure 1. Intra-renal infiltrates, their microanatomical localization, and content of T and B lymphocytes. (**A**) shows intra-renal infiltrate expansion, which was measured using Histoquest software and was expressed as the cumulative area of infiltrates/area of the renal cortex. (**B**) shows the microanatomical localization of infiltrates, which was recorded as perivascular, periglomerular, or interstitial. (**C**) shows the intra-renal content of $CD3^+$ T cells and $CD20^+$ B cells, which was determined using Histoquest software after immunohistochemical staining and normalized to the area of renal cortex. (**D**) shows the ratio of intra-renal B/T cells in arbitrary units (AU). NR, no rejection (black); CR, chronic rejection (pink); CR + AB, chronic rejection and anti-BAFF antibody (green). Data is shown as individual data points per rat and group means. Statistical significance is shown as * $p < 0.05$, ** $p < 0.01$, and *** $p < 0.001$.

2.2. Anti-BAFF Treatment Interfered with TLO Formation

B cells and T cells can organize into distinct zones within infiltrates to form TLOs. We assessed the microanatomical organization of intra-renal T and B cells into T and B cell zones using immunofluorescence microscopy. Figure 2A shows representative images of staining of $CD3^+$ T cells (red), $CD20^+$ B cells (yellow), and $Ki67^+$ proliferating cells (green). In NR, infiltrates were rare and small compared to the other groups. In CR, large infiltrates containing distinct B and T cell zones were found as shown in Figure 2A. Infiltrates after anti-BAFF treatment showed dense T cell zones but a lack of B cell zones. We determined the presence of T and B cell zones per infiltrate, and found that T cell zones were similarly frequent in all groups (Figure 2B), but the frequency of B cell zones within infiltrates was significantly higher in CR compared to NR (CR vs. NR: 0.44 ± 0.20 vs. 0.00 ± 0.00, $p = 0.0001$) but substantially lower with anti-BAFF treatment (CR vs. CR + AB: 0.44 ± 0.20 vs. 0.05 ± 0.06, $p = 0.0002$) (Figure 2B). TLOs were defined by the presence of T and B cell zones, and were absent in NR but significantly elevated in CR (CR vs. NR: 0.44 ± 0.20 vs. 0.00 ± 0.00, $p = 0.0001$) (Figure 2C). However, the frequency of TLO was significantly diminished after anti-BAFF treatment (CR vs. CR + AB: 0.44 ± 0.20 vs. 0.048 ± 0.06, $p = 0.0002$) (Figure 2C).

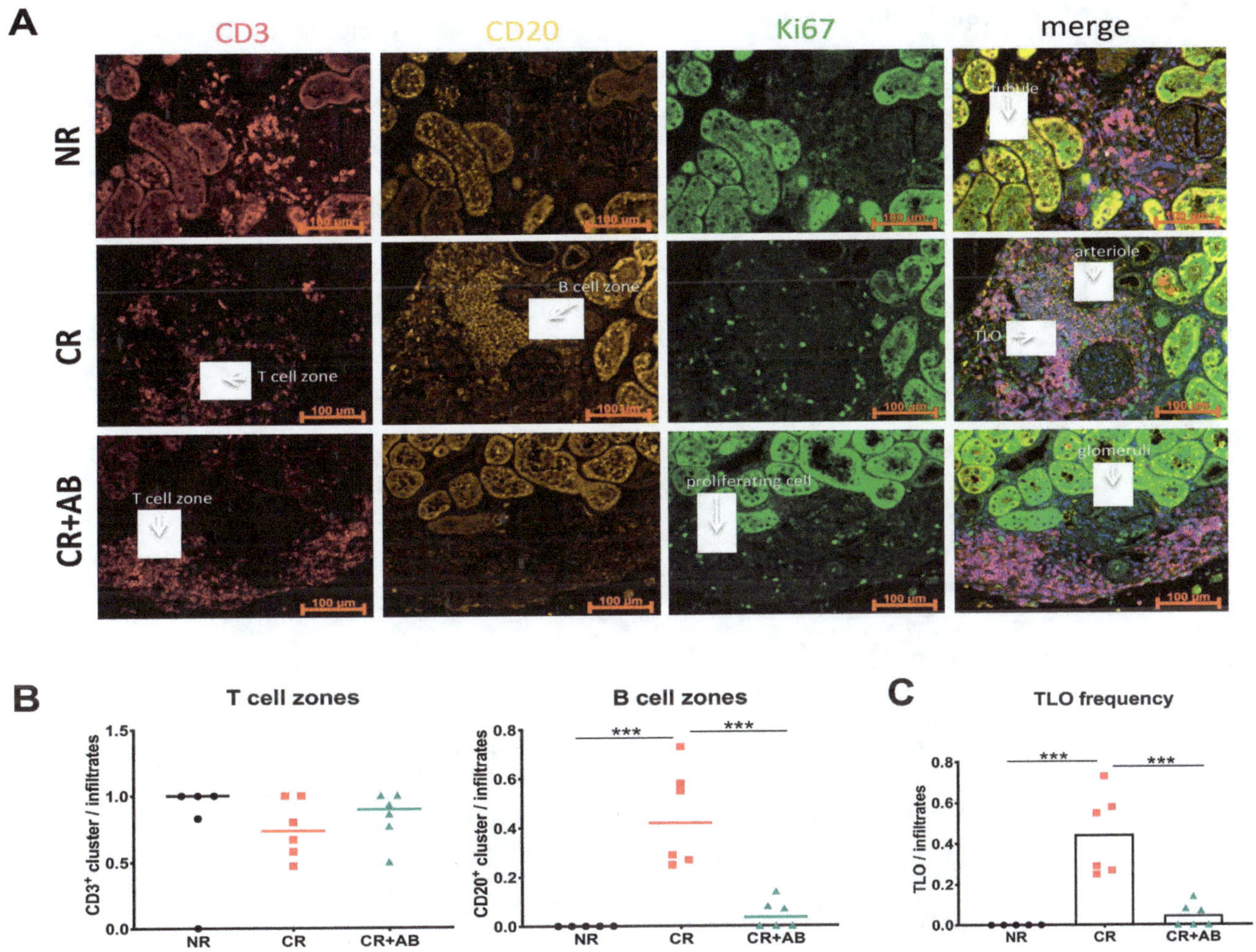

Figure 2. Effect of anti-BAFF treatment on intra-renal T and B cell zones and TLO formation. (**A**) shows representative allograft sections stained for CD3 (T cells, pink), CD20 (B cells, yellow), and Ki67 (proliferating cells, green) with distinct T and B cell zones. (**B**) shows the frequency of T cell ($CD3^+$) and B cell ($CD20^+$) zones, which were defined as dense clusters of predominantly one cell type. (**C**) shows the frequency of TLOs, which were defined as dense intra-renal infiltrates containing a T and a B cell zone. NR, no rejection (black); CR, chronic rejection (pink); CR + AB, chronic rejection and anti-BAFF antibody (green). Data is shown as group means and individual data points per rat. Statistical significance is shown as *** $p < 0.001$.

2.3. Proliferation of Intra-Renal T and B Cells Was Not Altered by Anti-BAFF Treatment

Since the number of B cells was significantly reduced within kidney allografts by anti-BAFF treatment, we were interested in whether anti-BAFF treatment had affected the local proliferation of intra-renal lymphocytes. We therefore analyzed the absolute numbers of proliferating T and B cells by co-staining for the proliferation marker $Ki67^+$. We found that proliferation of T cells was significantly increased in CR and CR + AB compared to NR (CR vs. NR: 31 ± 11 vs. 3 ± 3, $p = 0.0005$; CR + AB vs. NR: 25 ± 10 vs. 3 ± 3, $p = 0.0034$). In B cells, only CR + AB showed significantly increased proliferation compared to NR, while elevation of B cell proliferation in CR was not significant compared to NR (CR + AB vs. NR: 0.11 ± 0.04 vs. 0 ± 00, $p = 0.02$; CR vs. NR: 0.08 ± 0.03 vs. 0 ± 00, $p = 0.137$). However, anti-BAFF treatment did not change the number of proliferating T cells (Figure 3A) or B cells (Figure 3B).

Antigen-activated B cells may clonally proliferate in germinal centers (GCs) when given appropriate T helper cell signals. We analyzed infiltrates for the presence of GCs within TLOs and found that GCs were rare but could be detected in CR, as shown in Figure 3C.

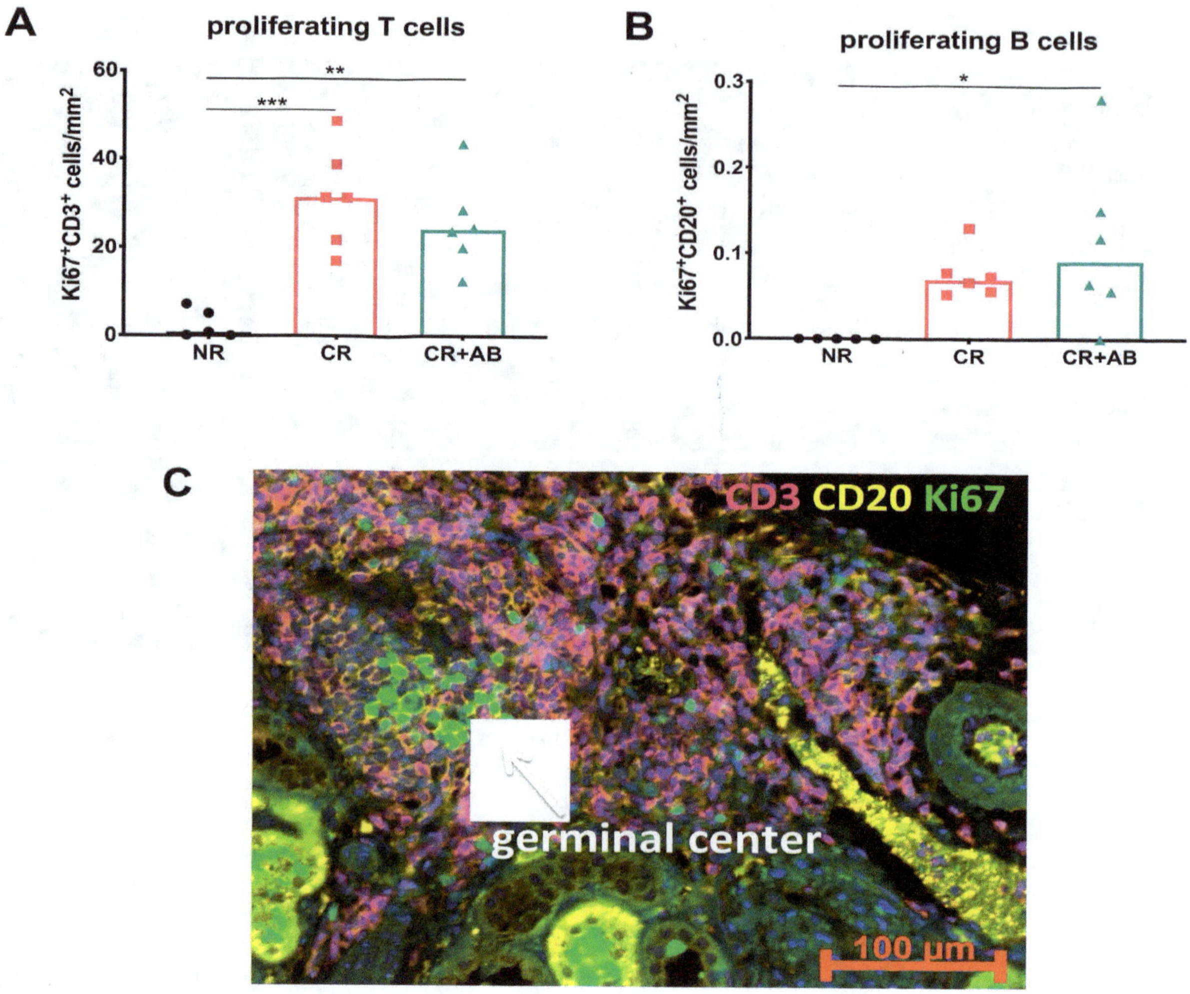

Figure 3. Intra-renal T and B cell proliferation and germinal center (GC) formation within TLOs. (**A**) shows the intra-renal content of proliferating Ki67$^+$CD3$^+$ T cells and (**B**) proliferating Ki67$^+$CD20$^+$ B cells, which were quantified using Histoquest software after immunohistochemical staining and normalized to the area of renal cortex. (**C**) shows a TLO with GC formation, which was defined as a dense cluster of Ki67$^+$ proliferating cells (green) within a CD20$^+$ B cell zone (yellow); the kidney section was from the CR group. NR, no rejection (black); CR, chronic rejection (pink); CR + AB, chronic rejection and anti-BAFF antibody (green). Data is shown as group means and individual data points per rat. Statistical significance is shown as * $p < 0.05$, ** $p < 0.01$, and *** $p < 0.001$.

2.4. *Effect of Anti-BAFF Treatment on Intra-Renal Plasma Cells*

Plasma cells are antibody-producing cells derived from B cells and have been found within kidney allograft infiltrates [24]. We therefore determined the amount of intra-renal plasma cells by staining for IgG$^+$ elliptical cells, as previously described [23]. Plasma cells were present in allografts from all groups and appeared increased in CR compared to NR and CR + AB, but the difference was not statistically significant (Figure 4).

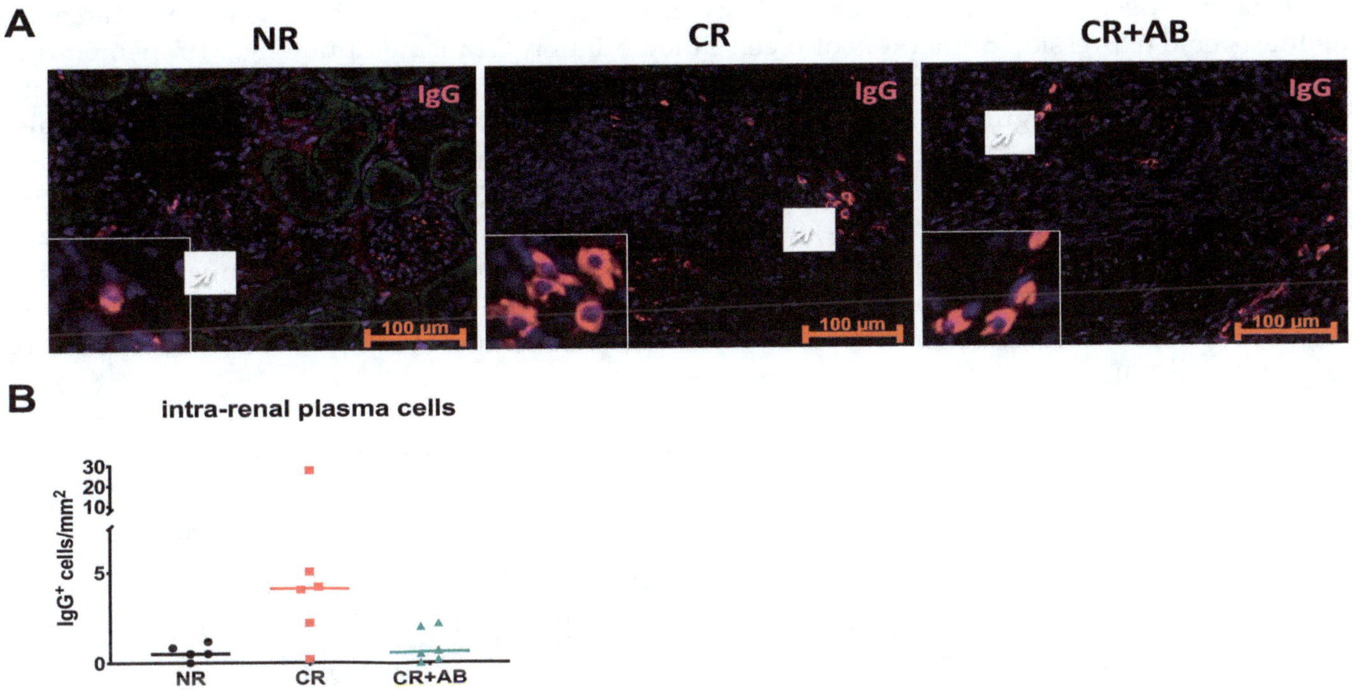

Figure 4. Effect of anti-BAFF treatment on intra-renal plasma cells. (**A**) shows immunofluorescence staining of IgG$^+$ plasma cells typically arranged in small nests within allografts. (**B**) shows the intra-renal content of IgG$^+$ plasma cells, which was determined by blinded manual counting of IgG$^+$ cells and normalized to the renal cortex area. NR, no rejection (black); CR, chronic rejection (pink); CR + AB, chronic rejection and anti-BAFF antibody (green). Data is shown as group means and individual data points per rat.

2.5. Anti-BAFF Treatment Regulated Expression of TLO-Promoting Factors and B Cell Differentiation Markers within Allografts

Since BAFF was required for TLO formation, we were interested in the expression of TLO-promoting factors and B cell activation and differentiation molecules. To this end, we used a heat-map to visualize normalized gene expression (Figure 5). We analyzed the intra-renal mRNA expression of BAFF, its homolog APRIL (a proliferation-inducing ligand), and their receptors, BAFF-R (BAFF receptor), TACI (transmembrane activator and calcium modulator and cyclophilin ligand interactor), and BCMA (B cell maturation antigen). We found that BAFF and its receptors were more strongly expressed in CR than NR, but anti-BAFF treatment led to decreased expression of BAFF-R, TACI, and to a lesser degree BCMA (Figure 5A).

TLO formation is driven by lymphoid chemokines and cytokines. We therefore measured intra-renal mRNA expression of the B cell chemokine CXCL13 and its receptor CXCR5, as well as lymphotoxin-β and the T cell chemokine CCL19 and its receptor CCR7. We found that expression of B cell chemokine CXCL13 and its receptors CXCR5, as well as lymphotoxin-β, was elevated in CR but reduced after anti-BAFF, while expression of T cell chemokine CCL19 and its receptor CCR7 was increased in CR + AB (Figure 5B).

We found evidence of germinal center formation in CR, but anti-BAFF treatment did not affect the number of proliferating B cells within allografts. We therefore analyzed the expression of molecules, which drive B cell proliferation. We found that expression of interleukin (IL)-21, an important T cell cytokine, which stimulates B cell proliferation, was elevated in CR + AB compared to CR (Figure 5C). Similarly, the expression of T cell costimulatory molecules, CD40L (CD40 ligand) and ICOS (inducible T cell costimulator), was higher in CR + AB compared to CR, while expression of corresponding B cell ligands CD40 and ICOS ligand was lower in CR + AB compared to CR (Figure 5C).

Finally, BAFF is a survival factor for B cells at different differentiation stages. Therefore, we assessed the intra-renal expression of markers of B cell differentiation. Transmembrane IgD (transmemIgD) is expressed by immature and naïve B cells and its expression was elevated in CR and substantially reduced in CR + AB (Figure 5D). Pax5 (paired box protein 5), a pan-B cell lineage factor, was also elevated in CR and reduced in CR + AB (Figure 5D). Bcl-6 (B cell lymphoma 6) is expressed by germinal center B cells after activation in B cell follicles and was elevated in CR but lower in CR + AB (Figure 5D). Finally, XBP-1 (X-box binding protein 1) is a transcription factor for differentiating plasma cells and its intra-renal expression was elevated in CR compared to NR, and anti-BAFF treatment reduced its expression compared to CR (Figure 5D). Overall, early B cell differentiation markers appeared to be increased in CR and more strongly reduced by anti-BAFF treatment than markers of later differentiation stages (Figure 5D).

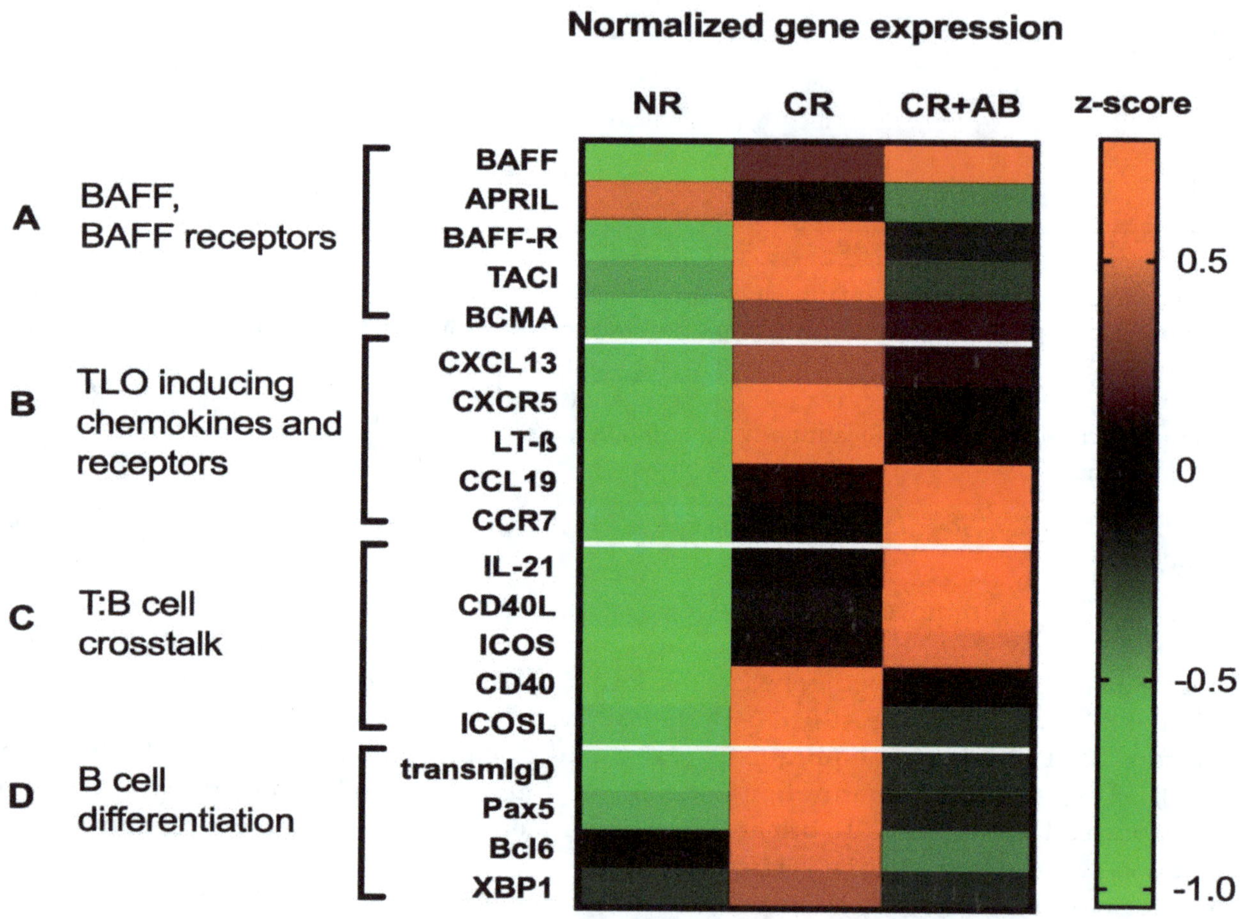

Figure 5. Effect of anti-BAFF treatment on intra-renal gene expression in chronic rejection. A heat-map was used to visualize relative mRNA expression of genes between groups. (**A**) BAFF, APRIL, and their receptors; (**B**) TLO-inducing chemokines and cytokines and receptors; (**C**) molecules of T:B cell crosstalk; (**D**) markers of B cell differentiation. MRNA expression of target genes was normalized to the house-keeper hypoxanthine-guanine-phosphoribosyl-transferase (HPRT,). The z-score was calculated from delta CT values per sample using the mean of all samples. Average z-scores from each group are shown using the indicated color scale for up- or downregulation.

Since we saw no significant difference in the amount of T cells present within allografts (Figure 1) or their proliferation rate (Figure 3) with or without anti-BAFF treatment, we analyzed the expression of molecules associated with T cell function by qPCR. We found no difference in the expression of interleukin-2, interferon-γ, interleukin-21, TGF-β, granzyme B, perforin, or foxp3 with or without anti-BAFF treatment (data not shown).

3. Discussion

TLOs are sites of adaptive alloimmune activation and have been detected in failed kidney allografts with chronic rejection [11]. We tested if BAFF is required for TLO formation in a model of chronic kidney allograft rejection in rats. Our results showed that intra-renal infiltrates were more frequent in chronic rejection than in non-rejecting allografts and included TLOs with distinct T and B cell zones. Furthermore, we observed B cell germinal center formation within TLOs. Anti-BAFF treatment diminished the number of intra-renal B cells and effectively blocked the formation of B cell zones and TLOs. Gene expression analysis showed that intra-renal expression of BAFF receptors and TLO-promoting factors was elevated in CR but diminished by anti-BAFF treatment. We found that B cells in early differentiation stages were particularly sensitive to anti-BAFF treatment. In summary, we showed that TLOs harbor local activation of alloresponses and that BAFF is required for TLO formation in chronic rejection.

In fully immunosuppressed non-rejecting allografts, intra-renal infiltrates were virtually absent; however, there was significant expansion of infiltrates within allografts in chronic rejection. Intra-renal infiltrates were most frequently found in the vicinity of arterioles, suggesting leukopedesis across existing blood vessels, rather than sprouting of high endothelial venules, which have been described in TLOs [14]. Anti-BAFF treatment did not affect the expansion of intra-renal infiltrates; it did, however, lead to a significant reduction in the number of intra-renal B cells and a lower B/T cell ratio.

Detailed analysis of the microanatomical organization of intra-renal T and B cells showed that a large portion of infiltrates consisted of distinct T and B cell zones forming lymphoid follicle-like structures or TLOs. Staining of the proliferation marker Ki67 revealed that germinal centers, or areas of clonal proliferation of antigen-specific B cells, could form within these TLOs in our model. Germinal centers are highly advanced structures, which arise from coordinated T:B cell crosstalk [25]. It is within germinal centers that B cells get fully activated, go through somatic hypermutation, get positively selected for the highest antibody affinity for alloantigens, and differentiate into antibody-secreting plasma cells and memory B cells [26]. Cheng et al. have previously shown that TLOs can harbor such diversification and clonal expansion of alloimmune responses in allografts [16]. Our results showed that anti-BAFF treatment can effectively prevent the formation of intra-renal TLOs, since B cell zones were mostly absent in anti-BAFF-treated rats. Although TLO formation has been observed in cardiac transplant models in mice [27], this is the first kidney transplant model showing TLO formation in chronic rejection. As such, the findings from our study may provide a basis for further investigation into the role of TLOs in kidney transplant rejection.

We were interested in the mechanism by which anti-BAFF treatment prevented TLO formation in allografts. There are three known receptors for BAFF and its homolog APRIL: BAFF-R, TACI, and BCMA, as reviewed by Parsons [28]. We found that the intra-renal expression of BAFF receptors was significantly lower after anti-BAFF treatment, which illustrated the dependency of BAFF receptor-expressing cells on the presence of BAFF as a survival factor. Whether there was a shortage of infiltrating B cells into allografts or intra-renal B cells locally succumbed to cell death in the absence of BAFF could not be determined by our experiments. CXCL13, a B cell chemokine that promotes TLO formation, was highly expressed during chronic rejection, but expression appeared lower after anti-BAFF treatment. The expression of CXCR5, the receptor for CXCL13, was also lower after anti-BAFF treatment. Furthermore, B cells are potent producers of lymphotoxin-β, an important factor for secondary and tertiary lymphoid organ formation [29,30]. The expression of lymphotoxin-β was elevated in chronic rejection but substantially diminished after anti-BAFF antibody. The regulation of these factors may have played in important role in preventing the development of TLO in anti-BAFF-treated rats in our model.

Intra-renal mRNA expression of B cell differentiation markers showed that anti-BAFF treatment strongly affected B cells at early differentiation stages and to a lesser extent reduced expression of advanced differentiation markers. Transmembrane IgD is expressed by immature transitional and naïve B cells. We found elevated transmembrane IgD expression in chronic rejection, reflecting the infiltration of these cells into allografts. Interestingly, expression of intra-renal transmembrane IgD was substantially reduced by anti-BAFF treatment. We also found increased expression of Pax5, a pan-B cell lineage transcription factor, within allografts with chronic rejection but a significant reduction of its expression after anti-BAFF treatment. Interestingly, the transcription factor Bcl-6 was also upregulated during chronic rejection but downregulated by anti-BAFF treatment. Bcl-6 is expressed in lymphoid follicles by germinal center B cells and T follicular helper cells, which provide essential activation signals to B cells, as reviewed by Vinuesa [31]. Bcl-6 is therefore a necessary factor for full activation of humoral alloresponses. Decreased Bcl-6 expression in rats treated with anti-BAFF antibody could reflect decreased humoral immune activation in allografts due to a lack of TLOs. Finally, expression of XBP-1, a transcription factor expressed during plasma cell differentiation [32], was elevated in chronic rejection. XBP-1 expression was also reduced in anti-BAFF, but the difference was much less pronounced compared with factors of early B cell differentiation. We investigated the presence of plasma cells within allografts in our model. Although the exact effector function of intra-renal plasma cells and their role in allograft rejection is not fully understood, intra-renal plasma cells have been associated with chronic allograft rejection and poor prognosis [24,33–36]. Although we have previously shown that anti-BAFF therapy reduced the number of splenic plasma cells [23], the difference in intra-renal plasma cells between groups was not statistically significant in this study. In summary, we found that intra-renal B cells during early differentiation stages were particularly sensitive to anti-BAFF treatment.

Signals required for B cell proliferation include antigen-activation, T cell help, and cytokines, but not BAFF, which was reflected by our data showing that B cell proliferation was not altered by anti-BAFF treatment. Analysis of B cell differentiation factors showed that early antigen-naïve B cells were particularly reduced by anti-BAFF treatment, suggesting that the remaining B cells were already antigen-activated. Proliferation of antigen-activated B cells depends on the expression of important signals by T helper cells, namely CD40L and IL-21. In line with this, we found that the relative expression of CD40L and IL-21 was not decreased by anti-BAFF treatment, demonstrating a potentially important gap in the mechanism of BAFF. This observation may point towards a shortcoming of BAFF-targeted therapy and raise interest in combining targets for therapy.

We demonstrated that TLOs are sites of humoral immune activation within allografts during chronic rejection, and that anti-BAFF treatment can hinder the formation of TLO in allografts. Belimumab®, a monoclonal anti-BAFF antibody, has been approved for treatment of lupus erythematodes and has been explored as an immunosuppressive agent in kidney transplant patients [37]. Our study shows that TLO formation may be prevented using an anti-BAFF antibody with a potential benefit to kidney transplant patients. We previously reported that anti-BAFF treatment interfered with systemic humoral responses and reduced formation of DSA of certain IgG subclasses in a Ktx model, but we found no direct evidence for any specific alteration in T cell function and it did not significantly affect allograft rejection according to Banff or allograft function [23]. A limitation of our study is the duration of our experiment. Extending experiments beyond d56 post-transplant may provide insight into the long-term effects of anti-BAFF treatment on cellular responses within allografts. To assess the long-term benefits of such an intervention, further investigation is needed.

4. Materials and Methods

4.1. Experimental Kidney Transplantation

Animal experiments were approved by the local inspecting authorities (Regierung von Unterfranken, No. 55.2-2532-2-47, 30-06-2015) and performed according to German animal protection laws and NIH's laboratory animal care principles. In brief, a previously described MHC-mismatched rat kidney transplantation model was used [22,23], in which male Brown Norway rats (BN) served as donors and male Lewis rats (LEW) as recipients (Charles River Laboratories, Sulzfeld, Germany, 200–250 g). Kidney transplantation was performed orthotopically as previously described [38].

Rats were either treated with daily cyclosporine A (CsA) at 10 mg/kg body weight (Neoral, Novartis, Basel, Switzerland), administered once daily by gavage (no rejection group, NR), or they received CsA 5 mg/kg daily until d6, then on every 2nd day to induce DSA and chronic rejection (CR). In addition, one group received CsA 5 mg/kg daily until d6, then on every 2nd day, and in addition a monoclonal anti-BAFF antibody (GSK, Hamburg, Germany) was injected in the peritoneal cavity on d3, d17, d31, and d45 after Ktx (CR + AB), as previously described [23]. Experimental groups are shown in Table 1 below. Rats were sacrificed on d56 after Ktx and allografts were harvested.

Table 1. Experimental groups.

Group	Abbreviation	n=
Ktx CsA 10 mg/kg/d d56 (no rejection)	NR	5
Ktx CsA 5 mg/kg/2nd d d56 (chronic rejection)	CR	6
Ktx CsA 5 mg/kg/2nd d d56 + anti-BAFF antibody (chronic rejection + anti-BAFF antibody)	CR + AB	6

4.2. Histology, Immunohistochemistry, and Immunofluorescence

Immunohistochemistry was performed on 3-µm formalin-fixed paraffin-embedded sections as previously described [39]. T cells were stained with rabbit anti-rat CD3 antibody (Abcam, ab5690, Cambridge, UK) and donkey anti-rabbit-Cy5 (Dianova, 711-175-152, Hamburg, Germany). B cells were stained with mouse anti-rat CD20 antibody (Santa Cruz, sc-393894, Heidelberg, Germany), goat anti-mouse-biotin (Thermofisher 31804), and Strep-Cy3 (Dianova, 016-160-084, Hamburg, Germany). Proliferation was stained using anti-Ki67-FITC (ebioscience, 11-5698), and plasma cells were stained using anti-rat-IgG-AlexaFluor647 (Thermofischer A21472, Waltham, MA, USA). Images were taken using a Zeiss observer Z.1 Fluorescence microscope at 20× magnification. Digital images from 10 high power fields (HPFs) per specimen were examined as previously described [39]. Using Histoquest® software (TissueGnostics GmbH, Vienna, Austria), the number of $CD20^+$, $CD3^+$, $Ki67^+CD20^+$, and $Ki67^+CD3^+$ cells were quantified within a defined section area. Intra-renal B cell ($CD20^+$) and T cell ($CD3^+$) zones were defined as dense clusters of predominantly one cell type (min. 20 cells/0.004 mm^2). TLO were defined as dense intra-renal infiltrates containing a T and B cell zone. Germinal centers (GCs) were defined as dense clusters of $Ki67^+$ proliferating cells within a B cell zone. The presence of T and B cell zones and GC was determined per infiltrate in a blinded manner. Intra-renal IgG^+ plasma cells, identified by strong intracellular IgG-positivity and typical cell shape, were counted manually in a blinded manner.

4.3. Real-Time PCR

Frozen tissue sections were homogenized using a RNeasy MiniKit® (cat. 74106, Qiagen, Hilden, Germany). Total RNA was extracted, and genomic DNA digested. Total RNA was reverse transcribed into cDNA. RT-PCR was performed on a ViiA7 detection system (Applied Biosystems, Darmstadt, Germany) using a QuantiTect SYBR Green PCR Kit (Qiagen, Hilden, Germany). The sequences of the primers are listed in Table S1). Copy numbers of target genes were normalized to the house-keeper gene hypoxanthine-guanine-phosphoribosyl-transferase (HPRT) and delta CT values were calculated. The z-score was calculated from delta CT values for each sample and target gene using the formula $z = (\chi - \mu)/\sigma$. Mean z-scores from each experimental group are shown in a heat map using a color scale for up- or downregulation of gene expression.

4.4. Statistical Analysis

Values are provided as individual data points and mean and SD. Statistical significance was calculated using Graphpad Prism software (Version 8.0, San Diego, CA, USA) using ANOVA; $p < 0.05$ was considered to be statistically significant.

Author Contributions: L.S. designed experiments, performed data analysis and interpretation and prepared the manuscript. H.P. performed rat operations and treatments. M.H. analyzed intra-renal cell proliferation. A.S. assisted in data analysis and reviewed the manuscript. B.B. contributed to data interpretation and reviewed the manuscript. T.B. designed experiments, interpreted data and reviewed the manuscript. All authors have read and agreed to the published version of the manuscript.

Acknowledgments: We thank Stefanie Ellmann and Alexandra Müller for their technical support.

Abbreviations

AB	antibody
ABMR	antibody-mediated rejection
APRIL	a proliferation inducing ligand
BAFF	B cell activating factor
BAFF-R	BAFF receptor
Bcl-6	B cell lymphoma 6
BCMA	B cell maturation antigen
BN	Brown Norway rat
CD	cluster of differentiation
CD40L	CD40 ligand
CR	chronic rejection
CR + AB	chronic rejection + anti-BAFF antibody
CsA	cyclosporine A
HPRT	hypoxanthine-guanine-phosphoribosyl-transferase
GC	germinal center
ICOS	inducible T cell costimulator
ICOSL	ICOS ligand
IFTA	interstitial fibrosis and tubular atrophy
Ig	immunoglobulin
IL	interleukin
Ktx	kidney transplantation
LEW	Lewis rat
MHC	major histocompatibility complex
NR	no rejection
Pax5	paired box protein 5
SLE	systemic lupus erythematosus
TACI	transmembrane activator and calcium modulator and cyclophilin ligand interactor
TLO	tertiary lymphoid organs
XBP-1	X-box binding protein 1

References

1. Gondos, A.; Dohler, B.; Brenner, H.; Opelz, G. Kidney graft survival in Europe and the United States: Strikingly different long-term outcomes. *Transplantation* **2013**, *95*, 267–274. [CrossRef] [PubMed]
2. Lefaucheur, C.; Loupy, A.; Hill, G.S.; Andrade, J.; Nochy, D.; Antoine, C.; Gautreau, C.; Charron, D.; Glotz, D.; Suberbielle-Boissel, C. Preexisting donor-specific HLA antibodies predict outcome in kidney transplantation. *J. Am. Soc. Nephrol.* **2010**, *21*, 1398–1406. [CrossRef] [PubMed]

3. Sellares, J.; Reeve, J.; Loupy, A.; Mengel, M.; Sis, B.; Skene, A.; de Freitas, D.G.; Kreepala, C.; Hidalgo, L.G.; Famulski, K.S.; et al. Molecular diagnosis of antibody-mediated rejection in human kidney transplants. *Am. J. Transplant.* **2013**, *13*, 971–983. [CrossRef] [PubMed]
4. Mannon, R.B.; Matas, A.J.; Grande, J.; Leduc, R.; Connett, J.; Kasiske, B.; Cecka, J.M.; Gaston, R.S.; Cosio, F.; Gourishankar, S.; et al. Inflammation in areas of tubular atrophy in kidney allograft biopsies: A potent predictor of allograft failure. *Am. J. Transplant.* **2010**, *10*, 2066–2073. [CrossRef] [PubMed]
5. Shishido, S.; Asanuma, H.; Nakai, H.; Mori, Y.; Satoh, H.; Kamimaki, I.; Hataya, H.; Ikeda, M.; Honda, M.; Hasegawa, A. The impact of repeated subclinical acute rejection on the progression of chronic allograft nephropathy. *J. Am. Soc. Nephrol.* **2003**, *14*, 1046–1052. [CrossRef] [PubMed]
6. Park, W.D.; Griffin, M.D.; Cornell, L.D.; Cosio, F.G.; Stegall, M.D. Fibrosis with inflammation at one year predicts transplant functional decline. *J. Am. Soc. Nephrol.* **2010**, *21*, 1987–1997. [CrossRef]
7. Tse, G.H.; Johnston, C.J.; Kluth, D.; Gray, M.; Gray, D.; Hughes, J.; Marson, L.P. Intrarenal B Cell Cytokines Promote Transplant Fibrosis and Tubular Atrophy. *Am. J. Transplant.* **2015**, *15*, 3067–3080. [CrossRef]
8. Sarwal, M.; Chua, M.S.; Kambham, N.; Hsieh, S.C.; Satterwhite, T.; Masek, M.; Salvatierra, O., Jr. Molecular heterogeneity in acute renal allograft rejection identified by DNA microarray profiling. *N. Engl. J. Med.* **2003**, *349*, 125–138. [CrossRef]
9. Hueso, M.; Navarro, E.; Moreso, F.; O'Valle, F.; Perez-Riba, M.; Del Moral, R.G.; Grinyo, J.M.; Seron, D. Intragraft expression of the IL-10 gene is up-regulated in renal protocol biopsies with early interstitial fibrosis, tubular atrophy, and subclinical rejection. *Am. J. Pathol.* **2010**, *176*, 1696–1704. [CrossRef]
10. Thaunat, O.; Field, A.C.; Dai, J.; Louedec, L.; Patey, N.; Bloch, M.F.; Mandet, C.; Belair, M.F.; Bruneval, P.; Meilhac, O.; et al. Lymphoid neogenesis in chronic rejection: Evidence for a local humoral alloimmune response. *Proc. Natl. Acad. Sci. USA* **2005**, *102*, 14723–14728. [CrossRef]
11. Thaunat, O.; Patey, N.; Caligiuri, G.; Gautreau, C.; Mamani-Matsuda, M.; Mekki, Y.; Dieu-Nosjean, M.C.; Eberl, G.; Ecochard, R.; Michel, J.B.; et al. Chronic rejection triggers the development of an aggressive intragraft immune response through recapitulation of lymphoid organogenesis. *J. Immunol.* **2010**, *185*, 717–728. [CrossRef] [PubMed]
12. Thaunat, O.; Graff-Dubois, S.; Brouard, S.; Gautreau, C.; Varthaman, A.; Fabien, N.; Field, A.C.; Louedec, L.; Dai, J.; Joly, E.; et al. Immune responses elicited in tertiary lymphoid tissues display distinctive features. *PLoS ONE* **2010**, *5*, e11398. [CrossRef]
13. Pitzalis, C.; Jones, G.W.; Bombardieri, M.; Jones, S.A. Ectopic lymphoid-like structures in infection, cancer and autoimmunity. *Nat. Rev. Immunol.* **2014**, *14*, 447–462. [CrossRef] [PubMed]
14. Luther, S.A.; Bidgol, A.; Hargreaves, D.C.; Schmidt, A.; Xu, Y.; Paniyadi, J.; Matloubian, M.; Cyster, J.G. Differing activities of homeostatic chemokines CCL19, CCL21, and CXCL12 in lymphocyte and dendritic cell recruitment and lymphoid neogenesis. *J. Immunol.* **2002**, *169*, 424–433. [CrossRef] [PubMed]
15. Ziegler, E.; Gueler, F.; Rong, S.; Mengel, M.; Witzke, O.; Kribben, A.; Haller, H.; Kunzendorf, U.; Krautwald, S. CCL19-IgG prevents allograft rejection by impairment of immune cell trafficking. *J. Am. Soc. Nephrol.* **2006**, *17*, 2521–2532. [CrossRef]
16. Cheng, J.; Torkamani, A.; Grover, R.K.; Jones, T.M.; Ruiz, D.I.; Schork, N.J.; Quigley, M.M.; Hall, F.W.; Salomon, D.R.; Lerner, R.A. Ectopic B-cell clusters that infiltrate transplanted human kidneys are clonal. *Proc. Natl. Acad. Sci. USA* **2011**, *108*, 5560–5565. [CrossRef] [PubMed]
17. Koenig, A.; Thaunat, O. Lymphoid Neogenesis and Tertiary Lymphoid Organs in Transplanted Organs. *Front. Immunol.* **2016**, *7*, 646. [CrossRef]
18. Thaunat, O.; Patey, N.; Gautreau, C.; Lechaton, S.; Fremeaux-Bacchi, V.; Dieu-Nosjean, M.C.; Cassuto-Viguier, E.; Legendre, C.; Delahousse, M.; Lang, P.; et al. B cell survival in intragraft tertiary lymphoid organs after rituximab therapy. *Transplantation* **2008**, *85*, 1648–1653. [CrossRef]
19. Mackay, F.; Figgett, W.A.; Saulep, D.; Lepage, M.; Hibbs, M.L. B-cell stage and context-dependent requirements for survival signals from BAFF and the B-cell receptor. *Immunol. Rev.* **2010**, *237*, 205–225. [CrossRef]
20. Irure-Ventura, J.; San Segundo, D.; Rodrigo, E.; Merino, D.; Belmar-Vega, L.; Ruiz San Millán, J.C.; Valero, R.; Benito, A.; López-Hoyos, M. High Pretransplant BAFF Levels and B-cell Subset Polarized towards a Memory Phenotype as Predictive Biomarkers for Antibody-Mediated Rejection. *Int. J. Mol. Sci.* **2020**, *21*, 779. [CrossRef]

21. Friebus-Kardash, J.; Wilde, B.; Keles, D.; Heinold, A.; Kribben, A.; Witzke, O.; Heinemann, F.M.; Eisenberger, U. Pretransplant serum BAFF levels are associated with pretransplant HLA immunization and renal allograft survival. *Transpl. Immunol.* **2018**, *47*, 10–17. [CrossRef] [PubMed]
22. Kuhne, L.; Jung, B.; Poth, H.; Schuster, A.; Wurm, S.; Ruemmele, P.; Banas, B.; Bergler, T. Renal allograft rejection, lymphocyte infiltration, and de novo donor-specific antibodies in a novel model of non-adherence to immunosuppressive therapy. *BMC Immunol.* **2017**, *18*, 52. [CrossRef] [PubMed]
23. Steines, L.; Poth, H.; Schuster, A.; Geissler, E.K.; Amann, K.; Banas, B.; Bergler, T. Anti-BAFF Treatment Interferes With Humoral Responses in a Model of Renal Transplantation in Rats. *Transplantation* **2020**, *104*, e16–e22. [CrossRef] [PubMed]
24. Hasegawa, J.; Honda, K.; Omoto, K.; Wakai, S.; Shirakawa, H.; Okumi, M.; Ishida, H.; Fuchinoue, S.; Hattori, M.; Tanabe, K. Clinical and Pathological Features of Plasma Cell-Rich Acute Rejection After Kidney Transplantation. *Transplantation* **2018**, *102*, 853–859. [CrossRef] [PubMed]
25. Kwun, J.; Manook, M.; Page, E.; Burghuber, C.; Hong, J.; Knechtle, S.J. Crosstalk Between T and B Cells in the Germinal Center After Transplantation. *Transplantation* **2017**, *101*, 704–712. [CrossRef]
26. Krautler, N.J.; Suan, D.; Butt, D.; Bourne, K.; Hermes, J.R.; Chan, T.D.; Sundling, C.; Kaplan, W.; Schofield, P.; Jackson, J.; et al. Differentiation of germinal center B cells into plasma cells is initiated by high-affinity antigen and completed by Tfh cells. *J. Exp. Med.* **2017**, *214*, 1259–1267. [CrossRef]
27. Baddoura, F.K.; Nasr, I.W.; Wrobel, B.; Li, Q.; Ruddle, N.H.; Lakkis, F.G. Lymphoid neogenesis in murine cardiac allografts undergoing chronic rejection. *Am. J. Transplant.* **2005**, *5*, 510–516. [CrossRef]
28. Parsons, R.F.; Vivek, K.; Redfield, R.R.; 3rd Migone, T.S.; Cancro, M.P.; Naji, A.; Noorchashm, H. B-lymphocyte homeostasis and BLyS-directed immunotherapy in transplantation. *Transplant. Rev.* **2010**, *24*, 207–221. [CrossRef]
29. Ngo, V.N.; Korner, H.; Gunn, M.D.; Schmidt, K.N.; Riminton, D.S.; Cooper, M.D.; Browning, J.L.; Sedgwick, J.D.; Cyster, J.G. Lymphotoxin alpha/beta and tumor necrosis factor are required for stromal cell expression of homing chemokines in B and T cell areas of the spleen. *J. Exp. Med.* **1999**, *189*, 403–412. [CrossRef]
30. Grabner, R.; Lotzer, K.; Dopping, S.; Hildner, M.; Radke, D.; Beer, M.; Spanbroek, R.; Lippert, B.; Reardon, C.A.; Getz, G.S.; et al. Lymphotoxin beta receptor signaling promotes tertiary lymphoid organogenesis in the aorta adventitia of aged ApoE-/- mice. *J. Exp. Med.* **2009**, *206*, 233–248. [CrossRef]
31. Vinuesa, C.G.; Linterman, M.A.; Yu, D.; MacLennan, I.C. Follicular Helper T Cells. *Annu. Rev. Immunol.* **2016**, *34*, 335–368. [CrossRef] [PubMed]
32. Reimold, A.M.; Iwakoshi, N.N.; Manis, J.; Vallabhajosyula, P.; Szomolanyi-Tsuda, E.; Gravallese, E.M.; Friend, D.; Grusby, M.J.; Alt, F.; Glimcher, L.H. Plasma cell differentiation requires the transcription factor XBP-1. *Nature* **2001**, *412*, 300–307. [CrossRef] [PubMed]
33. Wehner, J.R.; Fox-Talbot, K.; Halushka, M.K.; Ellis, C.; Zachary, A.A.; Baldwin, W.M., 3rd. B cells and plasma cells in coronaries of chronically rejected cardiac transplants. *Transplantation* **2010**, *89*, 1141–1148. [CrossRef] [PubMed]
34. Einecke, G.; Reeve, J.; Mengel, M.; Sis, B.; Bunnag, S.; Mueller, T.F.; Halloran, P.F. Expression of B cell and immunoglobulin transcripts is a feature of inflammation in late allografts. *Am. J. Transplant.* **2008**, *8*, 1434–1443. [CrossRef] [PubMed]
35. Desvaux, D.; Le Gouvello, S.; Pastural, M.; Abtahi, M.; Suberbielle, C.; Boeri, N.; Rémy, P.; Salomon, L.; Lang, P.; Baron, C. Acute renal allograft rejections with major interstitial oedema and plasma cell-rich infiltrates: High gamma-interferon expression and poor clinical outcome. *Nephrol. Dial. Transplant.* **2004**, *19*, 933–939. [CrossRef]
36. Hamada, A.M.; Yamamoto, I.; Kawabe, M.; Katsumata, H.; Yamakawa, T.; Katsuma, A.; Nakada, Y.; Kobayashi, A.; Koike, Y.; Miki, J.; et al. Clinicopathological features and outcomes of kidney allografts in plasma cell-rich acute rejection: A case series. *Nephrology* **2018**, *23*, 22–26. [CrossRef]
37. Banham, G.D.; Flint, S.M.; Torpey, N.; Lyons, P.A.; Shanahan, D.N.; Gibson, A.; Watson CJ, E.; O'Sullivan, A.M.; Chadwick, J.A.; Foster, K.E.; et al. Belimumab in kidney transplantation: An experimental medicine, randomised, placebo-controlled phase 2 trial. *Lancet* **2018**, *391*, 2619–2630. [CrossRef]
38. Bergler, T.; Hoffmann, U.; Bergler, E.; Jung, B.; Banas, M.C.; Reinhold, S.W.; Kramer, B.K.; Banas, B. Toll-like receptor 4 in experimental kidney transplantation: Early mediator of endogenous danger signals. *Nephron Exp. Nephrol.* **2012**, *121*, e59–e70. [CrossRef]

12

Toll-Like Receptor as a Potential Biomarker in Renal Diseases

Sebastian Mertowski [1,*], Paulina Lipa [2], Izabela Morawska [1], Paulina Niedźwiedzka-Rystwej [3,*], Dominika Bębnowska [3], Rafał Hrynkiewicz [3], Ewelina Grywalska [1,*], Jacek Roliński [1] and Wojciech Załuska [4]

1 Department of Clinical Immunology and Immunotherapy, Medical University of Lublin, 20-093 Lublin, Poland; izabelamorawska19@gmail.com (I.M.); jacek.rolinski@gmail.com (J.R.)

2 Department of Genetics and Microbiology, Institute of Microbiology and Biotechnology, Faculty of Biology and Biotechnology, Maria Curie-Skłodowska University, Akademicka 19 St., 20-033 Lublin, Poland; paulina.lipa56@gmail.com

3 Institute of Biology, University of Szczecin, Felczaka 3c, 71-412 Szczecin, Poland; bebnowska.d@wp.pl (D.B.); rafal.hrynkiewicz@gmail.com (R.H.)

4 Department of Nephrology, Medical University of Lublin, 20-954 Lublin, Poland; wojciech.zaluska@umlub.pl

* Correspondence: mertowskisebastian@gmail.com (S.M.); paulina.niedzwiedzka-rystwej@usz.edu.pl (P.N.-R.); ewelina.grywalska@gmail.com (E.G.)

Abstract: One of the major challenges faced by modern nephrology is the identification of biomarkers associated with histopathological patterns or defined pathogenic mechanisms that may assist in the non-invasive diagnosis of kidney disease, particularly glomerulopathy. The identification of such molecules may allow prognostic subgroups to be established based on the type of disease, thereby predicting response to treatment or disease relapse. Advances in understanding the pathogenesis of diseases, such as membranous nephropathy, minimal change disease, focal segmental glomerulosclerosis, IgA (immunoglobulin A) nephropathy, and diabetic nephropathy, along with the progressive development and standardization of plasma and urine proteomics techniques, have facilitated the identification of an increasing number of molecules that may be useful for these purposes. The growing number of studies on the role of TLR (toll-like receptor) receptors in the pathogenesis of kidney disease forces contemporary researchers to reflect on these molecules, which may soon join the group of renal biomarkers and become a helpful tool in the diagnosis of glomerulopathy. In this article, we conducted a thorough review of the literature on the role of TLRs in the pathogenesis of glomerulopathy. The role of TLR receptors as potential marker molecules for the development of neoplastic diseases is emphasized more and more often, as prognostic factors in diseases on several epidemiological backgrounds.

Keywords: acute kidney injury; biomarker; diabetic nephropathy; focal segmental glomerulosclerosis; innate immunity; membranous nephropathy; minimal change diseases; TLR

---

1. Introduction

The term "biological marker" in the literature refers to the objective health status of the patient, which can be observed from the outside, i.e., in a way that can be measured in an extremely accurate and, most importantly, repeatable manner. Various medical symptoms can often contrast with each other, or, on the contrary, correlations between them are observed, which may contribute to a better and faster diagnosis of the disease or the effectiveness of the treatment process. A joint project of the World Health Organization together with the United Nations under the name of the International Program on Chemical Safety has attempted to standardize the term biomarker used in the literature.

Currently, a biomarker is defined as "any substance, structure or process that can be measured in the body or its products and that can influence or predict the occurrence of an outcome or disease" [1], which means that the modern definition of biomarkers covers every response of the body, whether functional, physiological, or biochemical, to the occurrence of a potential threat (physical, chemical, or biological) that may modify the body's reactions at the cellular or molecular level. Usually, biomarker is used with two meanings: (1) A biomarker is a component (analyte) of a human biological system (i.e., plasma, urine, etc.); or (2) a biomarker is a biological property (i.e., mass concentration of X in plasma) [2]. Currently, examples of biomarkers can be both simple parameters of heart rate and blood pressure, as well as the determination of complex constituent molecules present in our blood or tissues, which are indicative of health. Types and applications of biomarkers are constantly changing as it evaluates our knowledge about them. Thus, it has recently been shown that counts of urinary T-cell, renal tubular epithelial cells, and podocalyxin-positive cells provide an excellent biomarker for the detection of renal transplant rejection in routine clinical trials [3]. Currently, the role of TLR receptors as potential marker molecules for the development of neoplastic diseases is emphasized more and more often, e.g., TLR5 as a prognostic marker for gastric cancer [4]. It was also shown that the activity of TLR receptor is correlated with the state of injury of post-surgical patients who have a disorder of the immune response related to the interaction of TLR receptors with DAMP (damage-associated molecular pattern). Moreover, the analyses led to conclusions regarding the role of TLR receptors in predicting pathological conditions, including tissue damage, in these patients [5]. One of the increasing threats in today's world is chronic kidney disease, the cause of which may be both primary processes related to the kidneys, and secondary processes observed in the course of rheumatic, cardiological, or diabetic diseases. As indicated in the literature, one of the largest causes of the development of chronic kidney disease in highly developed countries as well as in developing countries is hypertension and type 2 diabetes, currently classified as diseases of civilization [6]. As far as type 2 diabetes and renal disorders are concerned, it was shown that polypharmacy has a great impact on the occurrence, course, and treatment of the disease [7].

Genetic, epigenetic, or environmental factors that play a more or less important role in different regions of the world may lead to diseases associated with kidney glomerular damage, which leads to their chronic hypofunction and subsequent renal failure. Research conducted by O'Shaughnessy et al. [6], aimed to analyze the data from centers dealing with chronic kidney diseases, where several types of nephropathy were considered. Analysis shows that there is a difference in the incidence of individual nephropathy depending on the region. It turned out that focal segmental glomerulosclerosis (FSGS) and diabetic nephropathy are the most numerous in the USA because it occurred in 19% of diagnosed patients; the second type that dominated was IgA nephropathy (12%), another was membranous nephropathy (12%) and lupus nephritis (10%). Furthermore, FSGS was also common in Latin America (16%), although lupus nephritis strongly dominated the region (38%), while diabetic nephropathy (DN) (4%) and IgA nephropathy (IgAN) (6%) were relatively rare. A reverse dependence than in the USA has been observed in Europe and Asia. In Europe, IgA nephropathy dominated the diagnosis, and the second most common diagnosis was FSGS (15%), while in Asia, IgA glomerulopathy included 40% of diagnoses and the second most common diagnosis was lupus nephritis (17%) [8].

All of these diseases are the subject of intensive research by many scientists around the world. The following review of the literature focuses on the problems of diseases associated with glomerular dysfunction, in which there are answers to questions about the participation in the pathogenesis of diseases on TLR, which may become a potential marker molecule.

2. Classification of Biomarkers

There are many different ways to classify biological molecules as biomarkers in the literature. One of the basic methods is division according to the type of marker molecule. These are DNA, mitochondrial DNA, RNA, or mRNA molecules that belong to the genomic biomarker category, but also proteins, peptides, or antibodies that are classified as proteomic biomarkers. The third group is metabolic markers (metabolomics), which includes lipids, carbohydrates, enzymes, and products of metabolism (metabolites). Our attention was drawn to a slightly different classification of these unusual molecules, i.e., classification based on genetics and molecular biology, due to the usefulness of biomarkers in diagnostic processes and due to their application (Figure 1). The first group includes three types of biomarkers. Type 0 are biomarkers that correlate over time with known clinical indications and show the natural course and history of the disease. Type I relates to biomarkers of drug activity, which can be divided into biomarkers of efficacy (taking into account the therapeutic effect of a given drug), mechanism (providing information about the drug's mechanism of action), and toxicity (including the toxic effect of a given drug). Type II is known as surrogate biomarkers to help evaluate and predict the effect of therapy [9].

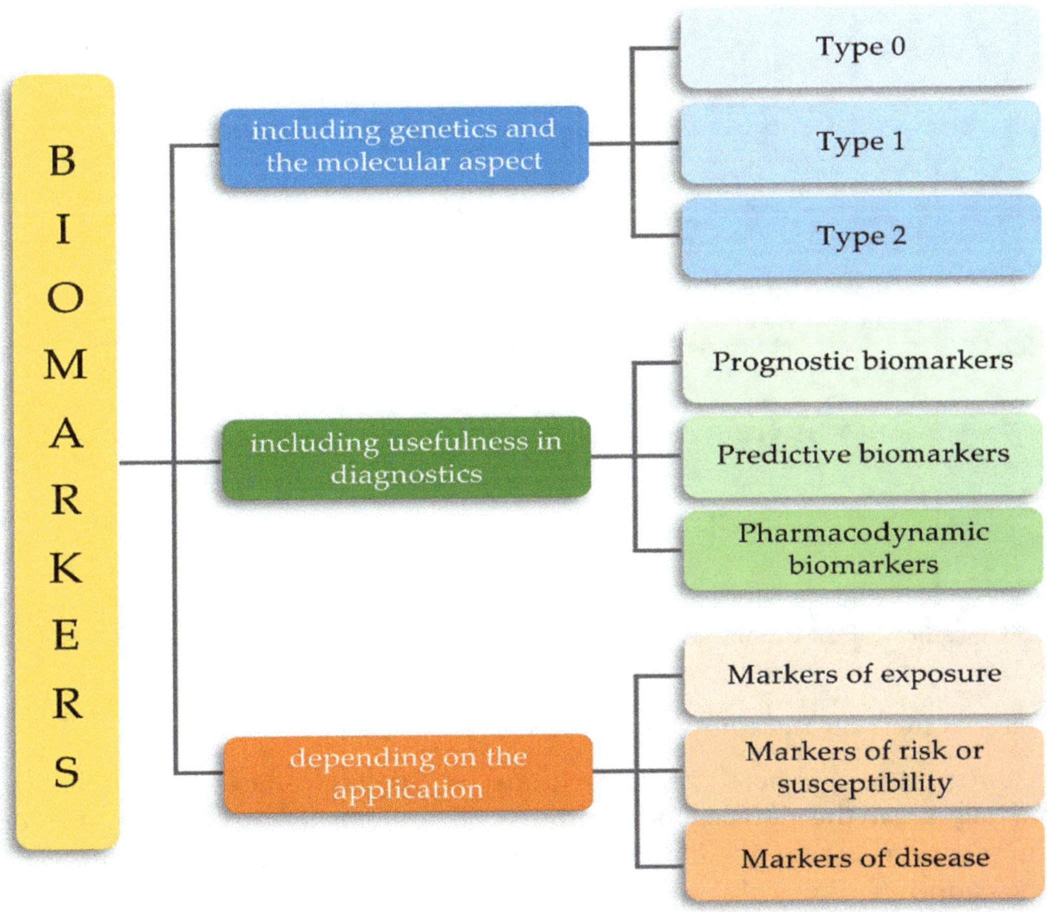

Figure 1. Classification of biomarkers due to the genetic and molecular aspect, the usefulness of biomarkers in diagnostic processes, and application.

Due to the usefulness of biomarkers in diagnostics, we can distinguish prognostic biomarkers; in other words, those that suggest the probable outcome of the disease in an untreated individual, and predictive biomarkers, the purpose of which is to identify patients for whom a specific therapy is most effective. Lastly, we can distinguish pharmacodynamic biomarkers that determine the pharmacological action of a given drug [10]. Another classification is based on the use of biomarkers. We distinguish here exposure markers and doses that are used to reconstruct and predict past accidental or occupational exposures. Risk or vulnerability markers, which relate to the identification of vulnerable individuals (or future patients) at increased risk of developing a disease, and disease markers represent the initial cellular or molecular changes that occur during the development of a particular disease entity. It is the latter group that includes TLR receptors [11,12]. However, what characteristics does an ideal biomarker need to meet? Is there an "ideal biomarker"? What features should a biomarker have to be close to the ideal? Well, according to the FDA, an ideal biomarker must meet the following six characteristics (Figure 2). First, it must be specific in the course of a particular disease entity and easy to differentiate between different physiological conditions of the patient. Secondly, such a biomarker must above all be easy to measure and safe. Then, the speed of its detection is also important, as it enables a quick diagnosis as well as the repeatability and accuracy of the results obtained. Attention is also paid to the cost of detecting such biomarkers, which must be relatively cheap. The advantage of such a biomarker is also the consistency between ethnic groups and genders of patients [13].

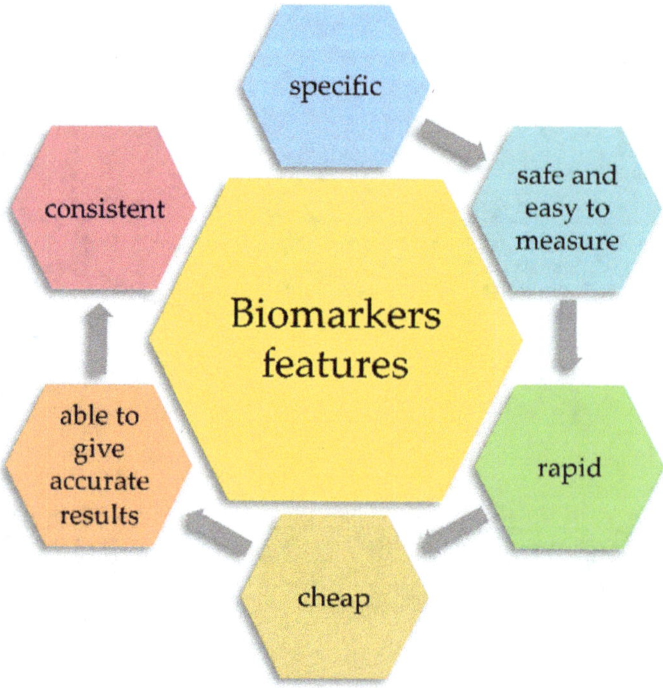

Figure 2. Classification of biomarkers due to the genetic and molecular aspect, the usefulness of biomarkers in diagnostic processes, and application.

3. Characteristic of the TLR Receptors

Glomerulonephritis is a heterogeneous group of diseases whose common denominator is inflammation, ongoing in the glomerulus, resulting from systemic (secondary glomerulonephritis) or only glomerulonephritis (primary glomerulonephritis) [14–19]. The etiopathogenesis and the cause of the variable course of glomerulopathy is the subject of numerous studies but remains unknown. Although the pathogenesis is not unequivocally elucidated, the literature data clearly indicate the involvement of various immune mechanisms in the etiopathogenesis of glomerulopathy. Researchers indicate the role of the immune system in the development of chronic kidney disease on the basis of primary and secondary disorders of the glomerular functions, and AKI (acute kidney injury) resulting from the above-mentioned entities and other disease states, e.g., sepsis [20]. The main elements involved in promoting kidney damage are dendritic cells, NK (natural killer) cells, macrophages, and proinflammatory cytokines. A critical role is played by the complement system, which can both protect and promote damage to the glomeruli [21].

Literature data suggest the contribution of innate immunity to TLRs in these processes. These receptors are a classic example of pattern recognition receptors (PRRs). Signals received by these receptors by recruiting specific molecules lead to activation of the transcription factors NF-κB (nuclear factor kappa-light-chain-enhancer of activated B cells) and IRF (interferon regulatory factor) and affect various elements of the host's innate immune response [22]. TLR mechanisms are based on the ability to recognize twofold signals. The first one is based on the detection of pathogen-associated molecular patterns (PAMPs), while the second reads molecules related to damage to the body's own cells (DAMPs; danger-associated molecular patterns) [23]. However, the origin of the signal, in the case of PAMP, is compounds of exogenous origin, while DAMP receives endogenous information. The result of receiving signals from both pathways is the effector reaction in which the production of costimulatory molecules and cytokines takes place. The location of TLRs is the cell surface or intracellular compartments, including ER (endoplasmic reticulum), lysosomes, and endosomes. It is pointed out that intracellular localization is important not only for ligand recognition but also for avoiding TLR contact with self-nucleic acids, which could cause autoimmunity. A high number of TLR receptors on cells of the immune system, such as monocytes, macrophages, dendritic cells, or lymphocytes, enables the thesis that they constitute a network allowing rapid cooperation of leukocytes and cells present at the site of infection or in the immediate vicinity of damaged host cells [23,24]. TLR synthesis begins in the rough endoplasmic reticulum, from where it goes to the Golgi apparatus and then to its destinations, in other words to the cell surface or to the intercellular compartments [22].

At present, there are 10 types of TLR receptors in humans and three additional types in mice, whereas others species may have more of these receptors (Table 1). Based on the amino acid sequence homology, TLRs occurring in vertebrates were divided into six subfamilies: TLR 1/2/6/10, TLR3, TLR4, TLR5, followed by TLR 7/8/9, and TLR 11 to the last 12/13 (Table 2). However, not all vertebrates have all types of receptors. PRRs have a specific structure in the form of transmembrane proteins, being an integral component of the cell membrane, in which the N-terminal part is responsible for ligand binding, whereas the C-terminal end is equipped with a signaling domain for IL-1 (TIR; toll IL-1 receptor), being part of the signal induction cascade for the production of anti-inflammatory mediators [23]. The transmembrane domain of TLRs contains about 20, mostly hydrophobic, amino acid residues. The N-terminal end (ECDs (extracellular domain) N-terminal ectodomains) is a glycoprotein of 500–800 amino acid residues. In their structure, we distinguish the presence of leucine-rich tandem repeats (LRRs), the number of which depends on the receptor type and ranges from 20–29 repeats (Table 1).

Table 1. Characteristics of individual TLRs (toll-like receptors).

Name	Location of Coding Genes	Location in the Cell	The Number of Amino Acids	Molecular Weight (kDa)	Number of LLR	Reference
TLR1	Chromosome 4	Golgi apparatus, Phagosome, Cell membrane	786aa	90.31	19	[25–27]
TLR2	Chromosome 4	Phagosome	784aa	89.83	19	[25,28,29]
TLR3	Chromosome 4	Early endosome, ER	904aa	103.82	23	[25,30,31]
TLR4	Chromosome 9	Cell membrane, Early endosome	839aa	95.68	21	[25,32,33]
TLR5	Chromosome 1	No data	858aa	97.83	20	[25,34,35]
TLR6	Chromosome 4	Golgi apparatus, Cell membrane, Phagosome	796aa	91.88	19	[25,36,37]
TLR7	Chromosome X	Endosomes, Lysosomes, ER, Phagosome	1049aa	120.92	25	[25,38]
TLR8	Chromosome X	No data	1041aa	119.82	25	[25,39,40]
TLR9	Chromosome 3	Endosomes, Lysosomes, ER, Phagosome	1032aa	115.86	25	[25,41]
TLR10	Chromosome 4	No data	811aa	94.56	19	[25,42,43]

Table 1. *Cont.*

Name	Location of Coding Genes	Location in the Cell	The Number of Amino Acids	Molecular Weight (kDa)	Number of LLR	Reference
TLR11	Expression in mice	No data	926aa	105.83	10	[44]
TLR12	Expression in mice	No data	906aa	99.94	17	[45]
TLR13	Expression in mice	Endosomes	991aa	114.44	25	[46]

TLRs also differ in the cell site. TLR 1/2/4/5/6/10/11/12 receptors are located on the outer membrane of cells, while 3/7/8/9 receptors are located inside of them. Several literature reports have identified specific PAMP and DAMP ligands, which are bound by particular TLRs (Table 2).

Table 2. Location and ligands bound by TLR.

Name	Occurrence	Ligand PAMP	The Origin of PAMP	Ligand DAMP	Reference
		Extracellular			
TLR1	Macrophages Neutrophils B lymphocytes Dendritic cells	Lipopeptides Soluble factors (lipoproteins)	Bacteria	No data	[47,48]
TLR2	Macrophages Neutrophils B lymphocytes Dendritic cells NK cells	Bacterial lipopeptides Teichoic acids, LAM Moduline, Glycolipids of bacteria, Porins, LPS,	Bacteria	Apolipoprotein CIII, Heparin sulphate, Hyaluronic acid, Hsp60, Hsp70, Peroxiredoxin	[47–50]
		Glycosinositolphospholipids	Protozoa, e.g., Trypanosoma cruzi		
		Zymosan	Fungi		
		Hemagglutinin	Measles virus		
		Protein	Herpesvirus		
		Hsp70 proteins	Host organism		
TLR4	Macrophages Neutrophils B lymphocytes Dendritic cells NK cells Treg cells	LPS	Bacteria	C-reactive protein, Fibronectin, Fibrinogen, Heparin sulphate, Neutrophil, Elastase, Angiotensin II, Hsp60	[48–51]
		Fusion proteins, Proteins present in the coating	Viruses, e.g., RSV virus		
		Taxol	Plants		
		Hsp60 protein Hsp70 protein A fragment of the A domain of fibronectin Hyaluronic acid oligosaccharide Fibrinogen Heparan sulphate	Host organism		
TLR5	Macrophages B lymphocytes Dendritic cells Treg cells	Flagellin	Bacteria (Gram-negative)	No data	[48,52]
TLR6	Macrophages Neutrophils Dendritic cells	Diacyl lipopeptides Lipoteichoic acids Zymosan	Bacteria Fungi	Versican	[47–50,53]
TLR10	Dendritic cells	No data	No data	No data	[54]
TLR11	Macrophages Dendritic cells	Flagellin Profilin	Bacteria Protozoa, e.g., Toxoplasma gondii	No data	[55,56]
TLR12	Dendritic cells	Profilin	Protozoa, e.g., Toxoplasma gondii	No data	[55]

Table 2. *Cont.*

Name	Occurrence	Ligand PAMP	The Origin of PAMP	Ligand DAMP	Reference
		Intracellular			
TLR3	Macrophages Neutrophils B lymphocytes Dendritic cells	Double-stranded RNA	Viruses	Own double-stranded RNA	[57,58]
TLR7	Macrophages Neutrophils Dendritic cells Treg cells	Single-stranded RNA Antiviral and anticancer compounds	Viruses Synthetic	Own single-stranded RNA	[48,59]
TLR8	Dendritic cells Treg cells	Single-stranded RNA Antiviral compounds	Viruses Synthetic	Own single-stranded RNA	[48,60]
TLR9	Macrophages Neutrophils Dendritic cells	Double-stranded DNA (containing unmethylated CpG sequences)	Bacteria, viruses and synthetic	HMGB1 Mitochondrial DNA	[48–50,61]

4. The Role of TLRs in Glomerulonephritis

Tissue damage glomerulonephritis predisposes many factors and individual characteristics. Most often, the first reveals hereditary predispositions in response to emerging environmental factors that can lead to a nephrogenic immune response. Then, there is a direct exposure to infectious etiological factors occurring in the environment (PAMP and DAMP), which may be subject to specific modification due to many epigenetic factors (such as physical exercise, microbes, environmental toxins, lifestyle, etc.) [62]. As a consequence of these changes, the innate immune system is activated as a result of interaction with TLRs present on circulating inflammatory cells (neutrophils, macrophages, basophils, and NK cells), as well as on resident glomerular cells and the complement system, which triggers a cascade of antigen-specific non-specific reactions [63]. These receptors are displayed on cells found inside the glomerulus (mesangial cells, monocytes, or dendritic cells) as well as in the renal interstitium (tubular epithelial cells, monocytes), where they interfere with potential ligands [63]. Part of the ligands, such as peptides, structural elements, or genetic material of both bacteria and viruses can be transmitted through the bloodstream to the inside of the nephron, in particular to the glomerulus. In the case of interstitial cells, in addition to the ligands of infectious origin, the potential ligands may also be fibrinogen, fibronectin, defensin 2, or necrotic cells (Figure 3).

In order to prevent over-activity of the immune system, TLRs are downregulated by numerous molecules and various mechanisms. Existing negative regulators target specific key molecules in TLR signaling, such as SOCS1 (suppressor of cytokine signaling 1), SOCS3 (suppressor of cytokine signaling 3), SARM (sterile α-and armadillo-motif containing protein), TANK (TRAF family member associated NF-κB activator), A20, and others [64–69]. Additionally, there are molecules that directly influence the inhibition of NF-kB and IRF-3 [70]. In addition, numerous mi-RNAs were discovered that affect the stability of mRNA encoding signaling molecules and mRNA for cytokines [69,71].

Activation of TLR releases the NF-κB transcription factor, which results in the production of inflammatory mediators (such as IL-1, IL-2, IL-6, IL-12, TNF-α (tumor necrosis factor alpha)), [72,73], and can cause glomerular damage. The next step is the conversion of the innate immune response that begins the antigen-specific reaction cycle. The transformation of the immune response includes several possible mechanisms, such as regulation of natural autoimmunity, conformational changes of epitopes, molecular mimicry, or the autoantigen complementarity phenomenon. TLRs are also required to activate the adaptive immune system by antigen-presenting cells that promote CD4 helper cell differentiation, B cell activation, and antibody production. Antibodies lead to the trapping of the circulating complex or the formation of in situ immune complexes that can activate both TLRs and complement components of the innate immune system [74]. CD4 Th1 and Th2 cells cause damage to the glomerular tissues indirectly, mainly through macrophages and basophils, whereas Th17 cells may directly mediate damage to kidney structures in particular diseases (Figure 4).

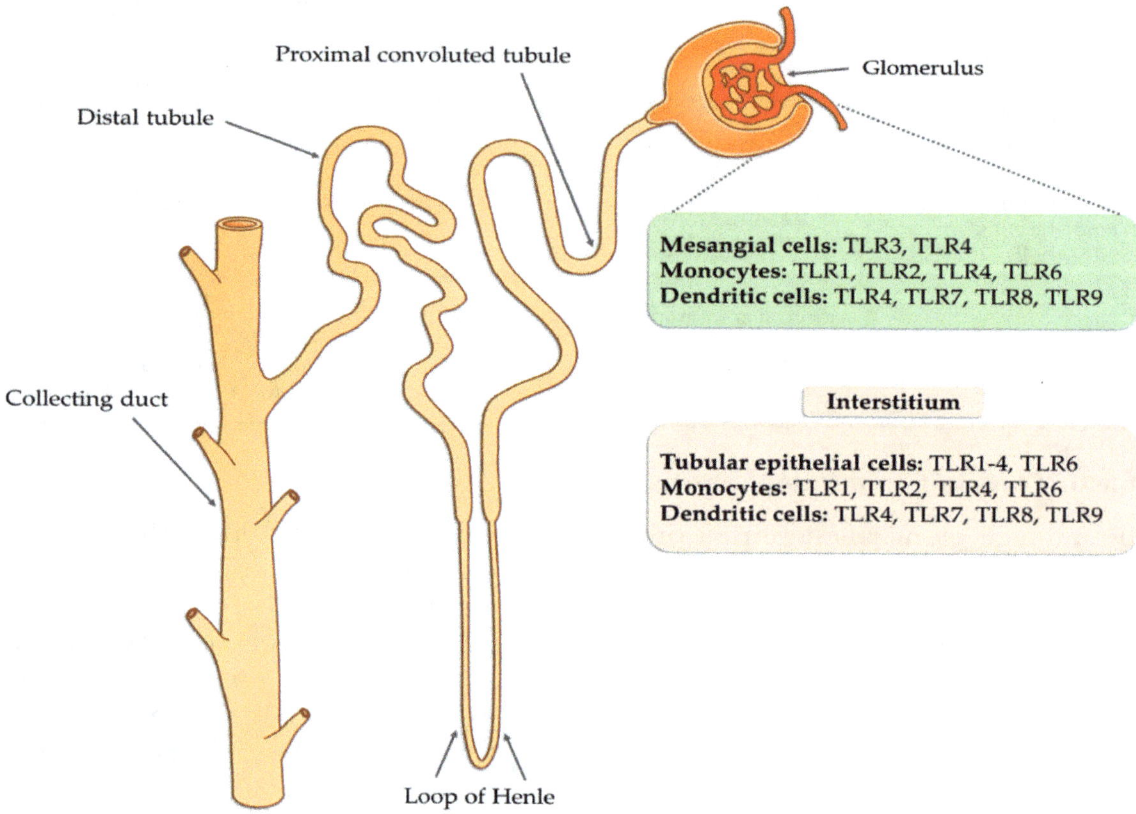

Figure 3. The potential occurrence of TLR receptors within the nephron (modified, based on [63]).

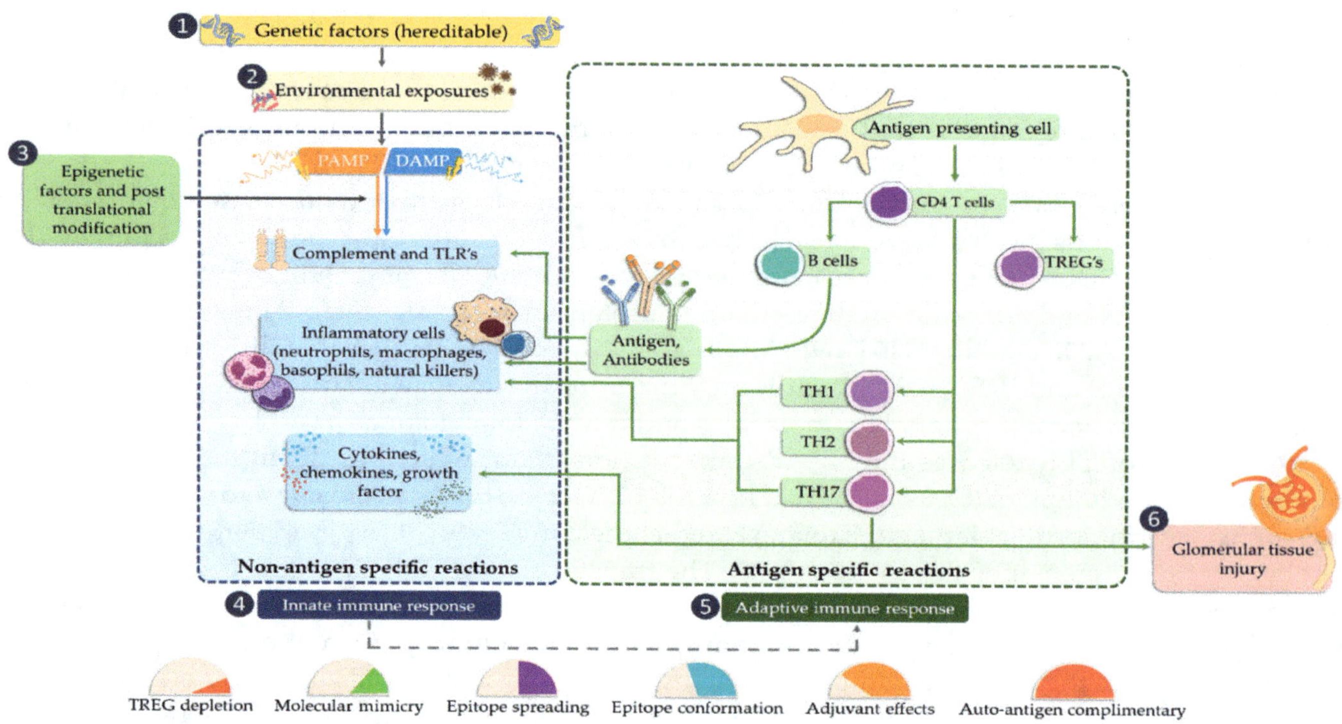

Figure 4. The potential occurrence of TLR receptors within the nephron (modified, based on [24]).

Various clinical situations affecting the kidneys, such as ischemic damage, toxic AKI, nephropathies secondary to diabetes mellitus, hypertension, or crystal deposition, are associated with aseptic inflammation caused, among others, by DAMP molecules [75,76]. These molecules can be released from dying parenchyma cells or during remodulation of the extracellular matrix. The presence of cells in the kidney capable of expressing TLR receptors makes it possible to initiate an immune response and inflammation [77,78]. In order to approximate the mode of action of these receptors in the disease state, their involvement in the most frequently diagnosed pathological conditions associated with glomerular dysfunction is presented in the further part of the material [8].

5. Biomarkers and Importance of the TLRs in Selected Glomerular Diseases

The literature classification divides the occurring nephropathies into two categories: Primary nephropathies, which are defined as those in which the systemic disease responsible for the condition cannot be established, and secondary nephropathies in which renal lesions appear as a result of other diseases accompanied by characteristic extrarenal symptoms. The first group includes diseases, such as: minimal change nephropathy (MCN), focal segmental glomerulosclerosis (FSGS), and membranous nephropathy (MN), which are also included in the nephrotic syndrome. The second group is primarily diabetic nephropathy and lupus nephropathy. In addition, the studies of our research group have resulted in the finding that the TLR-2 receptor may play an important role as a biomarker of primary non-proliferative nephropathies [79].

6. The Role of TLRs in Primary Non-Proliferative Nephropathies

6.1. Focal Segmental Glomerulosclerosis (FSGS)

FSGS is a diverse syndrome that arises after damage to podocytes for various reasons, some known and unknown. The sources of podocyte injury are diverse (circulating factors (primary FSGS), genetic abnormalities, viral infections, and medications) [80,81]. Most of the mutual interactions between these factors probably result in FSGS. There is a hypothesis about multistage pathogenic activation of autoimmunity in some forms of idiopathic FSGS [81]. Through the interaction of macrophages involved in kidney damage with many chemokines, the migration of monocytes to the site of damage occurs, which initiates the process of fibrosis. These macrophages also have the ability to self-spread and change into myofibroblasts that produce the extracellular matrix. Therefore, it can be assumed that excessive organ infiltration by monocytes and macrophages will cause an intensified fibrosis effect and, consequently, intensification of FSGS symptoms [82,83]. Currently, known biomarkers of FSGS are soluble urokinase-type plasminogen activator receptor (suPAR), soluble IL-2 receptor (sIL-2R), and ATP-binding cassette subfamily B member 1 glycoprotein-P (Figure 5). Damage to podocytes can release molecular patterns of proteins that are recognized by TLR as signals of danger. TLRs stimulate adapter proteins that activate a cascade of kinases, which amplify the signal and transmit it to the transcription factors regulating inflammatory genes. In the inflammatory microenvironment, the podocytes, acting as antigen-presenting cells, have a CD40 and CD80 receptor on their surface, thanks to which they capture antigens and present them to competent T-cells. However, in the case of abnormal expression of CD40 and CD80, they disorganize the cytoskeleton and filtration slit. In addition, CD40 can be identified as a foreign antigen, consequently leading to the production of anti-CD40 auto-antigen. Abnormal expression of CD40, CD80, and autoantibodies may lead to apoptosis of the podocytes, detachment of the podocytes from the glomerular basal membrane, proliferation of parietal epithelial cells, and attack on the glomeruli, and induction of segmental sclerosis [81]. In turn, other literature reports indicate the involvement of fibrinogen (Fg) in an inflammatory process mediated by the toll-like 4 receptor (TLR4) [84]. Fibrinogen is a protein that plays a proinflammatory role in vascular disorders, rheumatoid arthritis, glomerulonephritis, and certain cancers, e.g., myeloproliferative neoplasms [84,85]. Positive correlations have been noted between oxidative stress markers and, among others, fibrinogen, which may impact the course of several disorders [85]. Găman et al. [86] showed that obesity and diabetes are associated with increased levels of ROS (reactive oxygen species), accompanied by a simultaneous deficiency of antioxidants. The authors showed that the results of the free oxygen radical defense (FORT) and free oxygen radical defense (FORD) tests correlated with anthropometric/biochemical parameters in patients with obesity and diabetes. In studies carried out by Wang et al. [84], Fg has been shown to disrupt the actin cytoskeleton and induce apoptosis in podocytes via the TLR4-p38 MAPK-NF-κB p65 pathway in vitro and that co-expression of Fg and TLR4 is elevated in podocytes of Adriamycin-treated mice. It was also indicated that the level of fibrinogen in the urine may reflect the disease activity in patients with FSGS [84]. Literature data show that the use of synthetic small molecules lecinoxoids, which are inhibitors of TLR-2 and TLR-4, affects the activation and recruitment of monocytes in a rat model. The authors indicate [87] that the data demonstrate that targeting TLR-2-TLR-4 and/or monocyte migration directly affects the priming phase of fibrosis and may consequently perturb disease pathogenesis.

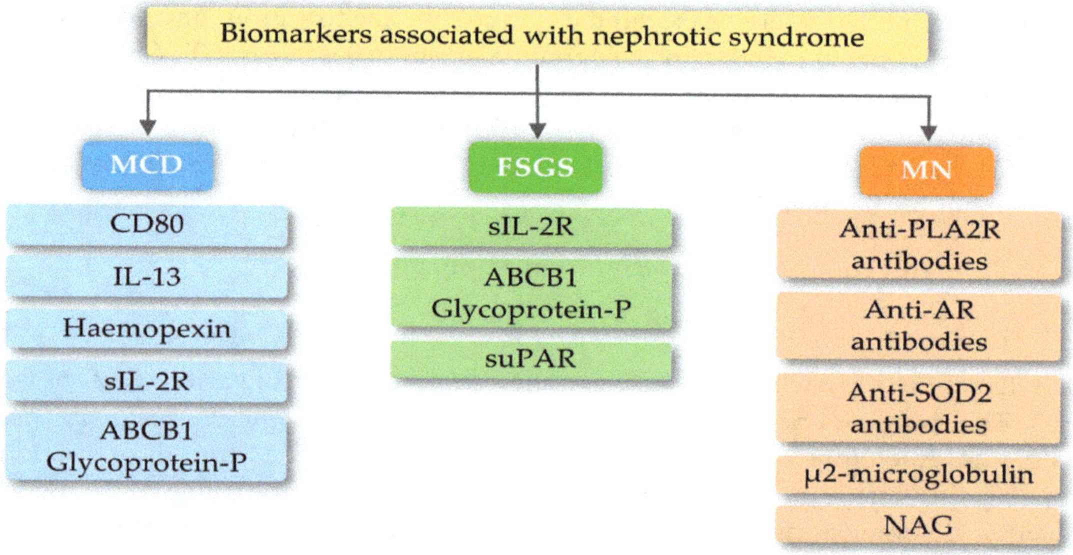

Figure 5. Biomarkers associated with nephrotic syndrome based on minimal change disease (MCD), focal segmental glomerulosclerosis (FSGS), and membranous nephropathy (MN) change based on [88]). CD80-Cluster of differentiation 80; IL-13-interleukin 13; sIL-2R-soluble IL-2 receptor; ABCB1 Glycoprotein-P-ATP-binding cassette subfamily B member 1 Glycoprotein-P; suPAR-soluble urokinase-type plasminogen activator receptor; PLA2R-M-type phospholipase A2 receptor; SOD2-manganese superoxide-dismutase 2; AR-Androgen Receptor; NAG-N-Acetyl-β-D Glucosaminidase.

6.2. Minimal Change Disease (MCD)

MCD is one of the most common glomerular kidney diseases in children and a common cause of nephrotic syndrome in adults. This disease entity is characterized by an outbreak of edema, selective proteinuria, and a clinical response to glucocorticoid therapy, as T-cell mechanisms are involved in the pathogenesis of the disease [89]. The pathogenesis is due to abnormalities in the functioning of podocytes, with the latest literature data suggesting the hypothesis that there are two initiating events. First, there are changes in the cytoskeleton of podocytes and, second, there are regulatory changes in T-cells that exacerbate abnormalities in podocytes [89,90]. Currently known biomarkers in MCD are urine levels and podocyte expression of CD80 (B7.1), interleukin 13, serum levels and protease activity of circulating hemopexin, serum levels of soluble interleukin 2 receptor, and ABCB1 and glycoprotein-P (Figure 5). The development of MCD may be significantly influenced by the body's innate immunity, in which TLRs are involved. Podocytes in the kidney glomeruli, due to their function and place of occurrence, are also equipped with the above receptors. In research conducted by Srivastava et al. [91], the presence of TLR receptors and their potential activity were checked on cell cultures stimulated with LPS (lipopolysaccharides) and the amino nucleoside puromycin (PAN). In the above studies, it was found that cultured human podocytes constitutively express TLR 1-6 and TLR-10 but not TLR 7–9.

Quantitative analysis using the RT-PCR method indicated that LPS at various concentrations and to varying degrees increased the expression of TLR (1–6) genes, the adapter molecule MyD88, and the transcription factor NF-κB within one hour. LPS also caused elevated levels of IL-6, IL-8, and MCP-1 (monocyte chemoattractant protein-1) without exerting any effect on TNF-α, IFN-α, or TGF-β1 after 24 h. It has also been shown that an increase in TLR 1 expression may attenuate the effect of TLR-4 activation, which is thought to be an indirect factor in LPS-induced podocyte damage [91]. Moreover, the increase in TLR-1 expression by LPS suggests that LPS damage to podocytes is associated with an increase in TLR-1 levels and its specific endogenous ligands (heat shock protein, heparin sulphate, and fibronectin). These results allow the conclusion that the main TLR4 ligand, which is LPS, can induce the expression of the genes of many TLR receptors, and thus may lead to changes being induced in podocytes, which may be related to the loss of receptor selectivity and stimulation of receptor interaction in podocytes [91]. An additional possibility indicating the involvement of TLRs in the development of MCD is the increase in the amount of the CD80 receptor in podocytes, after stimulation with ligands for TLR-and TLR-4 receptors. TLR ligands are usually microbial products and can be combined with a well-known association of viral infections as a causative agent of minimal lesion disease [92,93].

6.3. Membranous Nephropathy (MN)

MN is a common cause of nephrotic syndrome in adults. Patients with MN usually develop severe proteinuria, edema, hypoalbuminemia, and hyperlipidemia [94]. It is the most common cause of idiopathic nephrotic syndrome in non-diabetic white adults. About 80% of cases are restricted to the kidneys (primary MN, PMN, idiopathic membranous nephropathy) and 20% are related to other systemic diseases or exposure (secondary MN) [95]. MN is associated with a pathological alteration of the glomerular basement membrane. This change is due to the build-up of immune complexes that appear as granular immunoglobulin (Ig)G deposits after immunofluorescence imaging and as electron-dense deposits of high electron density. Deposits of these immune complexes between podocytes and the basement membrane have a complex that attacks the complement membrane (C5b-9) [96]. The formation of glomerular sub-epithelial immune complex deposits in the IMN is mediated by specific intrinsic podocyte antigens and their corresponding autoantibodies in humans. These include compounds, such as neutral endopeptidase (NEP), type M receptor for secretory phospholipase A2 (PLA2R1), and type 1 7A thrombospondin (THSD7A) (containing domain 8–10) [94–96]. The above-mentioned markers constitute the core of the research into the pathogenesis of membranous nephropathy. However, there are reports of a genetic susceptibility to idiopathic membranous nephropathy. This type of study was conducted in a high-prevalence area in Taiwan [97]. In these studies, the association of the *IL-6, NPHS1 (nephrin), TLR-4, TLR-9, STAT4 (signal transducer and activator of transcription)* and *MYH (mutY DNA glycosylase)*, genes with susceptibility to primary membranous nephropathy in Taiwan was established. In the case of the TLR4 receptor gene, the gene polymorphism indicated a significant single nucleotide difference in the rs10983755 A/G region ($p < 0.001$) and rs1927914 A/G ($p < 0.05$) between the control group and MN patients. In addition, the distributions of rs10759932 C/T and rs11536889 C/T polymorphisms differed significantly [97].

6.4. IgA Nephropathy (IgAN)

The development of IgA nephropathy consists of many mechanisms not yet fully understood. Literature data breaks down biomarkers for IgA nephropathy into a diagnostic and prognostic marker. The first group includes biomarkers detected in serum and urine, such as uromodulin, CD71, IL-6, complement components, and serum BAFF (B-cell activating factor) [98]. However, the group of prognostic markers includes urine kidney injury molecule-1, fractional excretion of IgG, soluble CD89, urinary angiotensinogen, and inflammatory cytokines (Figure 6). The above markers may indicate or predict the main cause of nephropathy development, which is the overproduction of anti-IgA complexes. One of the reasons for stimulating the body to produce IgA-related complexes may be signaling disorders associated with TLRs [99–101]. Ligands of bacterial or viral origin are recognized by toll-like receptors that trigger the process of chemokine release and recruitment of macrophages and neutrophils at the site of infection [102]. In numerous studies on IgAN pathogenesis, various types of receptors that could influence the development of this disease have been analyzed. These receptors were TLR3, mainly recognizing viral dsDNA [103]; TLR7 receptor [104]; binding to ssRNA viruses and TLR4 [105,106]; and binding of a variety of ligands, including LPS Gram-negative bacteria and DAMP (Table 2). Numerous observations of patients with diagnosed IgAN suggest the involvement of pathogens of viral origin, which is also confirmed by experimental models. There is an unexpected increase in the level of TLR4 activation, which is involved in the diagnosis of exogenous bacterial factors (LPS from Gram-negative bacteria, *Chlamydia pneumoniae*, HSP (heat shock proteins) proteins) and endogenous origin (HSP-60, additional fibronectin A domain, low-molecular LDL fractions, acid oligosaccharides hyaluronic acid, heparan sulphate), as well as factors derived from the breakdown of host cells [107–113]. To fully explain kidney damage in IgAN, it is necessary to fully understand the effects of TLR4 in the development of glomerulopathy, involving both glomerular cells and circulating leukocytes. Studies have shown that the administration of LPS activates TLR4 receptors on mesangial cells, and causes the release of chemokines (CXCs), which promotes neutrophil infusion and the development of glomerulonephritis [114–116]. In addition, the IFN-γ and IFN-α responses induced by TLR activation induce overexpression of the B-cell activation factor (BAFF) in dendritic cells, favoring the expansion of B-cells and increasing IgA synthesis [117–121]. It was also shown that in kidney biopsies of patients with IgAN, CD19+/CD5+ B cell infiltration is present, which in the progressive forms of this disease produce significant amounts of IFN-γ and IgA and are more resistant to apoptosis compared to cells obtained from healthy donors [122,123]. Moreover, Hitoshi Suzuki et al. [101] showed that there is an association between gene polymorphisms for TLR-9 and disease progression. Stimulation with ligands for TLR-9 led to the deterioration of kidney function in mice and influenced the shift of the balance towards Th1 lymphocytes. These findings led to the conclusion that activation of pathways related to this particular type of receptor may influence the severity of IgA nephropathy [101]. Moreover, Coppo et al. [124] showed that in patients diagnosed with IgA nephropathy, higher levels of TLR-4 in mononuclear cells and transcriptional mRNA were observed than in the control group. An important fact is that there is a statistical difference in the level of the above markers in patients with severe disease and those who do not have proteinuria and hematuria [124]. TLR-4 can be activated by many ligands, such as HLPs and LPS and DAMPs [106].

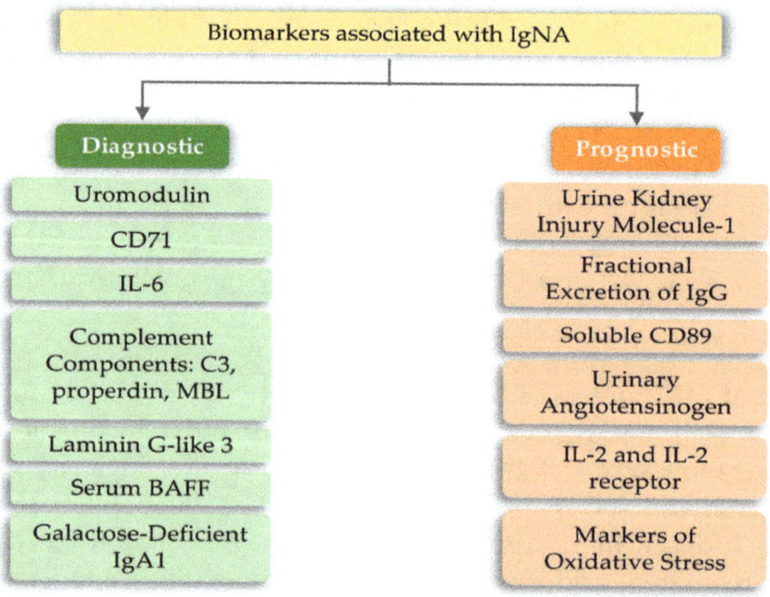

Figure 6. Biomarkers in IgA (immunoglobulin A) nephropathy.

7. The Role of TLR Receptors in Secondary Nephropathies

7.1. Lupus Nephritis

Systemic lupus erythematosus (SLE) is one example of systemic autoimmune diseases. SLE relies on the loss of tolerance to autoantigens, which is caused by the malfunctioning of acquired immunity cells [109,125–127]. In the case of SLE, clinical studies indicate that the most common source of biomarker searches is a urine sample. Due to this, numerous proteins, such as cytokines, chemokines, complement proteins, adhesive molecules, and autoantibodies, have been identified as potential biomarkers of disease activity in cross-sectional studies (Figure 7) [128].

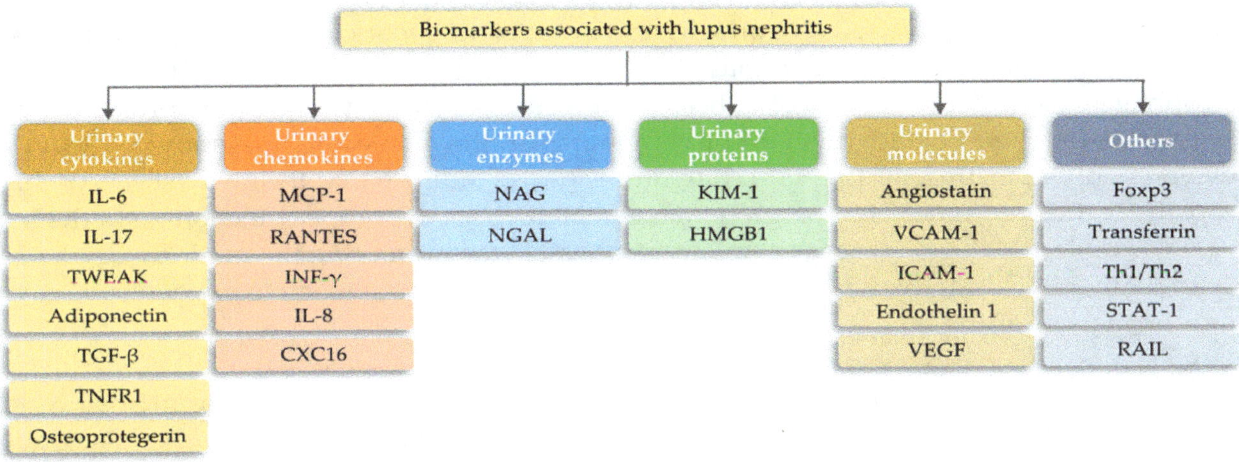

Figure 7. Biomarkers associated with lupus nephritis [128]; CXC16—C-X-C motif chemokine 16; FOXP3—forkhead box protein P3; HMGB1—High mobility group box 1; ICAM—Intercellular Adhesion Molecule 1; IL-6—Urinary Interleukin 6; IL-8—Interleukin 8; IL-17—Urinary Interleukin 17; KIM-1—Urinary kidney injury molecule-1; MCP-1—Monocyte chemoattractant protein-1; NAG—N-Acetyl-β-D Glucosaminidase; NGAL—neutrophil gelatinase-associated lipocalin; RAIL—Renal Activity Index for Lupus; RANTES—Regulated upon Activation, Normal T-cell Expressed, and Secreted; STAT-1—Signal transducer and activator of transcription 1; TGF-β—transforming growth factor beta; Th1—T helper 1; Th2—T helper 2; TNFR1—Tumor necrosis factor receptor 1; TWEAK—Urinary TNF-like weak inducer of apoptosis; VCAM—vascular cell adhesion molecule 1; VEGF—Vascular Endothelial Growth Factor.

Literature data of recent years indicate a special contribution to the etiopathogenesis of this disease of innate immunity elements, mainly TLR. External and endogenous ligands may interact with TLRs present on monocytes, dendritic cells, and B lymphocytes, infiltrating the glomeruli, and resulting in increased cytokine secretion [129,130]. In addition, mesangial cells and other cells of the parenchyma express TLR1-4 and TLR6 receptors and secrete interleukins and chemokines [15,129,131–134]. Studies show that most deposits of immune complexes contain TLR agonists that have the ability to activate mesangial cells and contribute to the development of lupus nephropathy [135]. Pawar et al. [136] summarized the literature data, indicating that microbial nucleic acids can constitute a universal PAMP. As a result, it is possible to activate various mechanisms, such as lymphoproliferation, production of autoantibodies, type I interferon, secretion of numerous cytokines, and promotion of lupus development, in genetically predisposed individuals [136].

TLR2 and TLR4 are expressed not only in parenchymal cells but also in infiltrating neutrophils and mononuclear phagocytes, including macrophages and dendritic cells [137]. The HMGB1 (high mobility group box 1) protein, which binds DNA and the lupus autoantigen released under inflammation, can induce the activation of NF-κB in a TLR2-dependent and TLR4-RAGE-dependent manner in mononuclear phagocytes and neutrophils [138–143] as well as in mesangial cells [144]. Mesangial cells and podocytes in humans are characterized by the expression of TLR4 [145]. Mesangial cells isolated from mice with autoimmune diseases have significantly higher TLR4 expression and produce much more proinflammatory chemokines both after LPS stimulation and spontaneously [146]. Other studies also indicate that the necrotic cell debris-enhanced endogenous TLR ligands stimulate cytokine release by TLR2/MyD88 from mesangial cells, which implies the expression of TLR2 in different cell populations, and kidney-building structure [147–150]. Intracellular expression of TLR2 and TLR4 is multiplied in the kidneys of CD32b receptor-deficient mice suffering from glomerulonephritis associated with cryoglobulinemia [145,151,152].

7.2. Diabetic Nephropathy (DN)

One of the most serious complications for patients diagnosed with type I or II diabetes is diabetic nephropathy, which can be caused by both environmental and genetic factors [18,153]. The diabetic nephropathy is important to the inflammatory process in which, besides an increase in the activity of macrophages and overproduction of adhesion molecules of leukocyte cells, the proximal tubular kidney releases cytokine chemoattractant protein matrix to the interstitium, thereby contributing to the development of the disease [154–156]. Literature studies indicate that the greatest risk of diabetic nephropathy is the occurrence of hyperglycemia, which disrupts the proper functioning of the human body. On the molecular level, hyperglycemia is responsible for promoting the mitochondrial electron transport chain, which causes the formation of excessive amounts of reactive oxygen species (ROS) (through formation of the advanced glycation end products (AGEs) and activation of the polyol pathway, hexosamine pathway, protein kinase C (PKC), and angiotensin II). ROS occurring in the cell initiate or also intensify the formation of oxidative stress, which causes the intensification of inflammation and formation of fibrosis. Abnormalities in the lipid metabolism pathway, activation of the renin-angiotensin-aldosterone system (RAAS), as well as systemic and glomerular hypertension are also involved in the progression of this disease. Impairment of insulin signaling, an increase in growth factors and proinflammatory cytokines, and activation of the intracellular signaling pathway also play a role in the development of this disease [157]. Therefore, the currently known DN biomarkers focus on three areas: Detection of oxidative stress, the occurrence of inflammation, and activation of the RAAS system (Figure 8).

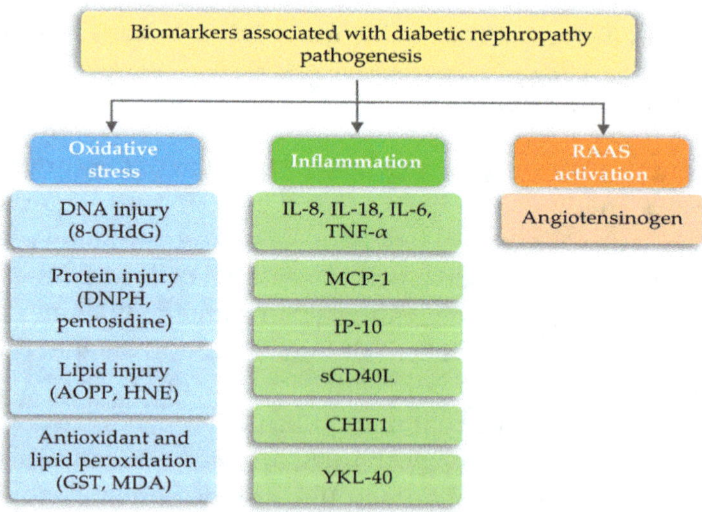

Figure 8. Biomarkers associated with diabetic nephropathy pathogenesis (based on [157]). 8-OHdG—8-hydroxy-2′-deoxyguanine; AOPP—advanced oxidation protein product; CHIT1—chitotriosidase; DNPH—2,4-dinitrophenylhydrazine; GS—Glutathione s-transferase; HNE—4-hydroxy-nonenal; IL-6—interleukin 6; IL-8—interleukin 8; IL-18—interleukin 18; IP-10—interferon-inducible protein-10; MCP-1—Monocyte chemoattractant protein-1; MDA—malondialdehyde; sCD40L—soluble CD40 ligand; TNF-α—Tumor necrosis factor alpha; YKL-40—cartilage glycoprotein 40.

Literature data from recent years indicate that an important role in diabetic nephropathy etiopathogenesis may be played by signal transduction pathways that are dependent on TLR2, TLR9, and TLR4 receptors. However, it is not clear which receptor is more pathogenic [154,158–160]. Studies of many research teams indicate increased expression of TLR2 and the presence of endogenous ligands HMGB1 [161,162] and HSP70 [107,122,163], detected on the basis of research conducted on diabetic-induced rats. In addition, the expression of MyD88 and MCP-1, NF-κB, and infiltration of macrophages has been demonstrated [164–167]. High TLR2 expression was also observed in the glomeruli and renal tubules of people with diabetes. The results were confirmed in vitro in cultures of NRK-52E cell lines in which a high glucose concentration induced TLR2 mRNA expression [168–170]. The pathogenic role of TLR4 in diabetic nephropathy has also been found. In vitro studies have shown that activation of NF-κB and the expression of proinflammatory cytokines was reduced when TLR4 expression was silenced or its signaling was inhibited. During mouse studies, higher TLR4 activity and expression of the NF-κB p65 subunit in the kidney cortex of mice with experimental diabetes was demonstrated [171]. In vitro, researchers also observed increased TLR4 expression and proinflammatory cytokine synthesis when podocytes and adipocytes were exposed to both high glucose and NEFA (non-esterified "free" fatty acids), suggesting a key role of TLR4 in supporting inflammation in diabetic nephropathy [171–173]. In addition, another research team [174] showed an increase in the expression of TLR4 and signaling proteins for this receptor along with the activation of NF-κB, but not TLR2, in a mouse mesangium that was exposed to high glucose concentrations. It was also observed that hyperglycemia stimulated the expression of TLR4 in glomerular renal endothelial cells in a mouse model of type 1 and type 2 diabetes, which underlines the relationship of the discussed receptor with diabetic nephropathy [174,175]. In addition, clinical data indicate that in patients with type 1 diabetes, ligands, endotoxins, heat shock proteins 60 (Hsp60), and high mobility groups 1 (HMGB1) of both TLR2 and TLR4 [176,177] are increased. Increased expression of mRNA was also observed. TLR2, MyD88, and proinflammatory cytokines in leukocytes of patients with type 1 diabetes mellitus suggests that the inflammatory process is mediated by TLR2 [176]. However, in patients with type 2 diabetes and confirmed biopsy, diabetic kidney disease has been found to increase TLR4 expression on renal tubules as opposed to TLR2. In addition, in patients with type II diabetes and confirmed diabetic kidney disease, microalbuminuria, mRNA, and TLR4 protein were overexpressed 4 to 10 times more in glomeruli and tubules compared to the control group. However, both TLR2 and TLR4 expression was increased on monocytes in patients with type II diabetes [176]. Although the literature data indicate a key role of TLR2 and TLR4 in the pathophysiology of diabetic nephropathy, the participation of other receptors is not excluded. There is evidence to suggest the involvement of TLR3, TLR7, and TLR9 receptors in the pathogenesis of type 1 diabetes by destroying pancreatic islets induced by viral infection [114,178,179].

7.3. Acute Kidney Injury (AKI) to Chronic Kidney Disease (CKD) Development

The 2019 definition published by Ronco in The Lancet says that AKI: "is defined by a rapid increase in serum creatinine, decrease in urine output, or both". The authors indicate that acute kidney injury accounts for up to 15% of the reasons for admission to hospital and occurs in as much as 50% of patients treated in intensive care units [180]. Therefore, it is argued that AKI is still associated with high morbidity and mortality [181]. There are many causes of AKI, including acute ischemia, analgesic nephropathy, sepsis, and severe glomerulopathies. Meta-analyses and cohort studies confirm the role of acute kidney injury in the development of chronic kidney disease and, as a complication of AKI, the more frequent need for chronic renal replacement therapy in the form of dialysis therapy [182–184]. The literature does not indicate clear causes and markers of the transition of acute kidney injury to chronic kidney disease, although it is known that this process involves numerous immune mechanisms. Inflammation, induced death, and fibrosis are likely contributors to the progression of AKI to CKD [185]. The renal epithelium plays an important role in promoting inflammation after damage by attracting leukocytes to the site of damage, which is seen as a strong role for TLR-4 [186]. The role of TLR2 and TLR4 in reperfusion after ischemic kidney injury is significant, where their expression increases significantly and enhances the proinflammatory response of tissues, with the participation of numerous cytokines and chemokines [187,188]. It is also noteworthy that the TLR-3 receptor system is involved in ischemia/reperfusion injury in the kidney. Studies have been carried out that showed rapid activation of these receptors, resulting in significant kidney damage, which was associated with elevated rates of apoptosis and necrosis in the renal tubes of mice [189]. Both TLR2 and TLR4 are also involved in sepsis-induced kidney damage [190], caused by Gram-positive and G-negative bacteria; nevertheless, the roles of single TLRs are differing [191]. There is also the TLR4-IL-22 pathway, which probably has regenerative functions in opposition to the above, and more research is needed on this topic [192]. After the action of a harmful factor, the repair process takes place, the element of which is sterile ignition [193]. In the first stage of inflammation, neutrophilic exudate appears, which over time is replaced by a monocytic-lymphocytic infiltrate [194,195]. The presence of monocytes is regarded as a mechanism promoting fibrosis and fibroblast proliferation [196]. The influx of cells of the immune system leads to cell apoptosis and the formation of a large amount of breakdown products and other substances that act as DAMPs, which can activate receptors, including TLRs [78,197]. It then promotes and strengthens the inflammatory response, attracting more cells of the immune system and subsequent fibrosis. Kidney infiltration by monocytes is recognized as a feature of chronic kidney disease [198] and the degree of monocyte infiltration correlates with the severity of kidney damage [199]. The above data indicate that it is the intensified process of fibrosis, mediated largely by the elements of the immune system, that can lead to permanent damage to the kidney function and the progression of AKI to CKD.

8. Conclusions

The innate immunity system in which TLRs participate, among others, cells, such as monocytes, macrophages, and NK (natural killer) cells, expressing TLR and lectin receptors are the body's first line of defense. TLRs identify the pathogen based on the specific pattern of the molecule and therefore stimulate the immune system acquired, including T and B lymphocytes to fight pathogens [15]. Long-term continuous antigenic stimulation, increasing the work of TLRs, can lead to the development of serious diseases, organ specific or systemic. In an increasing number of studies, the role of TLRs has become more important. Recognition receptors are certainly of importance in the pathogenesis of diseases associated with nephropathy, for example, glomerulopathy, diabetic, lupus IgA, or FSGS [1,16]. However, further research is necessary to clarify the possible involvement of TLR in the development of other disease entities associated with kidney damage.

Author Contributions: S.M., P.L., E.G., W.Z.; conceptualization, S.M., P.L., D.B., I.M., P.N.-R., E.G., R.H.; writing—original draft preparation; S.M., P.L., D.B., I.M., P.N.-R., E.G., R.H., W.Z., J.R.; writing—review and editing. All authors have read and agreed to the published version of the manuscript.

Abbreviations

8-OHdG	8-hydroxy-2′-deoxyguanine
ABCB1 Glycoprotein-P	ATP-binding cassette subfamily B member 1 Glycoprotein-P
AKI	Acute kidney injury
AOPP	Advanced oxidation protein product
AR	Androgen Receptor
BAFF	B-cell activation factor
CD80	Cluster of differentiation 80
CHIT1	Chitotriosidase; DNPH-2,4-dinitrophenylhydrazine
CKD	Chronic kidney disease

CXC16	C-X-C motif chemokine 16
DAMP	Damage-associated molecular patterns
DN	Diabetic nephropathy
FOXP3	Forkhead box protein P3
FSGS	Focal segmental glomerulosclerosis
GST	Glutathione s-transferase
HMGB1	High mobility group box 1
HNE	4-hydroxy-nonenal
HSP70	Heat shock proteins 70
ICAM	Intercellular Adhesion Molecule 1
IFN-α	Interferon alpha
IFN-γ	Interferon gamma
IgAN	IgA nephropathy
IL-17	Interleukin 13
IL-13	Interleukin 13
IL-2	Interleukin 2
IL-6	Interleukin 6
IL-7	Interleukin 7
IL-8	Interleukin 8
IP-10	Interferon-inducible protein-10
KIM-1	Urinary kidney injury molecule-1
LPS	Lipopolysaccharides
LRRs	Leucine-rich tandem repeats
MCN	Minimal change nephropathy
MCP-1	Monocyte chemoattractant protein-1
MDA	Malondialdehyde
MN	Membranous nephropathy
NAG	N-Acetyl-β-D Glucosaminidase
NAG	N-Acetyl-β-D Glucosaminidase
NF-κB	Nuclear factor kappa-light-chain-enhancer of activated B cells
NGAL	Neutrophil gelatinase-associated lipocalin
NK cells	Natural killer cells
PAMP	Pathogen-associated molecular patterns
PKC	Protein kinase C
PLA2R	M-type phospholipase A2 receptor
PRRs	Pattern recognition receptors
RAAS	Renin-angiotensin-aldosterone system
RAIL	Renal Activity Index for Lupus
RANTES	Regulated upon Activation, Normal T cell Expressed, and Secreted
ROS	Reactive oxygen species
sCD40L	Soluble CD40 ligand
sIL-2R	Soluble IL-2 receptor
SLE	Systemic lupus erythematosus
SOD2	manganese superoxide-dismutase 2
STAT-1	Signal transducer and activator of transcription 1
suPAR	Soluble urokinase-type plasminogen activator receptor
TGF-β1	Transforming growth factor beta 1
TLR	Toll-like receptor
TNF-a	Tumor necrosis factor alpha
TNFR1	Tumor necrosis factor receptor 1
TWEAK	Urinary TNF-like weak inducer of apoptosis
VCAM	Vascular cell adhesion molecule 1
VEGF	Vascular Endothelial Growth Factor
YKL-40	Cartilage glycoprotein 40

References

1. World Health Organization; International Programme on Chemical Safety. *Biomarkers in Risk Assessment: Validity and Validation*; World Health Organization: Geneva, Switzerland, 2001; ISBN 978-92-4-157222-4.
2. Fuentes-Arderiu, X. What is a biomarker? It's time for a renewed definition. *Clin. Chem. Lab. Med.* **2013**, *51*, 1689–1690. [CrossRef] [PubMed]
3. Goerlich, N.; Brand, H.A.; Langhans, V.; Tesch, S.; Schachtner, T.; Koch, B.; Paliege, A.; Schneider, W.; Grützkau, A.; Reinke, P.; et al. Kidney transplant monitoring by urinary flow cytometry: Biomarker combination of T cells, renal tubular epithelial cells, and podocalyxin-positive cells detects rejection. *Sci. Rep.* **2020**, *10*, 796. [CrossRef] [PubMed]
4. Kasurinen, A.; Hagström, J.; Laitinen, A.; Kokkola, A.; Böckelman, C.; Haglund, C. Evaluation of toll-like receptors as prognostic biomarkers in gastric cancer: High tissue TLR5 predicts a better outcome. *Sci. Rep.* **2019**, *9*, 12553. [CrossRef] [PubMed]
5. Darrabie, M.D.; Cheeseman, J.; Limkakeng, A.T.; Borawski, J.; Sullenger, B.A.; Elster, E.A.; Kirk, A.D.; Lee, J. Toll-like receptor activation as a biomarker in traumatically injured patients. *J. Surg. Res.* **2018**, *231*, 270–277. [CrossRef]
6. Webster, A.C.; Nagler, E.V.; Morton, R.L.; Masson, P. Chronic Kidney Disease. *Lancet* **2017**, *389*, 1238–1252. [CrossRef]
7. Dobrică, E.-C.; Găman, M.-A.; Cozma, M.-A.; Bratu, O.G.; Pantea Stoian, A.; Diaconu, C.C. Polypharmacy in Type 2 Diabetes Mellitus: Insights from an Internal Medicine Department. *Medicina* **2019**, *55*, 436. [CrossRef]
8. O'Shaughnessy, M.M.; Hogan, S.L.; Thompson, B.D.; Coppo, R.; Fogo, A.B.; Jennette, J.C. Glomerular disease frequencies by race, sex and region: Results from the International Kidney Biopsy Survey. *Nephrol. Dial. Transplant.* **2018**, *33*, 661–669. [CrossRef]
9. Naylor, S. Biomarkers: Current perspectives and future prospects. *Expert Rev. Mol. Diagn.* **2003**, *3*, 525–529. [CrossRef]
10. Sahu, P.; Pinkalwar, N.; Dubey, R.D.; Paroha, S.; Chatterjee, S.; Chatterjee, T. Biomarkers: An Emerging Tool for Diagnosis of a Disease and Drug Development. *Asian J. Res. Pharm. Sci.* **2011**, *1*, 9–16.
11. Drucker, E.; Krapfenbauer, K. Pitfalls and limitations in translation from biomarker discovery to clinical utility in predictive and personalised medicine. *EPMA J.* **2013**, *4*, 7. [CrossRef]
12. Mayeux, R. Biomarkers: Potential Uses and Limitations. *NeuroRx* **2004**, *1*, 182–188. [CrossRef] [PubMed]
13. FDA. About Biomarkers and Qualification. Available online: https://www.fda.gov/drugs/cder-biomarker-qualification-program/about-biomarkers-and-qualification (accessed on 10 August 2020).
14. Levin, A.; Tonelli, M.; Bonventre, J.; Coresh, J.; Donner, J.-A.; Fogo, A.B.; Fox, C.S.; Gansevoort, R.T.; Heerspink, H.J.L.; Jardine, M.; et al. Global kidney health 2017 and beyond: A roadmap for closing gaps in care, research, and policy. *Lancet* **2017**, *390*, 1888–1917. [CrossRef]
15. Devarapu, S.K.; Anders, H. Toll-like receptors in lupus nephritis. *J. Biomed. Sci.* **2018**, *25*, 35. [CrossRef]
16. Luyckx, V.A.; Tonelli, M.; Stanifer, J.W. The global burden of kidney disease and the sustainable development goals. *Bull. World Health Organ.* **2018**, *96*, 414–422D. [CrossRef] [PubMed]
17. Yeo, S.C.; Cheung, C.K.; Barratt, J. New insights into the pathogenesis of IgA nephropathy. *Pediatr. Nephrol.* **2018**, *33*, 763–777. [CrossRef] [PubMed]
18. Zheng, Z.; Zheng, F. Immune Cells and Inflammation in Diabetic Nephropathy. *J. Diabetes Res.* **2016**, *2016*, 1841690. [CrossRef]
19. Mohammad Hosseini, A.; Majidi, J.; Baradaran, B.; Yousefi, M. Toll-Like Receptors in the Pathogenesis of Autoimmune Diseases. *Adv. Pharm. Bull.* **2015**, *5*, 605–614. [CrossRef] [PubMed]
20. Imig, J.D.; Ryan, M.J. Immune and Inflammatory Role in Renal Disease. *Compr. Physiol.* **2013**, *3*, 957–976. [CrossRef]
21. Berger, S.P.; Daha, M.R. Complement in glomerular injury. *Semin. Immunopathol.* **2007**, *29*, 375–384. [CrossRef]
22. Kawasaki, T.; Kawai, T. Toll-Like Receptor Signaling Pathways. *Front. Immunol.* **2014**, *5*, 461. [CrossRef]
23. Eleftheriadis, T.; Lawson, B.R. Toll-like receptors and kidney diseases. *Inflamm. Allergy Drug Targets* **2009**, *8*, 191–201. [CrossRef] [PubMed]
24. Liu, Y.; Xue, G.; Li, S.; Fu, Y.; Yin, J.; Zhang, R.; Li, J. Effect of Intermittent and Mild Cold Stimulation on the Immune Function of Bursa in Broilers. *Animals* **2020**, *10*, 1275. [CrossRef] [PubMed]

25. Botos, I.; Segal, D.M.; Davies, D.R. The Structural Biology of Toll-Like Receptors. *Structure* **2011**, *19*, 447–459. [CrossRef] [PubMed]
26. UniProt. Toll-Like Receptor 1. Available online: https://www.uniprot.org/uniprot/Q15399 (accessed on 10 August 2020).
27. Protein Data Bank in Europe. Crystal Structure of the TLR1-TLR2 Heterodimer Induced by Binding of a tri-Acylatedlipopeptide. Available online: https://www.ebi.ac.uk/pdbe/entry/pdb/2z7x (accessed on 10 August 2020).
28. UniProt. Toll-Like Receptor 2. Available online: https://www.uniprot.org/uniprot/O60603 (accessed on 10 August 2020).
29. Protein Data Bank in Europe. Crystal Structure of TLR2-TLR6-Pam2CSK4 Complex. Available online: https://www.ebi.ac.uk/pdbe/entry/pdb/3a79 (accessed on 10 August 2020).
30. UniProt. Toll-Like Receptor 3. Available online: https://www.uniprot.org/uniprot/O15455 (accessed on 10 August 2020).
31. Protein Data Bank in Europe. Crystal Structure of the Complex of TLR3 and bi-Specific Diabody. Available online: https://www.ebi.ac.uk/pdbe/entry/pdb/5gs0 (accessed on 10 August 2020).
32. UniProt. Toll-Like Receptor 4. Available online: https://www.uniprot.org/uniprot/O00206 (accessed on 10 August 2020).
33. Protein Data Bank in Europe. The Crystal Structure of Mouse TLR4/MD-2/neoseptin-3. Available online: https://www.ebi.ac.uk/pdbe/entry/pdb/5ijc (accessed on 10 August 2020).
34. UniProt. Toll-Like Receptor 5. Available online: https://www.uniprot.org/uniprot/O60602 (accessed on 10 August 2020).
35. Protein Data Bank in Europe. Homology Model of Human Toll-Like Receptor 5 Fitted into an Electron Microscopy Single Particle Reconstruction. Available online: https://www.ebi.ac.uk/pdbe/entry/pdb/3j0a (accessed on 10 August 2020).
36. UniProt. Toll-Like Receptor 6. Available online: https://www.uniprot.org/uniprot/Q9Y2C9 (accessed on 10 August 2020).
37. Protein Data Bank in Europe. Crystal Structure of TIR Domain TLR6. Available online: https://www.ebi.ac.uk/pdbe/entry/pdb/4om7 (accessed on 10 August 2020).
38. UniProt. Toll-Like Receptor 7. Available online: https://www.uniprot.org/uniprot/Q9NYK1 (accessed on 10 August 2020).
39. UniProt. Toll-Like Receptor 8. Available online: https://www.uniprot.org/uniprot/Q9NR97 (accessed on 10 August 2020).
40. Protein Data Bank in Europe. Crystal Structure of Human TLR8 in Complex with XG-1-236. Available online: https://www.ebi.ac.uk/pdbe/entry/pdb/4qc0 (accessed on 10 August 2020).
41. UniProt. Toll-Like Receptor 9. Available online: https://www.uniprot.org/uniprot/Q9NR96 (accessed on 10 August 2020).
42. UniProt. Toll-Like Receptor 10. Available online: https://www.uniprot.org/uniprot/Q9BXR5 (accessed on 10 August 2020).
43. Protein Data Bank in Europe. The TIR Domain of Human Toll-Like Receptor 10 (TLR10). Available online: https://www.ebi.ac.uk/pdbe/entry/pdb/2j67 (accessed on 10 August 2020).
44. UniProt. Toll-Like Receptor 11. Available online: https://www.uniprot.org/uniprot/Q6R5P0 (accessed on 10 August 2020).
45. UniProt. Toll-Like Receptor 12. Available online: https://www.uniprot.org/uniprot/Q6QNU9 (accessed on 10 August 2020).
46. UniProt. Toll-Like Receptor 13. Available online: https://www.uniprot.org/uniprot/Q6R5N8 (accessed on 10 August 2020).
47. Farhat, K.; Riekenberg, S.; Heine, H.; Debarry, J.; Lang, R.; Mages, J.; Buwitt-Beckmann, U.; Röschmann, K.; Jung, G.; Wiesmüller, K.-H.; et al. Heterodimerization of TLR2 with TLR1 or TLR6 expands the ligand spectrum but does not lead to differential signaling. *J. Leukoc. Biol.* **2008**, *83*, 692–701. [CrossRef] [PubMed]
48. Zhao, S.; Zhang, Y.; Zhang, Q.; Wang, F.; Zhang, D. Toll-like receptors and prostate cancer. *Front. Immunol.* **2014**, *5*, 352. [CrossRef]
49. Goulopoulou, S.; McCarthy, C.G.; Clinton Webb, R. Toll-like receptors in the vascular system: Sensing the dangers within. *Pharmacol. Rev.* **2016**, *68*, 142–167. [CrossRef]

50. Schaefer, L. Complexity of danger: The diverse nature of damage-associated molecular patterns. *J. Biol. Chem.* **2014**, *289*, 35237–35245. [CrossRef]
51. Brubaker, S.W.; Bonham, K.S.; Zanoni, I.; Kagan, J.C. Innate immune pattern recognition: A cell biological perspective. *Annu. Rev. Immunol.* **2015**, *33*, 257–290. [CrossRef]
52. Miao, E.A.; Andersen-Nissen, E.; Warren, S.E.; Aderem, A. TLR5 and Ipaf: Dual sensors of bacterial flagellin in the innate immune system. *Semin. Immunopathol.* **2007**, *29*, 275–288. [CrossRef]
53. Takeuchi, O.; Kawai, T.; Sanjo, H.; Copeland, N.G.; Gilbert, D.J.; Jenkins, N.A.; Takeda, K.; Akira, S. TLR6: A novel member of an expanding Toll-like receptor family. *Gene* **1999**, *231*, 59–65. [CrossRef]
54. Oosting, M.; Cheng, S.C.; Bolscher, J.M.; Vestering-Stenger, R.; Plantinga, T.S.; Verschueren, I.C.; Arts, P.; Garritsen, A.; van Eenennaam, H.; Sturm, P.; et al. Human TLR10 is an anti-inflammatory pattern-recognition receptor. *Proc. Natl. Acad. Sci. USA* **2014**, *111*, E4478–E4484. [CrossRef] [PubMed]
55. Raetz, M.; Kibardin, A.; Sturge, C.R.; Pifer, R.; Li, H.; Burstein, E.; Ozato, K.; Larin, S.; Yarovinsky, F. Cooperation of TLR12 and TLR11 in the IRF8-Dependent IL-12 Response to Toxoplasma gondii Profilin. *J. Immunol.* **2013**, *191*, 4818–4827. [CrossRef] [PubMed]
56. Yarovinsky, F.; Zhang, D.; Andersen, J.F.; Bannenberg, G.L.; Serhan, C.N.; Hayden, M.S.; Hieny, S.; Sutterwala, F.S.; Flavell, R.A.; Ghosh, S.; et al. Immunology: TLR11 activation of dendritic cells by a protozoan profilin-like protein. *Science* **2005**, *308*, 1626–1629. [CrossRef] [PubMed]
57. Xiao, X.; Zhao, P.; Rodriguez-Pinto, D.; Qi, D.; Henegariu, O.; Alexopoulou, L.; Flavell, R.A.; Wong, F.S.; Wen, L. Inflammatory Regulation by TLR3 in Acute Hepatitis. *J. Immunol.* **2009**, *183*, 3712–3719. [CrossRef] [PubMed]
58. Negishi, H.; Osawa, T.; Ogami, K.; Ouyang, X.; Sakaguchi, S.; Koshiba, R.; Yanai, H.; Seko, Y.; Shitara, H.; Bishop, K.; et al. A critical link between Toll-like receptor 3 and type II interferon signaling pathways in antiviral innate immunity. *Proc. Natl. Acad. Sci. USA* **2008**, *105*, 20446–20451. [CrossRef]
59. Hemmi, H.; Kaisho, T.; Takeuchi, O.; Sato, S.; Sanjo, H.; Hoshino, K.; Horiuchi, T.; Tomizawa, H.; Takeda, K.; Akira, S. Small-antiviral compounds activate immune cells via the TLR7 MyD88-dependent signaling pathway. *Nat. Immunol.* **2002**, *3*, 196–200. [CrossRef] [PubMed]
60. Peng, G.; Guo, Z.; Kiniwa, Y.; Voo, K.S.; Peng, W.; Fu, T.; Wang, D.Y.; Li, Y.; Wang, H.Y.; Wang, R.F. Immunology: Toll-like receptor 8-mediated reversal of CD4+ regulatory T cell function. *Science* **2005**, *309*, 1380–1384. [CrossRef]
61. Notley, C.A.; Jordan, C.K.; McGovern, J.L.; Brown, M.A.; Ehrenstein, M.R. DNA methylation governs the dynamic regulation of inflammation by apoptotic cells during efferocytosis. *Sci. Rep.* **2017**, *7*, 1–10. [CrossRef]
62. Kanherkar, R.R.; Bhatia-Dey, N.; Csoka, A.B. Epigenetics across the human lifespan. *Front. Cell Dev. Biol.* **2014**, *2*, 49. [CrossRef]
63. Anders, H.-J.; Banas, B.; Schlöndorff, D. Signaling Danger: Toll-Like Receptors and their Potential Roles in Kidney Disease. *J. Am. Soc. Nephrol.* **2004**, *15*, 854–867. [CrossRef]
64. Verstak, B.; Stack, J.; Ve, T.; Mangan, M.; Hjerrild, K.; Jeon, J.; Stahl, R.; Latz, E.; Gay, N.; Kobe, B.; et al. The TLR signaling adaptor TRAM interacts with TRAF6 to mediate activation of the inflammatory response by TLR4. *J. Leukoc. Biol.* **2014**, *96*, 427–436. [CrossRef] [PubMed]
65. Kayagaki, N.; Phung, Q.; Chan, S.; Chaudhari, R.; Quan, C.; O'Rourke, K.M.; Eby, M.; Pietras, E.; Cheng, G.; Bazan, J.F.; et al. DUBA: A deubiquitinase that regulates type I interferon production. *Science* **2007**, *318*, 1628–1632. [CrossRef] [PubMed]
66. Han, C.; Jin, J.; Xu, S.; Liu, H.; Li, N.; Cao, X. Integrin CD11b negatively regulates TLR-triggered inflammatory responses by activating Syk and promoting degradation of MyD88 and TRIF via Cbl-b. *Nat. Immunol.* **2010**, *11*, 734–742. [CrossRef] [PubMed]
67. Skaug, B.; Chen, J.; Du, F.; He, J.; Ma, A.; Chen, Z.J. Direct, noncatalytic mechanism of IKK inhibition by A20. *Mol. Cell* **2011**, *44*, 559–571. [CrossRef] [PubMed]
68. Yuk, J.M.; Shin, D.M.; Lee, H.M.; Kim, J.J.; Kim, S.W.; Jin, H.S.; Yang, C.S.; Park, K.A.; Chanda, D.; Kim, D.K.; et al. The orphan nuclear receptor SHP acts as a negative regulator in inflammatory signaling triggered by Toll-like receptors. *Nat. Immunol.* **2011**, *12*, 742–751. [CrossRef] [PubMed]
69. Kondo, T.; Kawai, T.; Akira, S. Dissecting negative regulation of Toll-like receptor signaling. *Trends Immunol.* **2012**, *33*, 449–458. [CrossRef] [PubMed]

70. Saitoh, T.; Tun-Kyi, A.; Ryo, A.; Yamamoto, M.; Finn, G.; Fujita, T.; Akira, S.; Yamamoto, N.; Lu, K.P.; Yamaoka, S. Negative regulation of interferon-regulatory factor 3-dependent innate antiviral response by the prolyl isomerase Pin1. *Nat. Immunol.* **2006**, *7*, 598–605. [CrossRef]
71. Kawai, T.; Akira, S. The role of pattern-recognition receptors in innate immunity: Update on Toll-like receptors. *Nat. Immunol.* **2010**, *11*, 373–384. [CrossRef]
72. Kawai, T.; Akira, S. Signaling to NF-kappaB by Toll-like receptors. *Trends Mol. Med.* **2007**, *13*, 460–469. [CrossRef]
73. Liu, T.; Zhang, L.; Joo, D.; Sun, S.C. NF-κB signaling in inflammation. *Signal Transduct. Target. Ther.* **2017**, *2*, 1–9. [CrossRef]
74. Couser, W.G.; Johnson, R.J. The etiology of glomerulonephritis: Roles of infection and autoimmunity. *Kidney Int.* **2014**, *86*, 905–914. [CrossRef] [PubMed]
75. Rock, K.L.; Latz, E.; Ontiveros, F.; Kono, H. The sterile inflammatory response. *Annu. Rev. Immunol.* **2010**, *28*, 321–342. [CrossRef] [PubMed]
76. Yamanishi, Y.; Kitaura, J.; Izawa, K.; Kaitani, A.; Komeno, Y.; Nakamura, M.; Yamazaki, S.; Enomoto, Y.; Oki, T.; Akiba, H.; et al. TIM1 is an endogenous ligand for LMIR5/CD300b: LMIR5 deficiency ameliorates mouse kidney ischemia/reperfusion injury. *J. Exp. Med.* **2010**, *207*, 1501–1511. [CrossRef] [PubMed]
77. Anders, H.J. Toll-Like Receptors and Danger Signaling in Kidney Injury. *J. Am. Soc. Nephrol.* **2010**, *21*, 1270–1274. [CrossRef]
78. Rosin, D.L.; Okusa, M.D. Dangers Within: DAMP Responses to Damage and Cell Death in Kidney Disease. *J. Am. Soc. Nephrol.* **2011**, *22*, 416–425. [CrossRef] [PubMed]
79. Mertowski, S.; Grywalska, E.; Gosik, K.; Smarz-Widelska, I.; Hymos, A.; Dworacki, G.; Niedźwiedzka-Rystwej, P.; Drop, B.; Roliński, J.; Załuska, W. TLR2 Expression on Select Lymphocyte Subsets as a New Marker in Glomerulonephritis. *J. Clin. Med.* **2020**, *9*, 541. [CrossRef]
80. Rosenberg, A.Z.; Kopp, J.B. Focal Segmental Glomerulosclerosis. *Clin. J. Am. Soc. Nephrol.* **2017**, *12*, 502–517. [CrossRef]
81. Reggiani, F.; Ponticelli, C. Focal segmental glomerular sclerosis: Do not overlook the role of immune response. *J. Nephrol.* **2016**, *29*, 525–534. [CrossRef]
82. Eardley, K.S.; Kubal, C.; Zehnder, D.; Quinkler, M.; Lepenies, J.; Savage, C.O.; Howie, A.J.; Kaur, K.; Cooper, M.S.; Adu, D.; et al. The role of capillary density, macrophage infiltration and interstitial scarring in the pathogenesis of human chronic kidney disease. *Kidney Int.* **2008**, *74*, 495–504. [CrossRef]
83. Wu, X.; Dolecki, G.J.; Sherry, B.; Zagorski, J.; Lefkowith, J.B. Chemokines are expressed in a myeloid cell-dependent fashion and mediate distinct functions in immune complex glomerulonephritis in rat. *J. Immunol.* **1997**, *158*, 3917–3924.
84. Wang, H.; Zheng, C.; Xu, X.; Zhao, Y.; Lu, Y.; Liu, Z. Fibrinogen links podocyte injury with Toll-like receptor 4 and is associated with disease activity in FSGS patients. *Nephrology* **2018**, *23*, 418–429. [CrossRef] [PubMed]
85. Gaman, A.M.; Moisa, C.; Diaconu, C.C.; Gaman, M.A. Crosstalk between Oxidative Stress, Chronic Inflammation and Disease Progression in Essential Thrombocythemia. *Rev. Chim.* **2019**, *70*, 3486–3489. [CrossRef]
86. Găman, M.A.; Epîngeac, M.E.; Diaconu, C.C.; Găman, A.M. Evaluation of oxidative stress levels in obesity and diabetes by the free oxygen radical test and free oxygen radical defence assays and correlations with anthropometric and laboratory parameters. *World J. Diabetes* **2020**, *11*, 193–201. [CrossRef] [PubMed]
87. Yacov, N.; Feldman, B.; Volkov, A.; Ishai, E.; Breitbart, E.; Mendel, I. Treatment with lecinoxoids attenuates focal and segmental glomerulosclerosis development in nephrectomized rats. *Basic Clin. Pharmacol. Toxicol.* **2019**, *124*, 131–143. [CrossRef]
88. Segarra-Medrano, A.; Carnicer-Cáceres, C.; Arbós-Via, M.A.; Quiles-Pérez, M.T.; Agraz-Pamplona, I.; Ostos-Roldán, E. Biological markers of nephrotic syndrome: A few steps forward in the long way. *Nefrología* **2012**, *32*, 558–572. [CrossRef] [PubMed]
89. Shah, S.R.; Choi, M. Minimal Change Disease in Adults. In *Glomerulonephritis*; Trachtman, H., Herlitz, L.C., Lerma, E.V., Hogan, J.J., Eds.; Springer International Publishing: Cham, Switzerland, 2019; pp. 97–114. ISBN 978-3-319-49379-4.
90. Uwaezuoke, S.N. Biomarkers of Common Childhood Renal Diseases. In *Biomarker—Indicator of Abnormal Physiological Process*; IntechOpen: London, UK, 2018. [CrossRef]

91. Srivastava, T.; Sharma, M.; Yew, K.H.; Sharma, R.; Duncan, R.S.; Saleem, M.A.; McCarthy, E.T.; Kats, A.; Cudmore, P.A.; Alon, U.S.; et al. LPS and PAN-induced podocyte injury in an in vitro model of minimal change disease: Changes in TLR profile. *J. Cell Commun. Signal.* **2013**, *7*, 49–60. [CrossRef]
92. Mishra, O.P.; Kumar, R.; Narayan, G.; Srivastava, P.; Abhinay, A.; Prasad, R.; Singh, A.; Batra, V.V. Toll-like receptor 3 (TLR-3), TLR-4 and CD80 expression in peripheral blood mononuclear cells and urinary CD80 levels in children with idiopathic nephrotic syndrome. *Pediatr. Nephrol.* **2017**, *32*, 1355–1361. [CrossRef] [PubMed]
93. Ishimoto, T.; Shimada, M.; Araya, C.E.; Huskey, J.; Garin, E.H.; Johnson, R.J. Minimal Change Disease: A CD80 podocytopathy? *Semin. Nephrol.* **2011**, *31*, 320–325. [CrossRef]
94. Lai, W.L.; Yeh, T.H.; Chen, P.M.; Chan, C.K.; Chiang, W.C.; Chen, Y.M.; Wu, K.D.; Tsai, T.J. Membranous nephropathy: A review on the pathogenesis, diagnosis, and treatment. *J. Formos. Med. Assoc.* **2015**, *114*, 102–111. [CrossRef]
95. Couser, W.G. Primary Membranous Nephropathy. *Clin. J. Am. Soc. Nephrol.* **2017**, *12*, 983–997. [CrossRef]
96. Liu, W.; Gao, C.; Dai, H.; Zheng, Y.; Dong, Z.; Gao, Y.; Liu, F.; Zhang, Z.; Liu, Z.; Liu, W.; et al. Immunological Pathogenesis of Membranous Nephropathy: Focus on PLA2R1 and Its Role. *Front. Immunol.* **2019**, *10*, 1809. [CrossRef] [PubMed]
97. Chen, S.Y.; Chen, C.H.; Huang, Y.C.; Chan, C.J.; Chen, D.C.; Tsai, F.J. Genetic susceptibility to idiopathic membranous nephropathy in high-prevalence Area, Taiwan. *Biomedicine* **2014**, *4*, 9. [CrossRef] [PubMed]
98. Nafar, M.; Samavat, S. Biomarkers in IgA Nephropathy. In *Biomarkers in Kidney Disease*; Patel, V.B., Ed.; Springer: Dordrecht, The Netherlands, 2015; pp. 1–29. ISBN 978-94-007-7743-9.
99. Liu, Y.; Ma, X.; Lv, J.; Shi, S.; Liu, L.; Chen, Y.; Zhang, H. Risk factors for pregnancy outcomes in patients with IgA nephropathy: A matched cohort study. *Am. J. Kidney Dis.* **2014**, *64*, 730–736. [CrossRef] [PubMed]
100. Coppo, R.; Camilla, R.; Amore, A.; Peruzzi, L. Oxidative Stress in IgA Nephropathy. *Nephron Clin. Pract.* **2010**, *116*, c196–c199. [CrossRef]
101. Suzuki, H.; Suzuki, Y.; Narita, I.; Aizawa, M.; Kihara, M.; Yamanaka, T.; Kanou, T.; Tsukaguchi, H.; Novak, J.; Horikoshi, S.; et al. Toll-Like Receptor 9 Affects Severity of IgA Nephropathy. *J. Am. Soc. Nephrol.* **2008**, *19*, 2384–2395. [CrossRef]
102. Rollino, C.; Vischini, G.; Coppo, R. IgA nephropathy and infections. *J. Nephrol.* **2016**, *29*, 463–468. [CrossRef]
103. Merkle, M.; Ribeiro, A.; Köppel, S.; Pircher, J.; Mannell, H.; Roeder, M.; Wörnle, M. TLR3-dependent immune regulatory functions of human mesangial cells. *Cell. Mol. Immunol.* **2012**, *9*, 334–340. [CrossRef]
104. Coppo, R.; Amore, A.; Peruzzi, L.; Vergano, L.; Camilla, R. Innate immunity and IgA nephropathy. *J. Nephrol.* **2010**, *23*, 626–632.
105. Sheng, X.; Zuo, X.; Liu, X.; Zhou, Y.; Sun, X. Crosstalk between TLR4 and Notch1 signaling in the IgA nephropathy during inflammatory response. *Int. Urol. Nephrol.* **2018**, *50*, 779–785. [CrossRef]
106. Lim, B.J.; Lee, D.; Hong, S.W.; Jeong, H.J. Toll-Like Receptor 4 Signaling is Involved in IgA-Stimulated Mesangial Cell Activation. *Yonsei Med. J.* **2011**, *52*, 610–615. [CrossRef]
107. Chebotareva, N.; Bobkova, I.; Shilov, E. Heat shock proteins and kidney disease: Perspectives of HSP therapy. *Cell Stress Chaperones* **2017**, *22*, 319–343. [CrossRef] [PubMed]
108. Kaneko, T.; Mii, A.; Fukui, M.; Nagahama, K.; Shimizu, A.; Tsuruoka, S. IgA Nephropathy and Psoriatic Arthritis that Improved with Steroid Pulse Therapy and Mizoribine in Combination with Treatment for Chronic Tonsillitis and Epipharyngitis. *Intern. Med.* **2015**, *54*, 1085–1090. [CrossRef] [PubMed]
109. Brown, H.J.; Lock, H.R.; Wolfs, T.G.A.M.; Buurman, W.A.; Sacks, S.H.; Robson, M.G. Toll-like receptor 4 ligation on intrinsic renal cells contributes to the induction of antibody-mediated glomerulonephritis via CXCL1 and CXCL2. *J. Am. Soc. Nephrol.* **2007**, *18*, 1732–1739. [CrossRef] [PubMed]
110. Myllymäki, J.; Syrjänen, J.; Helin, H.; Pasternack, A.; Kattainen, A.; Mustonen, J. Vascular diseases and their risk factors in IgA nephropathy. *Nephrol. Dial. Transplant.* **2006**, *21*, 1876–1882. [CrossRef] [PubMed]
111. Feehally, J.; Barratt, J. The Genetics of IgA Nephropathy: An Overview from Western Countries. *Kidney Dis.* **2015**, *1*, 33–41. [CrossRef]
112. Takeda, K.; Kaisho, T.; Akira, S. Toll-Like Receptors. *Annu. Rev. Immunol.* **2003**, *21*, 335–376. [CrossRef] [PubMed]
113. Sano, N.; Kitazawa, K.; Sugisaki, T. Localization and roles of CD44, hyaluronic acid and osteopontin in IgA nephropathy. *Nephron* **2001**, *89*, 416–421. [CrossRef]

114. Zhang, Y.-M.; Zhou, X.-J.; Zhang, H. What Genetics Tells Us About the Pathogenesis of IgA Nephropathy: The Role of Immune Factors and Infection. *Kidney Int. Rep.* **2017**, *2*, 318–331. [CrossRef]
115. Cui, Y.; Liu, S.; Cui, W.; Gao, D.; Zhou, W.; Luo, P. Identification of potential biomarkers and therapeutic targets for human IgA nephropathy and hypertensive nephropathy by bioinformatics analysis. *Mol. Med. Rep.* **2017**, *16*, 3087–3094. [CrossRef]
116. Tycová, I.; Hrubá, P.; Maixnerová, D.; Girmanová, E.; Mrázová, P.; Straňavová, L.; Zachoval, R.; Merta, M.; Slatinská, J.; Kollár, M.; et al. Molecular profiling in IgA nephropathy and focal and segmental glomerulosclerosis. *Physiol. Res.* **2018**, *67*, 93–105. [CrossRef]
117. Wardle, E.N. B Lymphocyte Stimulator and Autoimmune Disease. *Saudi J. Kidney Dis. Transplant.* **2004**, *15*, 155.
118. Li, W.; Peng, X.; Liu, Y.; Liu, H.; Liu, F.; He, L.; Liu, Y.; Zhang, F.; Guo, C.; Chen, G.; et al. TLR9 and BAFF: Their expression in patients with IgA nephropathy. *Mol. Med. Rep.* **2014**, *10*, 1469–1474. [CrossRef] [PubMed]
119. Gao, R.; Wu, W.; Wen, Y.; Li, X. Hydroxychloroquine alleviates persistent proteinuria in IgA nephropathy. *Int. Urol. Nephrol.* **2017**, *49*, 1233–1241. [CrossRef] [PubMed]
120. Wu, M.Y.; Chen, C.S.; Yiang, G.T.; Cheng, P.W.; Chen, Y.L.; Chiu, H.C.; Liu, K.H.; Lee, W.C.; Li, C.J. The Emerging Role of Pathogenesis of IgA Nephropathy. *J. Clin. Med.* **2018**, *7*, 225. [CrossRef] [PubMed]
121. Coppo, R. Treatment of IgA nephropathy: Recent advances and prospects. *Nephrol. Ther.* **2018**, *14*, S13–S21. [CrossRef]
122. Yuling, H.; Ruijing, X.; Xiang, J.; Yanping, J.; Lang, C.; Li, L.; Dingping, Y.; Xinti, T.; Jingyi, L.; Zhiqing, T.; et al. CD19+CD5+ B Cells in Primary IgA Nephropathy. *J. Am. Soc. Nephrol.* **2008**, *19*, 2130–2139. [CrossRef]
123. Wang, Y.Y.; Zhang, L.; Zhao, P.W.; Ma, L.; Li, C.; Zou, H.B.; Jiang, Y.F. Functional implications of regulatory B cells in human IgA nephropathy. *Scand. J. Immunol.* **2014**, *79*, 51–60. [CrossRef]
124. Coppo, R.; Camilla, R.; Amore, A.; Peruzzi, L.; Daprà, V.; Loiacono, E.; Vatrano, S.; Rollino, C.; Sepe, V.; Rampino, T.; et al. Toll-like receptor 4 expression is increased in circulating mononuclear cells of patients with immunoglobulin A nephropathy. *Clin. Exp. Immunol.* **2010**, *159*, 73–81. [CrossRef]
125. Almaani, S.; Meara, A.; Rovin, B.H. Update on Lupus Nephritis. *Clin. J. Am. Soc. Nephrol.* **2017**, *12*, 825–835. [CrossRef]
126. Ruiz Irastorza, G.; Espinosa, G.; Frutos, M.A.; Jiménez Alonso, J.; Praga, M.; Pallarés, L.; Rivera, F.; Robles Marhuenda, A.; Segarra, A.; Quereda, C.; et al. Diagnosis and treatment of lupus nephritis. Consensus document from the systemic auto-immune disease group (GEAS) of the Spanish Society of Internal Medicine (SEMI) and Spanish Society of Nephrology (S.E.N.). *Nefrologia* **2012**, *32* (Suppl. 1), 1–35. [CrossRef]
127. Klonowska-Szymczyk, A.; Kulczycka-Siennicka, L.; Robak, T.; Smolewski, P.; Cebula-Obrzut, B.; Robak, E. The impact of agonists and antagonists of TLR3 and TLR9 on concentrations of IL-6, IL10 and sIL-2R in culture supernatants of peripheral blood mononuclear cells derived from patients with systemic lupus erythematosus. *Adv. Hyg. Exp. Med.* **2017**, *71*, 867–875. [CrossRef] [PubMed]
128. Aragón, C.C.; Tafúr, R.A.; Suárez-Avellaneda, A.; Martínez, M.D.T.; de las Salas, A.; Tobón, G.J. Urinary biomarkers in lupus nephritis. *J. Transl. Autoimmun.* **2020**, *3*, 100042. [CrossRef] [PubMed]
129. Patole, P.S.; Pawar, R.D.; Lech, M.; Zecher, D.; Schmidt, H.; Segerer, S.; Ellwart, A.; Henger, A.; Kretzler, M.; Anders, H.-J. Expression and regulation of Toll-like receptors in lupus-like immune complex glomerulonephritis of MRL-Fas(lpr) mice. *Nephrol. Dial. Transplant.* **2006**, *21*, 3062–3073. [CrossRef] [PubMed]
130. Pawar, R.D.; Patole, P.S.; Zecher, D.; Segerer, S.; Kretzler, M.; Schlöndorff, D.; Anders, H.J. Toll-Like Receptor-7 Modulates Immune Complex Glomerulonephritis. *J. Am. Soc. Nephrol.* **2006**, *17*, 141–149. [CrossRef] [PubMed]
131. Gao, R.; Yu, W.; Wen, Y.; Li, H. Beta2-glycoprotein I Expression in Lupus Nephritis Patients with Antiphospholipid-associated Nephropathy. *J. Rheumatol.* **2016**, *43*, 2026–2032. [CrossRef]
132. Kwok, S.K.; Tsokos, G.C. New insights into the role of renal resident cells in the pathogenesis of lupus nephritis. *Korean J. Intern. Med.* **2018**, *33*, 284–289. [CrossRef]
133. Urbonaviciute, V.; Starke, C.; Pirschel, W.; Pohle, S.; Frey, S.; Daniel, C.; Amann, K.; Schett, G.; Herrmann, M.; Voll, R.E. Toll-like Receptor 2 Is Required for Autoantibody Production and Development of Renal Disease in Pristane-Induced Lupus. *Arthritis Rheum.* **2013**, *65*, 1612–1623. [CrossRef]

134. Conti, F.; Spinelli, F.R.; Truglia, S.; Miranda, F.; Alessandri, C.; Ceccarelli, F.; Bombardieri, M.; Giannakakis, K.; Valesini, G. Kidney Expression of Toll Like Receptors in Lupus Nephritis: Quantification and Clinicopathological Correlations. *Mediat. Inflamm.* **2016**, *2016*, 7697592. [CrossRef]
135. Lorenz, G.; Lech, M.; Anders, H.J. Toll-like receptor activation in the pathogenesis of lupus nephritis. *Clin. Immunol.* **2017**, *185*, 86–94. [CrossRef]
136. Pawar, R.D.; Patole, P.S.; Ellwart, A.; Lech, M.; Segerer, S.; Schlondorff, D.; Anders, H.J. Ligands to Nucleic Acid–Specific Toll-Like Receptors and the Onset of Lupus Nephritis. *J. Am. Soc. Nephrol.* **2006**, *17*, 3365–3373. [CrossRef]
137. Lorenz, G.; Anders, H.J. Neutrophils, Dendritic Cells, Toll-Like Receptors, and Interferon-α in Lupus Nephritis. *Semin. Nephrol.* **2015**, *35*, 410–426. [CrossRef]
138. Chen, D.N.; Fan, L.; Wu, Y.X.; Zhou, Q.; Chen, W.; Yu, X.Q. A Predictive Model for Estimation Risk of Proliferative Lupus Nephritis. *Chin. Med. J.* **2018**, *131*, 1275–1281. [CrossRef] [PubMed]
139. Pisetsky, D.S. HMGB1: A smoking gun in lupus nephritis? *Arthritis Res. Ther.* **2012**, *14*, 112. [CrossRef] [PubMed]
140. Sun, F.; Teng, J.; Yu, P.; Li, W.; Chang, J.; Xu, H. Involvement of TWEAK and the NF-κB signaling pathway in lupus nephritis. *Exp. Ther. Med.* **2018**, *15*, 2611–2619. [CrossRef] [PubMed]
141. Watanabe, H.; Watanabe, K.S.; Liu, K.; Hiramatsu, S.; Zeggar, S.; Katsuyama, E.; Tatebe, N.; Akahoshi, A.; Takenaka, F.; Hanada, T.; et al. Anti-high Mobility Group Box 1 Antibody Ameliorates Albuminuria in MRL/lpr Lupus-Prone Mice. *Mol. Ther. Meth. Clin. Dev.* **2017**, *6*, 31–39. [CrossRef]
142. Ma, K.; Li, J.; Fang, Y.; Lu, L. Roles of B Cell-Intrinsic TLR Signals in Systemic Lupus Erythematosus. *Int. J. Mol. Sci.* **2015**, *16*, 13084–13105. [CrossRef] [PubMed]
143. Wirestam, L.; Schierbeck, H.; Skogh, T.; Gunnarsson, I.; Ottosson, L.; Erlandsson-Harris, H.; Wetterö, J.; Sjöwall, C. Antibodies against High Mobility Group Box protein-1 (HMGB1) versus other anti-nuclear antibody fine-specificities and disease activity in systemic lupus erythematosus. *Arthritis Res. Ther.* **2015**, *17*, 338. [CrossRef]
144. Qing, X.; Pitashny, M.; Thomas, D.B.; Barrat, F.J.; Hogarth, M.P.; Putterman, C. Pathogenic anti-DNA antibodies modulate gene expression in mesangial cells: Involvement of HMGB1 in anti-DNA antibody-induced renal injury. *Immunol. Lett.* **2008**, *121*, 61–73. [CrossRef]
145. Banas, M.C.; Banas, B.; Hudkins, K.L.; Wietecha, T.A.; Iyoda, M.; Bock, E.; Hauser, P.; Pippin, J.W.; Shankland, S.J.; Smith, K.D.; et al. TLR4 Links Podocytes with the Innate Immune System to Mediate Glomerular Injury. *J. Am. Soc. Nephrol.* **2008**, *19*, 704–713. [CrossRef]
146. Jończyk, M.; Kuliczkowska-Płaksej, J.; Mierzwicka, A.; Bolanowski, M. The polycystic ovarian syndrome and chronic inflammation: The role of Toll-like receptors. *Postepy Hig. Med. Dosw.* **2018**, *72*, 1199–1207. [CrossRef]
147. Lartigue, A.; Colliou, N.; Calbo, S.; François, A.; Jacquot, S.; Arnoult, C.; Tron, F.; Gilbert, D.; Musette, P. Critical role of TLR2 and TLR4 in autoantibody production and glomerulonephritis in lpr mutation-induced mouse lupus. *J. Immunol.* **2009**, *183*, 6207–6216. [CrossRef] [PubMed]
148. Horton, C.G.; Pan, Z.; Farris, A.D. Targeting toll-like receptors for treatment of SLE. *Mediat. Inflamm.* **2010**, *2010*, 498980. [CrossRef] [PubMed]
149. Wardle, E.N. Toll-Like Receptors and Glomerulonephritis. *Saudi J. Kidney Dis. Transpl.* **2007**, *18*, 159–172.
150. Lichtnekert, J.; Vielhauer, V.; Zecher, D.; Kulkarni, O.; Clauss, S.; Hornung, V.; Mayadas, T.; Beutler, B.; Akira, S.; Anders, H.-J. Trif is not required for immune complex glomerulonephritis: Dying cells activate mesangial cells via Tlr2/Myd88 rather than Tlr3/Trif. *Am. J. Physiol. Renal. Physiol.* **2009**, *296*, F867–F874. [CrossRef]
151. Pradhan, V.; Patwardhan, M.; Ghosh, K. Fc gamma receptor polymorphisms in systemic lupus erythematosus and their correlation with the clinical severity of the disease. *Indian J. Hum. Genet.* **2008**, *14*, 77–81. [CrossRef] [PubMed]
152. Mackay, M.; Stanevsky, A.; Wang, T.; Aranow, C.; Li, M.; Koenig, S.; Ravetch, J.V.; Diamond, B. Selective dysregulation of the FcγIIB receptor on memory B cells in SLE. *J. Exp. Med.* **2006**, *203*, 2157–2164. [CrossRef] [PubMed]
153. Lim, A.K. Diabetic nephropathy—Complications and treatment. *Int. J. Nephrol. Renovasc. Dis.* **2014**, *7*, 361–381. [CrossRef] [PubMed]

154. Mudaliar, H.; Pollock, C.; Panchapakesan, U. Role of Toll-like receptors in diabetic nephropathy. *Clin. Sci.* **2014**, *126*, 685–694. [CrossRef] [PubMed]
155. Conserva, F.; Gesualdo, L.; Papale, M. A Systems Biology Overview on Human Diabetic Nephropathy: From Genetic Susceptibility to Post-Transcriptional and Post-Translational Modifications. *J. Diabetes Res.* **2016**, *2016*, 7934504. [CrossRef] [PubMed]
156. Umanath, K.; Lewis, J.B. Update on Diabetic Nephropathy: Core Curriculum 2018. *Am. J. Kidney Dis.* **2018**, *71*, 884–895. [CrossRef]
157. Zhang, J.; Liu, J.; Qin, X.; Zhang, J.; Liu, J.; Qin, X. Advances in early biomarkers of diabetic nephropathy. *Rev. Assoc. Med. Bras.* **2018**, *64*, 85–92. [CrossRef] [PubMed]
158. Mansour, I.; Thajudeen, B. Overview of Diabetic Nephropathy. *J. R. Soc. Med.* **2017**, 1–21. [CrossRef]
159. Wifi, M.-N.A.; Assem, M.; Elsherif, R.H.; El-Azab, H.A.-F.; Saif, A. Toll-like receptors-2 and -9 (TLR2 and TLR9) gene polymorphism in patients with type 2 diabetes and diabetic foot. *Medicine* **2017**, *96*, e6760. [CrossRef] [PubMed]
160. Eknoyan, G. A Historical Overview of Diabetic Nephropathy. In *Diabetic Nephropathy*; Springer: Cham, Switzerland, 2019; pp. 3–19. [CrossRef]
161. Chen, X.; Ma, J.; Kwan, T.; Stribos, E.G.D.; Messchendorp, A.L.; Loh, Y.W.; Wang, X.; Paul, M.; Cunningham, E.C.; Habib, M.; et al. Blockade of HMGB1 Attenuates Diabetic Nephropathy in Mice. *Sci. Rep.* **2018**, *8*, 8319. [CrossRef]
162. Shi, H.; Che, Y.; Bai, L.; Zhang, J.; Fan, J.; Mao, H. High mobility group box 1 in diabetic nephropathy (Review). *Exp. Ther. Med.* **2017**, *14*, 2431–2433. [CrossRef]
163. Bellini, S.; Barutta, F.; Mastrocola, R.; Imperatore, L.; Bruno, G.; Gruden, G. Heat Shock Proteins in Vascular Diabetic Complications: Review and Future Perspective. *Int. J. Mol. Sci.* **2017**, *18*, 2709. [CrossRef]
164. Guo, C.; Zhang, L.; Nie, L.; Zhang, N.; Xiao, D.; Ye, X.; Ou, M.; Liu, Y.; Zhang, B.; Wang, M.; et al. Association of polymorphisms in the MyD88, IRAK4 and TRAF6 genes and susceptibility to type 2 diabetes mellitus and diabetic nephropathy in a southern Han Chinese population. *Mol. Cell. Endocrinol.* **2016**, *429*, 114–119. [CrossRef]
165. Wang, Y.; Li, Y.; Zhang, T.; Chi, Y.; Liu, M.; Liu, Y. Genistein and Myd88 Activate Autophagy in High Glucose-Induced Renal Podocytes In Vitro. *Med. Sci. Monit.* **2018**, *24*, 4823–4831. [CrossRef]
166. Murea, M.; Register, T.C.; Divers, J.; Bowden, D.W.; Carr, J.J.; Hightower, C.R.; Xu, J.; Smith, S.C.; Hruska, K.A.; Langefeld, C.D.; et al. Relationships between serum MCP-1 and subclinical kidney disease: African American-Diabetes Heart Study. *BMC Nephrol.* **2012**, *13*, 148. [CrossRef]
167. Suryavanshi, S.V.; Kulkarni, Y.A. NF-κβ: A Potential Target in the Management of Vascular Complications of Diabetes. *Front. Pharmacol.* **2017**, *8*, 798. [CrossRef]
168. Lu, Q.; Wang, W.-W.; Zhang, M.-Z.; Ma, Z.-X.; Qiu, X.-R.; Shen, M.; Yin, X.-X. ROS induces epithelial-mesenchymal transition via the TGF-β1/PI3K/Akt/mTOR pathway in diabetic nephropathy. *Exp. Ther. Med.* **2019**, *17*, 835–846. [CrossRef]
169. Tong, Y.; Chuan, J.; Bai, L.; Shi, J.; Zhong, L.; Duan, X.; Zhu, Y. The protective effect of shikonin on renal tubular epithelial cell injury induced by high glucose. *Biomed. Pharmacother.* **2018**, *98*, 701–708. [CrossRef]
170. Li, F.; Yang, N.; Zhang, L.; Tan, H.; Huang, B.; Liang, Y.; Chen, M.; Yu, X. Increased Expression of Toll-Like Receptor 2 in Rat Diabetic Nephropathy. *Am. J. Nephrol.* **2010**, *32*, 179–186. [CrossRef]
171. Cha, J.J.; Hyun, Y.Y.; Lee, M.H.; Kim, J.E.; Nam, D.H.; Song, H.K.; Kang, Y.S.; Lee, J.E.; Kim, H.W.; Han, J.Y.; et al. Renal protective effects of toll-like receptor 4 signaling blockade in type 2 diabetic mice. *Endocrinology* **2013**, *154*, 2144–2155. [CrossRef]
172. Stadler, K.; Goldberg, I.J.; Susztak, K. The Evolving Understanding of the Contribution of Lipid Metabolism to Diabetic Kidney Disease. *Curr. Diabetes Rep.* **2015**, *15*, 40. [CrossRef]
173. Cao, A.; Wang, L.; Chen, X.; Guo, H.; Chu, S.; Zhang, X.; Peng, W. Ursodeoxycholic Acid Ameliorated Diabetic Nephropathy by Attenuating Hyperglycemia-Mediated Oxidative Stress. *Biol. Pharm. Bull.* **2016**, *39*, 1300–1308. [CrossRef]
174. Kaur, H.; Chien, A.; Jialal, I. Hyperglycemia induces Toll like receptor 4 expression and activity in mouse mesangial cells: Relevance to diabetic nephropathy. *Am. J. Physiol. Renal Physiol.* **2012**, *303*, F1145–F1150. [CrossRef]
175. Takata, S.; Sawa, Y.; Uchiyama, T.; Ishikawa, H. Expression of Toll-Like Receptor 4 in Glomerular Endothelial Cells under Diabetic Conditions. *Acta Histochem. Cytochem.* **2013**, *46*, 35–42. [CrossRef]

176. Panchapakesan, U.; Pollock, C. The role of toll-like receptors in diabetic kidney disease. *Curr. Opin. Nephrol. Hypertens.* **2018**, *27*, 30–34. [CrossRef]
177. Aluksanasuwan, S.; Sueksakit, K.; Fong-Ngern, K.; Thongboonkerd, V. Role of HSP60 (HSPD1) in diabetes-induced renal tubular dysfunction: Regulation of intracellular protein aggregation, ATP production, and oxidative stress. *FASEB J.* **2017**, *31*, 2157–2167. [CrossRef]
178. Zyzak, J.; Matuszyk, J.; Siednienko, J. Multilevel maturation of Toll-like receptor 9. *Postepy Hig. Med. Dosw.* **2013**, *67*, 1034–1046. [CrossRef] [PubMed]
179. Zipris, D. Toll-like receptors and type 1 diabetes. *Adv. Exp. Med. Biol.* **2010**, *654*, 585–610. [CrossRef]
180. Ronco, C.; Bellomo, R.; Kellum, J.A. Acute kidney injury. *Lancet* **2019**, *394*, 1949–1964. [CrossRef]
181. Baer, P.C.; Koch, B.; Geiger, H. Kidney Inflammation, Injury and Regeneration. *Int. J. Mol. Sci.* **2020**, *21*, 1164. [CrossRef] [PubMed]
182. Coca, S.G.; Yusuf, B.; Shlipak, M.G.; Garg, A.X.; Parikh, C.R. Long-term risk of mortality and other adverse outcomes after acute kidney injury: A systematic review and meta-analysis. *Am. J. Kidney Dis.* **2009**, *53*, 961–973. [CrossRef]
183. Hsu, C.; Chertow, G.M.; McCulloch, C.E.; Fan, D.; Ordoñez, J.D.; Go, A.S. Nonrecovery of kidney function and death after acute on chronic renal failure. *Clin. J. Am. Soc. Nephrol.* **2009**, *4*, 891–898. [CrossRef]
184. Wald, R.; Quinn, R.R.; Luo, J.; Li, P.; Scales, D.C.; Mamdani, M.M.; Ray, J.G.; University of Toronto Acute Kidney Injury Research Group. Chronic dialysis and death among survivors of acute kidney injury requiring dialysis. *JAMA* **2009**, *302*, 1179–1185. [CrossRef]
185. Dong, Y.; Zhang, Q.; Wen, J.; Chen, T.; He, L.; Wang, Y.; Yin, J.; Wu, R.; Xue, R.; Li, S.; et al. Ischemic Duration and Frequency Determines AKI-to-CKD Progression Monitored by Dynamic Changes of Tubular Biomarkers in IRI Mice. *Front. Physiol.* **2019**, *10*, 153. [CrossRef]
186. Leemans, J.C.; Stokman, G.; Claessen, N.; Rouschop, K.M.; Teske, G.J.D.; Kirschning, C.J.; Akira, S.; van der Poll, T.; Weening, J.J.; Florquin, S. Renal-associated TLR2 mediates ischemia/reperfusion injury in the kidney. *J. Clin. Investig.* **2005**, *115*, 2894–2903. [CrossRef]
187. Kim, B.S.; Lim, S.W.; Li, C.; Kim, J.S.; Sun, B.K.; Ahn, K.O.; Han, S.W.; Kim, J.; Yang, C.W. Ischemia-reperfusion injury activates innate immunity in rat kidneys. *Transplantation* **2005**, *79*, 1370–1377. [CrossRef]
188. Wolfs, T.G.A.M.; Buurman, W.A.; van Schadewijk, A.; de Vries, B.; Daemen, M.A.R.C.; Hiemstra, P.S.; van't Veer, C. In vivo expression of Toll-like receptor 2 and 4 by renal epithelial cells: IFN-gamma and TNF-alpha mediated up-regulation during inflammation. *J. Immunol.* **2002**, *168*, 1286–1293. [CrossRef]
189. Paulus, P.; Rupprecht, K.; Baer, P.; Obermüller, N.; Penzkofer, D.; Reissig, C.; Scheller, B.; Holfeld, J.; Zacharowski, K.; Dimmeler, S.; et al. The early activation of toll-like receptor (TLR)-3 initiates kidney injury after ischemia and reperfusion. *PLoS ONE* **2014**, *15*, e94366. [CrossRef] [PubMed]
190. Good, D.W.; George, T.; Watts, B.A. Toll-like Receptor 2 Is Required for LPS-induced Toll-like Receptor 4 Signaling and Inhibition of Ion Transport in Renal Thick Ascending Limb. *J. Biol. Chem.* **2012**, *287*, 20208–20220. [CrossRef] [PubMed]
191. Good, D.W.; George, T.; Watts, B.A. Toll-like receptor 2 mediates inhibition of HCO_3^- absorption by bacterial lipoprotein in medullary thick ascending limb. *Am. J. Physiol. Renal Physiol.* **2010**, *299*, F536–F544. [CrossRef] [PubMed]
192. Vallés, P.G.; Lorenzo, A.G.; Bocanegra, V.; Vallés, R. Acute kidney injury: What part do toll-like receptors play? *Int. J. Nephrol. Renovasc. Dis.* **2014**, *7*, 241–251. [CrossRef]
193. Bonventre, J.V.; Yang, L. Cellular pathophysiology of ischemic acute kidney injury. *J. Clin. Investig.* **2011**, *121*, 4210–4221. [CrossRef]
194. Devarajan, P. Update on Mechanisms of Ischemic Acute Kidney Injury. *J. Am. Soc. Nephrol.* **2006**, *17*, 1503–1520. [CrossRef]
195. Kinsey, G.R.; Li, L.; Okusa, M.D. Inflammation in acute kidney injury. *Nephron Exp. Nephrol.* **2008**, *109*, e102–e107. [CrossRef]
196. Venkatachalam, M.A.; Griffin, K.A.; Lan, R.; Geng, H.; Saikumar, P.; Bidani, A.K. Acute kidney injury: A springboard for progression in chronic kidney disease. *Am. J. Physiol. Renal Physiol.* **2010**, *298*, F1078–F1094. [CrossRef]
197. Lee, S.; Huen, S.; Nishio, H.; Nishio, S.; Lee, H.K.; Choi, B.-S.; Ruhrberg, C.; Cantley, L.G. Distinct macrophage phenotypes contribute to kidney injury and repair. *J. Am. Soc. Nephrol.* **2011**, *22*, 317–326. [CrossRef]

13

Emerging Modes of Treatment of IgA Nephropathy

Dita Maixnerova * and Vladimir Tesar

1st Faculty of Medicine, General University Hospital, Department of Nephrology, Charles University, 128 08 Prague, Czech Republic; vladimir.tesar@vfn.cz

* Correspondence: ditama@centrum.cz

Abstract: IgA nephropathy is the most common primary glomerulonephritis with potentially serious outcome leading to end stage renal disease in 30 to 50% of patients within 20 to 30 years. Renal biopsy, which might be associated with risks of complications (bleeding and others), still remains the only reliable diagnostic tool for IgA nephropathy. Therefore, the search for non-invasive diagnostic and prognostic markers for detection of subclinical types of IgA nephropathy, evaluation of disease activity, and assessment of treatment effectiveness, is of utmost importance. In this review, we summarize treatment options for patients with IgA nephropathy including the drugs currently under evaluation in randomized control trials. An early initiation of immunosupressive regimens in patients with IgA nephropathy at risk of progression should result in the slowing down of the progression of renal function to end stage renal disease.

Keywords: IgAN; proteinuria; CKD; progression; ACEI; corticosteroids

---

1. Introduction, Diagnosis, Pathogenesis

IgA nephropathy (IgAN) is the most common primary glomerulonephritis worldwide with potentially serious renal outcome leading, in 30–50% of patients, to end stage renal disease (ESRD) within 20 to 30 years of follow-up [1,2].

Diagnosis of IgAN is currently based on evaluation of renal biopsy specimens with the demonstration of mesangial IgA1-dominant or co-dominant immunodeposits [3,4].

Clinical risk factors predicting poor renal outcome in patients with IgAN include time-averaged proteinuria, hypertension, decreased estimated glomerular filtration rate (eGFR) [2,5] at presentation or during follow up as well as histological findings evaluated using C-MEST classification [6,7].

IgAN is an autoimmune disease arising from a multi-hit pathophysiological process and is believed to be caused by the interaction of genetic and environmental contributing factors [2,8,9]. Genome-wide associated studies indicated a pathogenetic role of the intestinal immunity abnormalities in IgAN and confirmed a direct link of IgAN with the risk of inflammatory bowel disease or maintenance of the intestinal epithelial barrier [9].

A key role in the pathogenesis of IgAN is played by aberrantly glycosylated forms of IgA1 with galactose-deficient *O*-glycans (galactose-deficient IgA1; Gd-IgA1), which are recognized by antiglycan autoantibodies of IgG and/or IgA1 isotype, resulting in the formation of circulating immune complexes [10,11]. These complexes are deposited in the glomerular mesangium with subsequent mesangial-cell activation and local stimulation of the complement system, proliferation of mesangial cells, and production of extracellular matrix and cytokines, which could alter podocyte gene expression and glomerular permeability in clinical presentation of proteinuria and tubulointerstitial changes in IgAN [12–15]. If unabated, the damage progresses to glomerulosclerosis and interstitial fibrosis with impaired renal function with subsequent end-stage renal disease.

2. Treatment

Which goals do we have in treatment of patients with IgAN? We have to respect the possibility of induction of clinical remmission, reduction in proteinuria and hematuria, stabilization of renal parameters without further decline of GFR, a decrease in the rate of progression, prevention of the necessity of renal replacement therapy as well as the risk of adverse events in patients with corticosteroids and other immunosuppressive regimens. The balance of risks and benefits needs to be taken into account in all individual cases.

2.1. Low Risk Patients with IgAN

Low risk patients with minor urinary abnormalities (proteinuria < 0.5 g/d and/or isolated microhematuria), normal glomerular filtration rate (GFR), no hypertension and without histological activity are at low risk of progression, do not require treatment and should be checked annually for at least 10 years according to KDIGO guidelines (Table 1) [16]. Supportive management such as diet modification, weight optimisation and smoking cessation should be taken into consideration. The ideal treatment of the initial phase of IgAN is focused on the decrease in or inhibition of production of Gd-IgA1 by means of a low cost drug with minimal adverse effects. Intestinal-associated lymphoid tissue and mucosal immunity show attractive targets [17,18]. Intestinal microbiota and/or diet regimens including gluten-free diet were suggested in an experimental mice model and human pilot studies [17,19].

Low protein diets were reported to decrease renal function decline [20]. The restriction of sodium was associated with sodium sensitivity of blood pressure and correlated with renal ultrastructural damage [21]. The decrease in proteinuria was shown even in normotensive patients with IgAN due to low-sodium diets [21]. The damaging effects of heightened sodium sensitivity are mediated due to the renin-angiotensin system and it was confirmed that sodium restriction improves the antiproteinuric effects of RAS inhibition in patients with IgAN [22]. Increased morbidity and mortality in patients with chronic kidney disease were associated with extreme body mass index [23]. The relation between body mass index and the probability of end stage renal disease was shown in patients with IgAN in a Chinese study [23]. Increased body mass index associated with lower remission of proteinuria subsequent to treatment was confirmed in a Japanese study [24]. It was assumed that obesity increased proteinuria in connection with hypertension and other parts of metabolic syndrome. Moreover, the advantages of losing weight in overweight patients with IgAN through protein/sodium restriction, and by attaining maximal control of hypertension using treatment with inhibitors of the renin-angiotension system, were confirmed [25].

In addition, the benefits of quitting smoking on slowing down the progression of renal function decline in patients with IgAN were assessed [26].

2.2. Intermediate Risk Patients with IgAN

Intermediate risk IgAN patients with proteinuria > 0.5–1 g/d, and/or hypertension and a reduced GFR (without active histological findings in renal specimens) should obtain optimized supportive treatment with the inhibitors of the renin-angiotensin system (RAS) with up-titration of the drug depending on blood pressure to achieve proteinuria < 1 g/d, and should be thoroughly monitored [16]. The suggested therapeutic goals of blood pressure in patients with proteinuria < 1 g/d are <130/80 mmHg, and <125/75 mmHg in patients with initial proteinuria >1 g/d (Table 1) [16]. RAS inhibition was demonstrated to reduce proteinuria and may possibly also reduce the progression of chronic kidney disease in patients with IgAN; at least part of this effect is probably mediated by improved control of blood pressure. High risk of mortality of patients with IgAN might be caused by chronic kidney disease [27–29].

Table 1. KDIGO guidelines for the treatment of IgAN [16].

Intervention	Recommendation	Grade
Antiproteinuric and Antihypertensive Therapy	Long-term treatment of ACE inhibitors or ARBs is recommended for patients with proteinuria > 1 g/day, with up-titration of the drug depending on blood pressure to achieve proteinuria < 1 g/day.	**1B**
	A target blood pressure of < 130/80 mmHg is recommended for patients with proteinuria < 1 g daily, and <125/75 for patients with proteinuria >1 g daily.	**Not graded**
Corticosteroids	A 6 month course of corticosteroids is recommended in patients with persistent proteinuria of >1 g/day despite 3–6 months of optimal supportive care and GFR > 50 mL/min per 1.73 m^2.	**2C**
Other Immunosuppressive Agents	Patients with crescentic IgAN involving over 50% of glomeruli and rapidly progressive course should be treated with steroids and cyclophosphamide.	**2D**
	Not treating with corticosteroids combined with cyclophosphamide or azathioprine (unless crescentic forms with rapidly progressive course).	**2D**
	Not using immunosuppressive regimen in patients with GFR < 30 mL/min per 1.73 m^2 (unless crescentic forms with rapidly progressive course).	**2C**
	Not using MMF.	**2C**
Fish oils	Fish oils may be potentially useful in patients with persistent proteinuria ≥ 1 g/day, despite 3–6 months of optimized supportive care.	**2D**
Tonsilectomy, Antiplatelet Agents	Not recommended.	**2C**

It was suggested that patients with persistent proteinuria ≥ 1 g/d, despite 3–6 months of optimized supportive care (including RAS and blood pressure control), and GFR > 50 mL/min per 1.73 m^2, should receive a 6-month course of corticosteroid therapy (Table 1) [16]. The 10-year renal survival and median proteinuria were significantly better in patients who received a 6-month regimen of corticosteroids compared to patients with a symptomatic treatment (97% vs. 53%, $p = 0.0003$; median proteinuria 1.9 g/24 h at baseline, 1.1 g/24 h after six months and 0.6 g/24 h after a median of seven years) [30]. Other randomized and observational trials supported the potential effect of corticosteroids in IgAN [27,31]. The retrospective analysis of the VALIGA study showed, in patients treated with steroids and RAS blockers (RASB), significant reduction in proteinuria, renal function decline and increased renal survival, not only in patients with normal renal function but also in patients with eGFR < 50 mL/min per 1.73 m^2 (reaching proteinuria <1 g/day in 74% patients with corticosteroids and RASB vs. 37% in patients with RASB; slope of eGFR −0.3 ± 6.2 mL/min/1.73 m^2/year in patients with corticosteroids and RASB vs. −4.8 ± 7.4 mL/min/1.73 m^2/year in patients with RASB; $p = 0.001$) [32]. Nevertheless, little information is available about the doses, the duration of steroid treatment and the adverse events caused by corticosteroids [27].

The TESTING study, a randomized study by Lv et al., included 262 patients with persistent proteinuria 1 g/day and estimated GFR 20–120 mL/min/1.73 m^2, who were randomly assigned to receive 0.6–0.8 mg/kg/day of oral methylprednisolone or matching placebo [33]. The temporary results demonstrated a reduction in time-averaged proteinuria and a decreased rate of progression of CKD in the steroid-treated arm (1.37 vs. 2.36 g/day (42% lower), $p < 0.01$; −1.7 vs. −6.8 mL/min/1.73 m^2/year, $p = 0.031$) [33]. However, after a median follow-up of 1.5 years, serious adverse events occurred in patients with corticosteroids vs. placebo groups (14.7% vs. 3.2%, HR 4.95 (95% CI 1.87–17.0), $p = 0.03$) [33]. The additional long-term follow-up might reveal the balance of risks and benefits of steroid treatment [33]. Multiethnic trials such as the ongoing TESTING Low Dose trial (NCT01560052), should evaluate this issue further [34].

The recent STOP-IgAN Clinical Trial showed that the addition of immunosuppressive therapy (corticosteroids and cyclophosphamide followed by azathioprine) to intensive supportive care (ACEI-inhibitors or ARB) in patients with high-risk IgA nephropathy induced full remission of proteinuria (OR 4.82 (95% CI 1.43–16.30), $p = 0.01$) but did not significantly improve renal function (OR O.89 (95% CI 0.44–1.81), $p = 0.75$) and more adverse effects were observed among the patients with immunosuppressive regimens with no change in the rate of decrease in the eGFR (total number of infectious events in steroid treatment arm 182 vs. 111 in supportive care) [35]. However, of 309 patients who completed the 6-month supportive care run-in phase, 106 responded to supportive care (proteinuria level, <0.75 g of urinary protein excretion per day after the end of the run-in phase) and were not eligible for randomization. It needs to be highlighted that one third of patients were no longer suitable for randomization at the end of the run-in phase and the importance of RAS blockade was emphasized. The kidney function loss in the control group was 4 times slower in the STOP-IgAN trial than in the TESTING trial, suggesting a lower-risk population and/or differences in supportive therapy. Thus, it was assumed that low risk population of patients with IgAN with excellent prognosis with supportive care was selected in the STOP-IgAN trial. Nonetheless, detailed assessment of included patients with specific evaluation of histological renal findings and prolonged follow-up would be required for the elucidation of the results [35]. Included patients with inactive form of the disease might predominate in case of absent histological evaluation of renal specimens in the trials and the treatment of patients with inactive forms is useless. Recently, after ten years of follow-up from this study, the significant number of patients in both arms (supportive care plus immunosuppression and supportive care alone) reached the end-point with no benefits seen from the immunosuppression arm [36].

The enteric budesonide was evaluated for the treatment of IgAN in a European multicenter RCT [37]. In the NEFIGAN trial, a novel targeted-release formulation of budesonide was evaluated, designed to deliver the drug to the distal ileum with suspected suppression of B cells and inhibition of production of Gd-IgA1 moleculs transported to blood in patients with IgAN [37]. The results of the Nefigan study showed a significant reduction in proteinuria with full stabilization of eGFR without any serious side-effects [37]. A confirmatory phase 3 trial is currently underway (NCT 03643965). Other potential protease treatment with selective cleavage of IgA1 reverses mesangial deposits and hematuria in animal model and on human kidney biopsies [38,39].

Among patients with chronic kidney disease, regardless of the presence or absence of diabetes, the risk of a composite of a sustained decline in the estimated GFR of at least 50%, end-stage kidney disease, or death from renal or cardiovascular causes was significantly lower with dapagliflozin than with placebo. IgAN made up a significant proportion of the non-diabetic subgroup and the HR was an impressive 0.79 for IgAN. Unlike corticosteroid, the side effect profile is likely more favourable [40].

2.3. *High Risk Patients with IgAN*

Nevertheless, high risk patients with a rapid decrease in the GFR and crescentic glomerulonephritis should be treated in addition to supportive treatment with combined immunosuppression (corticosteroids and cyclophosphamide) in a regimen for induction treatment of ANCA vasculitides (Table 1) [16]. Extreme conditions with crescents involving >50% of glomeruli were considered by the KDIGO guidelines [16]. However, these cases are very rare. Just a few crescents are evaluated in majority of forms of crescentic IgAN, for which the need for aggressive treatment is doubtful. Moreover, a few glomeruli in biopsy specimens are sometimes detected with difficulties for calculation of a valid percentage of crescents. Furthermore, the percentage of glomeruli with crescents changes within a few days which makes comparison impossible among individual patients within cohort studies. Crescentic lesions were not found to have a prognostic value in the Oxford and VALIGA studies, but there was a bias in favour of using of corticosteroid/immunossupression treatment [4,41]. Another international study [7] demonstrated that C correlated with E1 and was associated with the use of CS/IS. The revised Oxford classification [42] suggested considering C1 (1–24% of glomeruli) and C2 (≥25% glomeruli with crescents). Crescents in 16% glomeruli increased the risk of renal function decline in untreated cases and crescents in 25% glomeruli predicted an unfavourable outcome independent of treatment.

Undoubtedly, crescents are a marker of histological activity but crescents can regress and do not require treatment in case of involvement of low percentages of glomeruli [43]. However in untreated patients, the negative effect of crescents on the renal function decline is well known [43]. Treatment with corticosteroids/immunossuppresion might to be initiated in case of involved crescents lesions >25% of the glomeruli (C2) and in patients with C1 involving >16% of glomeruli with other signs of disease activity such as endocapillary hypercellularity (E1 according to the Oxford classification) [43]. The importance of identifying patients at risk of progression was detailed mentioned and the task remains to avoid of exposure to immunosuppression regimen unnecessarily in patients with low risk of progression of renal function. The new international risk-prediction tool was recently developed in patients with IgAN [44,45].

Other immunosuppressive agents including calcineurin inhibitors, azathioprine, mycophenolate salts (MMF) or high-dose immunoglobulins failed to show an evident benefit or manifested with toxicity and therefore they were not recommended in clinical practice (Table 1) [46–49]. A Chinese trial randomized patients to 6 months of full dose steroids or lower dose steroid with MMF [50]. Complete proteinuria remission was similar between the two groups after one year but with fewer steroid-related adverse events in the arm with MMF [50]. Nevertheless, it was not a multiethnic study population, not all patients were treated by means of RAS-blockade and the time of follow-up was too short to evaluate the effect on renal parameters [50]. Although a possible positive effect of mycophenolate mofetil treatment in IgAN was noticed in a randomized controlled trial in China [51] with a significant reduction in the percentage of patients positive for histological change of E1 [50], the effect in Caucasian was not assessed [52] apart from the recent study on the effect of MMF therapy with a significant histological reduction in E1 score in repeated renal biopsies after 24 months ($p < 0.0001$) [53]. Further studies are needed for the assessment of treatment with mycophenolate mofetil in patients with IgAN. On the other hand several authors suggested potential benefits of rapamycin in animal and cell models of IgAN [54].

Moreover, Hydroxychloroquine in addition to optimized RAAS inhibition significantly reduced proteinuria in patients with IgAN over 6 months without evidence of adverse events. Undoubtadly, these findings require confirmation in larger treatment trials [55].

The question of the efficacy of fish oil in IgAN is uncertain (Table 1) [16]. Many randomizedclinical trials testing the efficacy of fish oil in patients with IgAN provided contrasting results [16]. It was reported that daily treatment with fish oil for 2 years may reduce the progression of renal function with few side effects in patients with IgAN [56]. Fish oil was also recommended by KDIGO guidelines if it was tolerated [16,34].

The role of adrenocorticotropic hormone (ACTH) was considered in the treatment of resistant glomerular diseases [57]. The potential involved mechanisms imagine stimulation of endogenous steroid production, activation of melanocortin receptors on inflammatory cells and direct binding to melanocortin receptors on the podocyte [57]. Administration of a 6-month course of ACTH gel in patients with IgAN at high risk of progression (proteinuria > 1 g per 24 h despite documented ACEI/ARB therapy and adequate blood pressure control for >3 months, 24-h creatinine clearance >30 mL/min/1.73 m^2) was prospectively investigated in an open-label pilot study (NCT 02282930). A significant decline in 24-h urinary protein (2.6 to 1.3 g; $p = 0.007$) with no significant changes in eGFR (65.5 to 61.1 mL/min, $p = 0.1$) was detected at 12-month follow-up in patients with IgAN treated with 6 months of ACTH [58].

A systematic review and meta-analysis of 14 studies indicated that tonsillectomy may induce clinical remission and decrease the rates of ESRD in IgAN patients [59]. Another multicenter controlled trial did not show a beneficial effect of tonsillectomy combined with steroid pulse therapy over steroid pulses alone to increase the incidence of clinical remission [60]. In the large VALIGA cohort (the European validation study of the Oxford classification of IgAN) of 1.147 European subjects with IgAN, no significant correlation was found between tonsillectomy and renal function decline [61].

A therapeutic option targeting B-cell pathway treatment against the production of Gd-IgA1 and its specific antibodies, such as rituximab, was involved [62,63]. A multicenter trial of 34 adult patients wih biopsy-proven IgA nephropathy and proteinuria > 1 g per day, maintained on ACEIs or ARBs with well-controlled blood pressure and eGFR < 90 mL/min/1.73 m^2, were randomized to receive supportive therapy either alone or with rituximab. Rituximab effectively depleted B cells (a monoclonal antiCD20 antibody) but neither serum levels of Gd-IgA1 nor its antibodies were reduced and the addition of rituximab failed to improve eGFR decline and proteinuria reduction [62]. CD20 positive B cells were targeted by rituximab but IgA positive plasma cells secreting antibodies were not affected therefore the treatment with rituximab was not efficient in patients with IgAN.

The activation of complement plays an important role in the pathogenesis of IgAN [64–70]. It was suggested that the process occurs both systemically on IgA-containing circulating immune complexes, and also locally in glomeruli, and is mediated through both the alternative and lectin pathways [13]. Pathway components were presented in the mesangial immunodeposits, including properdin and factor H (alternative pathway) and mannan-binding lectin, mannan-binding lectin-associated serine proteases 1 nad 2, and C4d (lectin pathway) [13]. Deletion of complement factor H-related genes 1 and 3 was identified as protective against the disease in GWAS [9,67].

C5a is a potent local inflammatory mediator and the presence of C5a in the kidney correlates with histological severity and proteinuria in IgAN [71]. Targeting C5a enables the suppression of local inflammation, contributing to progressive renal disease including the maintaining of the formation of C5b-9 (membrane attack complex), which plays a crucial role in the elimination of gram negative bacteria [71]. Avacopan (CCX 168), an inhibitor of the C5a receptor [72], was evaluated in an open-label Phase II trial in patients with IgAN. At the end of twelve weeks, proteinuria reduced in 6 of the 7 patients and a significant improvement of UPCR < 1 g/g was detected in 3 of the 7 patients. Undoubtedly, larger studies with longer follow up are needed in IgAN. Nevertheless, the efficacy of avacopan was confirmed in patients with ANCA-associated vasculitis where avacopan allowed the replacement of high-dose corticosteroids with respect of adverse effects of hepatic dysfunction and an increased risk of infection in a small amount of patients [73].

The alternative pathway forms an essential amplification mechanism for the activation of the classical and lectin pathways, resulting in enormous opsonisation and generation of the terminal lytic pathway [74]. The two proteases of Factor D and Factor B are elementary for this amplification process [74]. Selective reversible inhibitors of Factors B and D were developed to efficiently block the activation of alternative pathways [74]. A phase II trial of LNP023, a first in the class of oral inhibitor of Factor B, was recently recruited in patients with IgAN (Table 2). The key component of the lectin pathway demonstrates Mannose-binding lectin associated serine protease 2 (MASP-2), which elevates the production of C3 convertase and leads to further inflammatory consequences. Targeting MASP-2 seems to be promising in terms of reducing the activation of the glomerular lectin pathway and not affecting the formation of C3 convertase through the classical and alternative pathways. Presently, the MASP-2 inhibitor OMS 721 is being assessed in Phase II and Phase III studies in IgAN (Table 2).

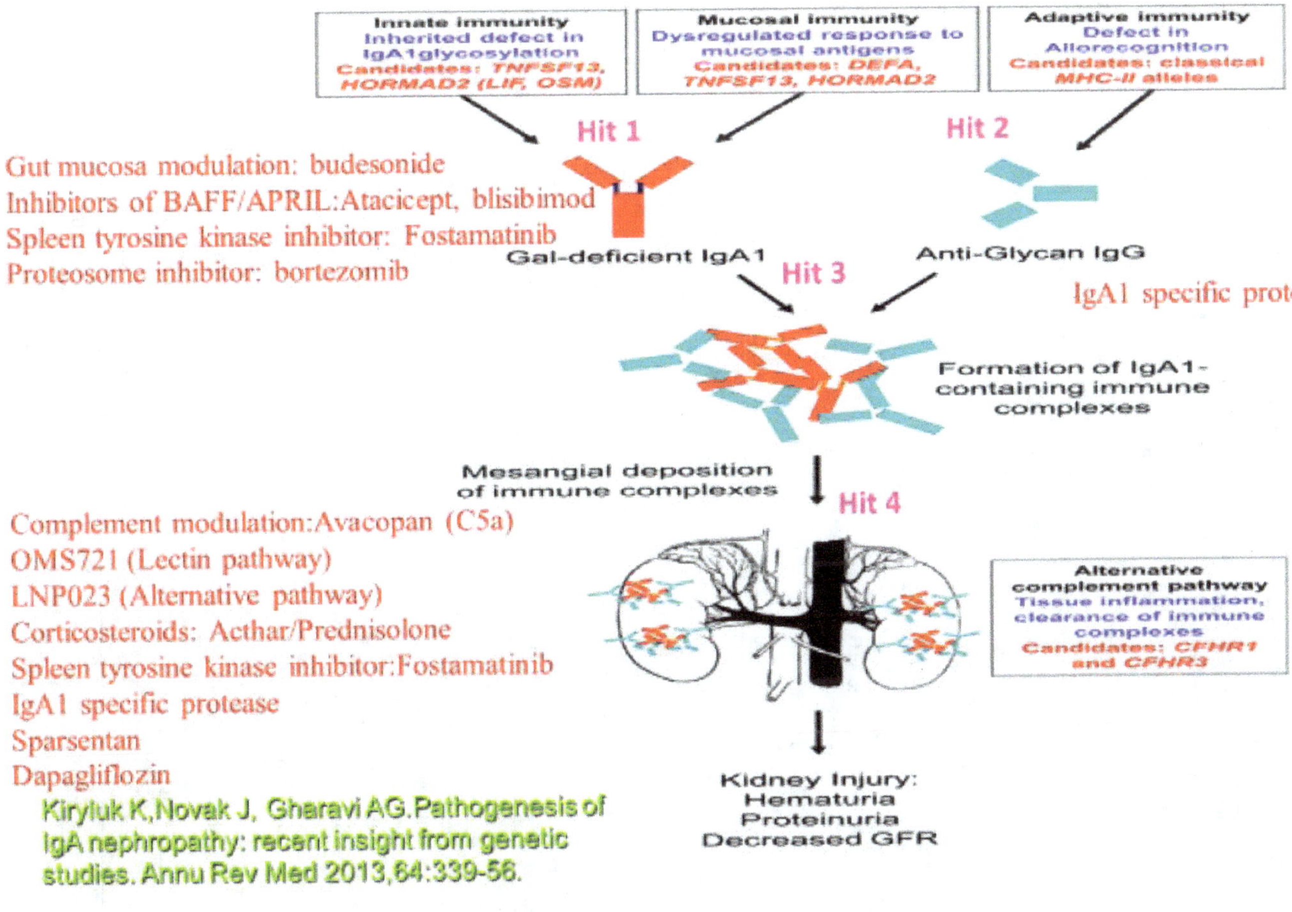

Figure 1. Therapeutic options related to the different targets. Target 1 **(Hit 1)**: B-lymphocyte activation results in the production of Gd-IgA1 (IgA1 poorly O-glycosylated at the hinge region). **Hit 2**: B-cell production of anti-Gd-IgA (IgG). Inhibitors of BAFF/APRIL:Atacicept, blisibimod; Spleen tyrosine kinase inhibitor: Fostamatinib;Gut mucosa modulation: budesonide; Proteosome inhibitor: bortezomib, microbiome modulation (may modulate B-lymphocyte activity with the reduction of Gd-IgA1). **Hit 3**: IgA1 specific protease. **Hit 4**:Spleen tyrosine kinase inhibitor:Fostamatinib; Corticosteroids: Acthar/Prednisolone, Complement mediation:Avacopan (C5a), OMS721 (Lectin pathway), LNP023 (Alternative pathway); IgA1 specific protease; Sparsentan; Dapagliflozin.

Table 2. Clinical trials in patients with IgA nephropathy—recruiting.

	Phase	Target	Clinical Trials in Patients with IgA Nephropathy—Recruiting	Estimated Enrollment				
				Number of pts	Inclusion Criteria	Treatment—Both Arms	Primary Endpoint	Time of Follow Up
Therapeutic options related to different targets of the pathogenesis (See Figure 1)								
NCT03633864	2	1	Fecal microbiota transplantation	30	eGFR:20–120 mL/min/1.73 m^2, PU > 1 g/d	Exp:FMT arm/Biol.FMT	Change of urinary protein for 24 h	8 wks
NCT04438603	NA	4	The Role of T/B Cell Repertoire in Non-invasive Diagnosis and Disease Monitoring in pts with IgAN	50	eGFR ≥ 30 mL/min/1.73/m^2	ACEI/ARB for non-progressive IgAN; Isu:CPA i.v./MMF p.o. for progressive IgAN	Urinary protein remission rate	2 yrs
NCT03001947	NA	others	Registration Initiative of High Quality (INSIGHT)	10,000	Biopsy proven IgAN	Observational/no intervention	Mortality, renal outcome (doubling of S-creat or ESRD)	10 yrs
NCT04042623	2	4	AVB-S6-500 (inhibitor of GAS6/AXL signaling pathway)	24	eGFR ≥ 45 mL/min/1.73 m^2, PU 1–3 g/d	Experimental: Treatment with AVB-S6-500	Incidence od AE, UPE (g/d)	14 wks
NCT03188887	3	4	TIGER study (Treatment of IgA nEphropathy according to Renal lesions)	122	Biopsy proven IgAN < 45 days, PCR ratio > 0.75 g/g (within 30 days the renal biopsy)	RAS blockade treatment/Corticotherapy + RAS blockade treatment	Change of PCR, decline of eGFR	2 yrs
NCT03945318	1	1	BION-1301, a humanized IgG4 anti-a proliferation-inducing ligand (APRIL) monoclonal antibody	92	Biopsy proven IgAN within the past 10 years, PU ≥ 0.5 g/24 h, eGFR ≥4 5 mL/min/1.73 m^2 or 30–45 mL/min/1.73 m^2 with RB within 2 years before day 1	Bion-1301/placebo	Incidence and severity of Treatment Emergent Adverse Events (TEAEs)	2 yrs
NCT04014335	2	4	IONIS-FB-LRx, an inhibitor of complement factor B	10	Biopsy proven IgAN	IONIS-FB-LRx	Percent reduction in 24-h urine protein excretion	29 wks
NCT02954419	NA	others	IgA nephropathy biomarkers evaluation study (INTEREST)	2000	Biopsy proven IgAN	no intervention	A doubling of serum creatinine level from baseline, progression to ESRD, death	10 yrs
NCT03418779	2, 3	4	Treatment effects of chinese medicine with immunosuppression therapies	56	Biopsy proven IgAN within 6 months before enrollment, PU > 1 g/24 h, eGFR 20–60 mL/min/1.73 m^2	herbal compound/Isu (Prednisolon, CPA)/optimized supportive care	Increase in GFR from the baseline at the 24th week and 48th week, ESRD	1 yr
NCT03373461	3	4	LNP023 (complement-factor-B-inhibitor)	146	eGFR ≥ 30 mL/min/1.73/m^2, PU > 1 g/d, v accination against Neisseria meningitis	LNP023/Placebo	Change of UPCR at baseline and day 90	180 days
NCT03608033	3	4	OMS 721 (mannan-binding lectin serine protease 2 (MASP2) protein inhibitor)	450	PU > 1 g/d within 6 months prior to screening, eGFR ≥ 30 mL/min/1.73/m^2	OMS 721/Placebo	Change from baseline in 24-h UPE in g/day at 36 weeks from beginning of treatment	3.5 yrs
NCT03643965	3	1	NefIgArd (Nefecon-budesonide modified-release capsules)	360	eGFR ≥ 35 mL/min/1.73/m^2 and ≤90 mL/min/1.73/m^2, PU >1 g/24 h or UPCR ≥ 0.8 g/g	Nefecon/Placebo	Change of UPCR at baseline and 9 months	25 mth
NCT03762850	3	4	PROTECT (Sparsentan-a dual inhibitor of AT1 and ETA receptor)	280	eGFR ≥ 30 mL/min/1.73/m^2, PU > 1 g/24 h	Sparsentan/Irbesartan	Change of UPCR at baseline and week 36	110 wks

Abbreviation: wks—weeks, yrs—years, mth—months.

The clinical effect of atacicept was investigated for treating systemic autoimmune diseases [75]. Studies in patients with IgA nephropathy investigate the contribution of dysregulation of IgA1 secretion in the intestinal epithelium to see if intestinal immunity or mucosal immunity inhibitors of overexpression of APRIL and B cell-activating factor would have a clinical effect [17,76,77]. Additional potential immunosuppressive regimens (such as blisibimod(NCT02062684)—A selective antagonist of the B-cell activating factor, atacicept (NCT02808429)—An inhibitor of B-cell activating factor (BLyS) and a proliferation-inducing ligand (APRIL), bortezomib—A proteasome inhibitor, fostamatinib–an inhibitor of spleen tyrosine kinase, leflunomide—A pyrimidine synthesis inhibitor) are currently being tested in ongoing trials (Table 2) [78–83].

BAFF (B-cell activating factor) and April (a proliferation inducing ligand) are members of the tumour necrosis factor family which mediate B-cell function and survival [84]. BAFF and April levels are elevated in the serum of patients with IgAN and correlate with the disease activity [85]. BAFF and April are bound by TACI (transmembrane activator and calcium-modulator and cyclophilin ligand interactor), which mediates their downflow effects through the NF-kB pathway. Blisibimod is a selective antagonist of BAFF and atacicept is a fusion protein containing the extracellular ligand binding domain of TACI and is able to block the downflow effects of BAFF and April.

The clinical effects of atacicept and blisibimod were investigated for treating systemic autoimmune diseases, including SLE and rheumatoid arthritis [75,86,87]. Studies in patients with IgAN investigate the contribution of dysregulation of IgA1 secretion in the intestinal epithelium to see if intestinal immunity or mucosal immunity inhibitors of overexpression of APRIL and B cell-activating factor would have a clinical effect [17,76,77].

Bortezomib, a plasma cell proteasome inhibitor, is applied in the treatment of multiple myeloma [88]. Proteasomes are indispensable intracellular protein complexes which destroy useless and impaired proteins by proteolysis [88]. Proteasomes are switched to immunoproteasomes but the dysregulation of the proteasome:immunoproteasome axis was confirmed in mononuclear cells in patients with IgAN with overexpression of the immunoproteasome, increased nuclear translocation of factors related to the NF-kB pathway, and more severe disease symptoms including higher proteinuria [89]. Nowadays, the treatment with bortezomib is more common in amyloidosis, lymphomas, tumours and antibody mediated allograft rejection [90]. A clinical trial to assess the safety and efficacy of bortezomib in patients with IgAN is currently underway (Table 2) but the use of bortezomib in mostly young asymptomatic patients with IgAN would probably be limited by the adverse effects of bortezomib (thrombocytopenia, rash, peripheral neuropathy, fatigue and anorexia) [90].

Tyrosine kinase pathways were asserted in the homeostasis of many diseases, and targeting of the tyrosine kinase signalling pathways was considered for treatment of immune-mediated glomerulonephritides [91]. Spleen tyrosine kinase is a non-receptor tyrosine kinase which might regulate the amount of key pathogenic pathways in IgAN [80]. Spleen tyrosine kinase is a signal transducer following B-cell receptor activation, arranging downflow signalling and promoting B-cell maturation and survival [80]. Spleen tyrosine kinase phosphorylation with the release of pro-inflammatory mediators was activated by stimulation of mesangial cells in vitro with IgA1 acquired from patients with IgAN [80].

Moreover, higher renal expression of spleen tyrosine kinase was confirmed in patients with endocapillary hypercellularity compared to patients without this sign in renal biopsy [92]. Fostamatinib, a selective inhibitor of spleen tyrosine kinase, was investigated in patients with rheumatoid artritis with a favourable effect on disease activity compared to placebo but with frequent adverse effects mostly involving diarrhoea and hypertension [93]. A Phase II trial of fostamatinib in patients with IgAN was recently completed.

Endothelin-1 (ET-1) is a growth factor for mesangial cells [94] and was shown to play a role in the progression of kidney disease in transgenic animals. In human subjects, urinary excretion of endothelin-1 correlates with the severity of kidney disease [95]. Expression of endothelin-1 and endothelin B receptor (mediating vasodilation and natriuresis), but not endothelin A receptor (mediating vasoconstriction and cell proliferation) was demonstrated in patients with IgAN and high-grade proteinuria [96] suggests that activation of the endothelin system in renal tubular cells may partly be a response to protein overload. We demonstrated association of the progresson of IgAN with polymorphisms of the ET-1 gene [97]. Association of ET-1 expression with the progression of IgAN was also confirmed using molecular profiling [98]. A specific ET-receptor antagonist (FR 139317) was shown to suppress the development of histologic lesions and proteinuria in ddY mice with IgAN [99]. Sparsentan, a dual inhibitor of the angiotensin II type 1 (AT1) and endothelin type A (ET-A) receptors was recently shown to significantly decrease proteinuria compared to irbesartan in patients with focal segmental glomerulosclerosis [100] and is currently tested in patients with FSGS in a phase 3 trial [101]. Recently, the PROTECT Study (Phase 3 NCT 03762850) evaluating the long-term nephroprotective potential of sparsentan for the treatment of IgAN was initiated. Activation of Nrf2/Keap 1 by bardoxolone methyl results in the suppression of the main proinflammatory transcription factor NFkappaB and activation of some antioxidative pathways [102]. In patients with type 2 diabetes and CKD4 bardoxolone, methyl was shown to increase the glomerular filtration rate by almost 50% [103]. Recently released data (PHOENIX–NCT03366337) demonstrated a significant increase in eGFR of 8 mL/min/1.73 m^2 in patients with IgAN treated with bardoxolone [104]. The increase in eGFR is, however, associated with a proportional increase in albuminuria with uncertain impact on the long-term outcome of the patients [105]. The updated KDIGO guideline will soon be released [34] and the current recommendation from KDIGO came from 2012 prior to STOP-IgAN, TESTING, Nefigan and DAPA-CKD. This is a rapidly evolving field and hence the importance of this review on currently recruiting trials was emphasized.

3. Conclusions

In conclusion, IgAN is a disease with variable clinical course. Validated urinary or serum biomarkers, able to provide information on the activity of the disease and the extent of fibrosis, are needed to stratify high risk patients with the necessity of use of immunossuppressive regimens with respect to possible adverse events. Nevertheless, IgAN patients with proteinuria < 1 g/d, and/or hypertension and a reduced GFR should obtain optimized supportive treatment with the inhibitors of the RAS. In IgAN patients with persistent proteinuria ≥ 1 g/d, despite 3–6 months of optimized supportive care (including RAS and blood pressure control), and GFR > 50 mL/min per 1.73 m^2, a 6-month course of corticosteroid treatment is indicated. Combined immunosuppression with corticosteroids and cyclophosphamide is reserved for high risk patients with a rapid decrease in the GFR and crescentic glomerulonephritis. Nowadays, many specific biological regimens in RCT are evaluated with expected common use in the future (Table 2). The search for an effective and well tolerated treatment of IgAN, directly targeting its pathogenetic mechanisms, continues (Figure 1).

References

1. Moriyama, T.; Tanaka, K.; Iwasaki, C.; Oshima, Y.; Ochi, A.; Kataoka, H.; Itabashi, M.; Takei, T.; Uchida, K.; Nitta, K. Prognosis in IgA nephropathy: 30-year analysis of 1012 patients at a single center in Japan. *PLoS ONE* **2014**, *9*, e91756. [CrossRef] [PubMed]
2. Wyatt, R.J.; Julian, B.A. IgA nephropathy. *N. Engl. J. Med.* **2013**, *368*, 2402–2414. [CrossRef] [PubMed]
3. Cattran, D.C.; Coppo, R.; Cook, H.T.; Feehally, J.; Roberts, I.S.; Troyanov, S.; Alpers, C.E.; Amore, A.; Barratt, J.; Berthoux, F.; et al. Working Group of the International IgA Nephropathy Network and the Renal

Pathology Society, The Oxford classification of IgA nephropathy: Rationale, clinicopathological correlations, and classification. *Kidney Int.* **2009**, *76*, 534–545. [CrossRef] [PubMed]

4. Coppo, R.; Troyanov, S.; Camilla, R.; Hogg, R.J.; Cattran, D.C.; Cook, T.H.; Feehally, J.; Roberts, I.S.D.; Amore, A.; Alpers, C.E.; et al. Working Group of the International IgA Nephropathy Network and the Renal Pathology Society, The Oxford IgA nephropathy clinicopathological classification is valid for children as well as adults. *Kidney Int.* **2010**, *77*, 921–927. [CrossRef]
5. Reich, H.N.; Troyanov, S.; Scholey, J.W.; Cattran, D.C.; Toronto Glomerulonephritis Registry. Remission of proteinuria improves prognosis in IgA nephropathy. *J. Am. Soc. Nephrol.* **2007**, *18*, 3177–3183. [CrossRef]
6. Barbour, S.J.; Espino-Hernandez, G.; Reich, H.N.; Coppo, R.; Roberts, I.S.D.; Feehally, J.; Herzenberg, A.M.; Cattran, D.C. Oxford Derivation, North American Validation and VALIGA Consortia, The MEST score provides earlier risk prediction in lgA nephropathy. *Kidney Int.* **2016**, *89*, 167–175. [CrossRef]
7. Barbour, S.J.; Espino-Hernandez, G.; Reich, H.; Coppo, R.; Roberts, I.S.D.; Feehally, J.; Herzenberg, A.M.; Cattran, D.; Bavbek, N.; Cook, T.M.; et al. A multicenter study of the predictive value of crescents in IgA nephropathy. *J. Am. Soc. Nephrol.* **2017**, *28*, 691–701.
8. Haas, M.; Verhave, J.C.; Liu, Z.-H.; Alpers, C.E.; Barratt, J.; Becker, J.U.; Cattran, D.; Cook, H.T.; Coppo, R.; Feehally, J.; et al. Geographic differences in genetic susceptibility to IgA nephropathy: GWAS replication study and geospatial risk analysis. *PLoS Genet* **2012**, *8*, e1002765.
9. Kiryluk, K.; Li, Y.; Sanna-Cherchi, S.; Rohanizadegan, M.; Suzuki, H.; Eitner, F.; Snyder, H.J.; Choi, M.; Hou, P.; Scolari, F.; et al. Discovery of new risk loci for IgA nephropathy implicates genes involved in immunity against intestinal pathogens. *Nat. Genet* **2014**, *46*, 1187–1196. [CrossRef]
10. Tomana, M.; Matousovic, K.; Julian, B.A.; Radl, J.; Konecny, K.; Mestecky, J. Galactose-deficient IgA1 in sera of IgA nephropathy patients is present in complexes with IgG. *Kidney Int.* **1997**, *52*, 509–516. [CrossRef]
11. Tomana, M.; Novak, J.; Julian, B.A.; Matousovic, K.; Konecny, K.; Mestecky, J. Circulating immune complexes in IgA nephropathy consist of IgA1 with galactose-deficient hinge region and antiglycan antibodies. *J. Clin. Investig.* **1999**, *104*, 73–81. [CrossRef] [PubMed]
12. Novak, J.; Kafkova, L.R.; Suzuki, H.; Tomana, M.; Matousovic, K.; Brown, R.; Hall, S.; Sanders, J.T.; Eison, T.M.; Moldoveanu, Z.; et al. IgA1 immune complexes from pediatric patients with IgA nephropathy activate cultured human mesangial cells. *Nephrol. Dial Transpl.* **2011**, *26*, 3451–3457. [CrossRef] [PubMed]
13. Maillard, N.; Wyatt, R.J.; Julian, B.A.; Kiryluk, K.; Gharavi, A.; Fremeaux-Bacchi, V.; Novak, J. Current understanding of the role of complement in IgA nephropathy. *J. Am. Soc. Nephrol.* **2015**, *26*, 1503–1512. [CrossRef] [PubMed]
14. Schmitt, R.; Stahl, A.L.; Olin, A.; Kristoffersson, A.Ch.; Rebetz, J.; Novak, J.; Lindahl, G.; Karpman, D. The combined role of galactose-deficient IgA1 and streptococcal IgA-binding M protein in inducing IL-6 and C3 secretion from human mesangial cells: Implications for IgA nephropathy. *J. Immunol.* **2014**, *193*, 317–326. [CrossRef] [PubMed]
15. Lai, K.N.; Leung, J.C.K.; Chan, L.Y.Y.; Saleem, M.A.; Mathieson, P.W.; Lai, F.M.; Tang, S.C.W. Activation of podocytes by mesangial-derived TNF-alpha: Glomerulo-podocytic communication in IgA nephropathy. *Am. J. Physiol. Renal Physiol.* **2008**, *294*, F945–F955. [CrossRef]
16. KDIGO. KDIGO clinical practice guideline for glomerulonephritis. *Kidney Int.* **2012**, *2*, 139–274.
17. Coppo, R. The gut-kidney axis in IgA nephropathy: Role of microbiota and diet on genetic predisposition. *Pediatr. Nephrol.* **2018**, *33*, 53–61. [CrossRef]
18. Monteiro, R.C. Recent advances in the physiopathology of IgA nephropathy. *Nephrol. Ther.* **2018**, *14* (Suppl. 1), S1–S8. [CrossRef]
19. Papista, C.; Lechner, S.; Mkaddem, S.B.; LeStang, M.B.; Abbad, L.; Bex-Coudrat, J.; Pillebout, E.; Chemouny, J.M.; Jablonski, M.; Flamant, M.; et al. Gluten exacerbates IgA nephropathy in humanized mice through gliadin-CD89 interaction. *Kidney Int.* **2015**, *88*, 276–285. [CrossRef]
20. Koulouridis, E.; Koulouridis, I. Is the dietary protein restriction achievable in chronic kidney disease? The impact upon quality of life and the dialysis delay. *Hippokratia* **2011**, *15* (Suppl. 1), 3–7.
21. Konishi, Y.; Okada, N.; Okamura, M.; Morikawa, T.; Okumura, M.; Yoshioka, K.; Imanishi, M. Sodium sensitivity of blood pressure appearing before hypertension and related to histological damage in immunoglobulin a nephropathy. *Hypertension* **2001**, *38*, 81–85. [CrossRef] [PubMed]

22. Suzuki, T.; Miyazaki, Y.; Shimizu, A.; Ito, Y.; Okonogi, H.; Ogura, M. Sodium-sensitive variability of the antiproteinuric efficacy of RAS inhibitors in outpatients with IgA nephropathy. *Clin. Nephrol.* **2009**, *72*, 274–285. [CrossRef] [PubMed]
23. Ouyang, Y.; Xie, J.; Yang, M.; Zhang, X.; Ren, H.; Wang, W.; Chen, N. Underweight is an independent risk factor for renal function deterioration in patients with IgA nephropathy. *PLoS ONE* **2016**, *11*, e0162044. [CrossRef] [PubMed]
24. Shimamoto, M.; Ohsawa, I.; Suzuki, H.; Hisada, A.; Nagamachi, S.; Honda, D.; Inoshita, H.; Shimizu, Y. Impact of Body Mass Index on progression of IgA nephropathy among Japanese patients. *J. Clin. Lab. Anal.* **2015**, *29*, 353–360. [CrossRef] [PubMed]
25. Kittiskulnam, P.; Kanjanabuch, T.; Tangmanjitjaroen, K.; Chancharoenthana, W.; Praditpornsilpa, K.; Eiam-Ong, S. The beneficial effects of weight reduction in overweight patients with chronic proteinuric immunoglobulin a nephropathy: A randomized controlled trial. *J. Ren. Nutr.* **2014**, *24*, 200–207. [CrossRef] [PubMed]
26. Cha, Y.J.; Lim, B.J.; Kim, B.S.; Kim, Y.; Yoo, T.H.; Han, S.H.; Kang, S.W.; Choi, K.H. Smoking-related renal histologic injury in IgA nephropathy patients. *Yonsei Med. J* **2016**, *57*, 209–216. [CrossRef]
27. Ponticelli, C.; Glassock, R.J. IgA Nephritis with Declining Renal Function: Treatment with Corticosteroids May Be Worthwhile. *J. Am. Soc. Nephrol.* **2015**, *26*, 2071–2073. [CrossRef]
28. Sharma, P.; Blackburn, R.C.; Parke, C.L.; McCullough, K.; Marks, A.; Black, C. Angiotension-converting enzyme inhibitors and angiotensin receptor blockers for adults with early (stage 1 to 3)non-diabetic chronic kidney disease. *Cochrane Database Syst. Rev.* **2011**, *10*, CD007751.
29. Jarrick, S.; Lundberg, S.; Welander, A.; Carrero, J.J.; Höijer, J.; Bottai, M.; Ludvigsson, J.F. Mortality in IgA nephropathy: A nationwide population-based cohort study. *J. Am. Soc. Nephrol.* **2019**, *30*, 866–876. [CrossRef]
30. Pozzi, C.; Andrulli, S.; Del Vecchio, L.; Melis, P.; Fogazzi, G.B.; Altieri, P.; Ponticelli, C.; Locatelli, F. Corticosteroid effectiveness in IgA nephropathy: Long-term results of a randomized, controlled trial. *J. Am. Soc. Nephrol.* **2004**, *15*, 157–163. [CrossRef]
31. Lv, J.; Xu, D.; Perkovic, V.; Ma, X.; Johnson, D.W.; Woodward, M.; Levin, A.; Zhang, H. TESTING Study Group. Corticosteroid therapy in IgA nephropathy. *J. Am. Soc. Nephrol.* **2012**, *23*, 1108–1116. [CrossRef] [PubMed]
32. Tesar, V.; Troyanov, S.; Bellur, S.; Verhave, J.C.; Cook, H.T.; Feehally, J.; Roberts, I.S.D.; Cattran, D. VALIGA study of the ERA-EDTA Immunonephrology Working Group. Corticosteroids in IgA Nephropathy: A Retrospective Analysis from the VALIGA Study. *J. Am. Soc. Nephrol.* **2015**, *26*, 2248–2258. [CrossRef]
33. Lv, J.; Zhang, H.; Wong, M.G.; Jardine, M.J.; Hladunewich, M.; Jha, V.; Monaghan, H.; Zhao, M. TESTING Study Group. Effect of Oral Methylprednisolone on Clinical Outcomes in Patients With IgA Nephropathy: The TESTING Randomized Clinical Trial. *JAMA* **2017**, *318*, 432–442. [CrossRef]
34. Floege, J.; Barbour, S.J.; Cattran, D.C.; Hogan, J.J.; Nachman, P.H.; Tang, S.C.W.; Wetzels, J.F.M. Management and treatment of glomerular diseases (part 1): Conclusions from a Kidney Disease: Improving Global Outcomes (KDIGO) Controversies Conference. *Kidney Int.* **2019**, *95*, 268–280. [CrossRef] [PubMed]
35. Rauen, T.; Eitner, F.; Fitzner, C.; Sommerer, C.; Zeier, M.; Otte, B.; Panzer, U.; Peters, H. STOP-IgAN Investigators. Intensive Supportive Care plus Immunosuppression in IgA Nephropathy. *N. Engl. J. Med.* **2015**, *373*, 2225–2236. [CrossRef] [PubMed]
36. Rauen, T.; Wied, S.; Fitzner, C.; Eitner, F.; Sommerer, C.; Zeier, M.; Otte, B.; Panzer, U. After ten years of follow-up, no difference between supportive care plus immunosuppression and supportive care alone in IgA nephropathy. *Kidney Int.* **2020**, *98*, 1044–1052. [CrossRef] [PubMed]
37. Fellström, B.C.; Barratt, J.; Cook, H.; Coppo, R.; Feehally, J.; de Fijter, J.W.; Floege, J.; Hetzel, G. NEFIGAN Trial Investigators. Targeted-release budesonide versus placebo in patients with IgA nephropathy (NEFIGAN): A double-blind, randomised, placebo-controlled phase 2b trial. *Lancet* **2017**, *389*, 2117–2127. [CrossRef]
38. Lechner, S.M.; Abbad, L.; Boedec, E.; Papista, C.; LeStang, M.B.; Moal, C.; Maillard, J.; Jamin, A.; Bex-Coudrat, J.; Wang, Y.; et al. IgA1 Protease Treatment Reverses Mesangial Deposits and Hematuria in a Model of IgA Nephropathy. *J. Am. Soc. Nephrol.* **2016**, *27*, 2622–2629. [CrossRef]
39. Berthelot, L.; Papista, C.; Maciel, T.T.; Biarnes-Pelicot, M.; Tissandie, E.; Wang, P.H.M.; Tamouza, H.; Jamin, A.; Bex-Coudrat, J.; Gestin, A.; et al. Transglutaminase is essential for IgA nephropathy development acting through IgA receptors. *J. Exp. Med.* **2012**, *209*, 793–806. [CrossRef]

40. Heerspink, H.J.L.; Stefánsson, B.V.; Correa-Rotter, R.; Chertow, G.M.; Greene, T.; Hou, F.F.; Mann, J.F.E.; McMurray, J.J.V.; Lindberg, M.; Rossing, P.; et al. Dapagliflozin in Patients with Chronic Kidney Disease. *N. Engl. J. Med.* **2020**, *383*, 1436–1446. [CrossRef]
41. Roberts, I.S.; Cook, H.T.; Troyanov, S.; Alpers, C.E.; Amore, A.; Barratt, J.; Berthoux, F.; Bonsib, S.; Bruijn, J.A.; Cattran, D.C.; et al. The Oxford classification of IgA nephropathy: Pathology definitions, correlations, and reproducibility. *Kidney Int.* **2009**, *76*, 546–556. [CrossRef] [PubMed]
42. Trimarchi, H.; Barratt, J.; Cattran, D.C.; Cook, H.T.; Coppo, R.; Haas, M.; Liu, Z.H.; Roberts, I.S.; Yuzawa, Y.; Zhank, H.; et al. Oxford classification of IgA nephropathy 2016: An update from the IgA Nephropathy Classification Working Group. *Kidney Int.* **2017**, *91*, 1014–1021. [CrossRef] [PubMed]
43. Coppo, R. Towards a personalized treatment for IgA nephropathy considering pathology and pathogenesis. *Nephrol. Dial Transpl.* **2019**, *34*, 1832–1838. [CrossRef] [PubMed]
44. Barbour, S.J.; Coppo, R.; Zhang, H.; Liu, Z.H.; Suzuki, Y.; Matsuzaki, K.; Katafuchi, R.; Er, L.; Espino-Hernandez, G.; Kim, S.J.; et al. Evaluating a new international risk-prediction tool in IgA nephropathy. *JAMA Int. Med.* **2019**, *179*, 942–952. [CrossRef] [PubMed]
45. Barbour, S.J.; Canney, M.; Coppo, R.; Zhang, H.; Liu, Z.H.; Suzuki, Y.; Matsuzaki, K.; Katafuchi, R.; Induruwage, D.; Er, L.; et al. Improving treatment decisions using personalized risk assessment from the international IgA nephropathy prediction tool. *Kidney Int.* **2020**, *98*, 1009–1019. [CrossRef]
46. Sarcina, C.; Tinelli, C.; Ferrario, F.; Pani, A.; De Silvestri, A.; Scaini, P.; De Silvestri, A.; Scaini, P.; Del Vecchio, L.; Alberghini, E.; et al. Changes in Proteinuria and Side Effects of Corticosteroids Alone or in Combination with Azathioprine at Different Stages of IgA Nephropathy. *Clin. J. Am. Soc. Nephrol.* **2016**, *11*, 973–981. [CrossRef]
47. Pozzi, C.; Andrulli, S.; Pani, A.; Scaini, P.; Del Vecchio, L.; Fogazzi, G.; Vogt, B.; Cristofaro, V.D.; Allegri, L.; Cirami, L.; et al. Addition of azathioprine to corticosteroids does not benefit patients with IgA nephropathy. *J. Am. Soc. Nephrol.* **2010**, *21*, 1783–1790. [CrossRef]
48. Liu, H.; Xu, X.; Fang, Y.; Ji, J.; Zhang, X.; Yuan, M.; Liu, C.; Ding, X. Comparison of glucocorticoids alone and combined with cyclosporine a in patients with IgA nephropathy: A prospective randomized controlled trial. *Intern Med.* **2014**, *53*, 675–681. [CrossRef]
49. Xu, L.; Liu, Z.C.; Guan, G.J.; Lv, X.A.; Luo, Q. Cyclosporine A combined with medium/low dose prednisone in progressive IgA nephropathy. *Kaohsiung J. Med. Sci* **2014**, *30*, 390–395. [CrossRef]
50. Hou, J.H.; Le, W.B.; Chen, N.; Wang, W.M.; Liu, Z.S.; Liu, D.; Chen, J.H.; Tian, J.; Fu, P.; Hu, Z.X.; et al. Mycophenolate mofetil combined with prednisone versus full-dose prednisone in IgA nephropathy with active proliferative lesions: A randomized controlled trial. *Am. J. Kidney Dis.* **2017**, *69*, 788–795. [CrossRef]
51. Tang, S.C.; Tang, A.W.; Wong, S.S.; Leung, J.C.; Ho, Y.W.; Lai, K.N. Long-term study of mycophenolate mofetil treatment in IgA nephropathy. *Kidney Int.* **2010**, *77*, 543–549. [CrossRef] [PubMed]
52. Hogg, R.J.; Bay, R.C.; Jennette, J.C.; Sibley, R.; Kumar, S.; Fervenza, F.C.; Appel, G.; Cattran, D.; Fischer, D.; Hurley, R.M.; et al. Randomized controlled trial of mycophenolate mofetil in children, adolescents, and adults with IgA nephropathy. *Am. J. Kidney Dis.* **2015**, *66*, 783–791. [CrossRef] [PubMed]
53. Beckwith, H.; Medjeral-Thomas, N.; Galliford, J.; Griffith, M.; Levy, J.; Lightstone, L.; Palmer, A.; Roufosse, C.; Pusey, C.; Cook, H.T.; et al. Mycophenolate mofetil therapy in immunoglobulin a nephropathy: Histological changes after treatment. *Nephrol. Dial Transpl.* **2017**, *32*, 123–128. [CrossRef] [PubMed]
54. Liu, D.; Liu, Y.; Chen, G.; He, L.; Tang, C.; Wang, C.; Yang, D.; Li, H.; Dong, Z.; Liu, H. Rapamycin Enhances Repressed Autophagy and Attenuates Aggressive Progression in a Rat Model of IgA Nephropathy. *Am. J. Nephrol.* **2017**, *45*, 293–300. [CrossRef]
55. Liu, L.J.; Yang, Y.Z.; Shi, S.F.; Bao, Y.F.; Yang, C.; Zhu, S.N.; Sui, G.L.; Chen, Y.Q.; Lv, J.C.; Zhang, H. Effects of Hydroxychloroquine on Proteinuria in IgA Nephropathy: A Randomized Controlled Trial. *Am. J. Kidney Dis.* **2019**, *74*, 15–22. [CrossRef]
56. Donadio, J.V., Jr. Use of fish oil to treat patients with immunoglobulin a nephropathy. *Am. J. Clin. Nutr.* **2000**, *71*, 373S–375S. [CrossRef]
57. Bomback, A.S.; Canetta, P.A.; Beck, L.H., Jr.; Ayalon, R.; Radhakrhisnan, J.; Appel, G.B. Treatment of resistant glomerular diseases with adrenocorticotropic hormon gel: A prospective trial. *Am. J. Nephrol.* **2012**, *36*, 58–67. [CrossRef]
58. Zand, L.; Canetta, P.; Lafayette, R.; Aslam, N.; Novak, J.; Sethi, S.; Fervenza, C.F. An open-label pilot study of adrenocorticotrophic hormone in the treatment of IgA nephropathy at high risk of progression. *KI Rep.* **2020**, *5*, 58–65. [CrossRef]

59. Zand, L.; Canetta, P.; Lafayette, R.; Aslam, N.; Jan, N.; Sethi, S.; Fervenza, F.C. Tonsillectomy for IgA nephropathy: A meta-analysis. *Am. J. Kidney Dis.* **2015**, *65*, 80–87.
60. Kawamura, T.; Yoshimura, M.; Miyazaki, Y.; Okamoto, H.; Kimura, K.; Hirano, K.; Matsushima, M.; Utsunomiya, Y.; Ogura, M.; Yokoo, T.; et al. A multicenter randomized controlled trial of tonsillectomy combined with steroid pulse therapy in patients with immunoglobulin a nephropathy. *Nephrol. Dial Transpl.* **2014**, *29*, 1546–1553. [CrossRef]
61. Feehally, J.; Coppo, R.; Troyanov, S.; Bellur, S.S.; Cattran, D.; Cook, T.; Roberts, I.S.D.; Verhave, J.C.; Camilla, R.; Vergano, L.; et al. VALIGA study of ERA-EDTA Immunonephrology Working Group. Tonsillectomy in a European Cohort of 1,147 Patients with IgA Nephropathy. *Nephron* **2016**, *132*, 15–24. [CrossRef] [PubMed]
62. Lafayette, R.A.; Canetta, P.A.; Rovin, B.H.; Appel, G.B.; Novak, J.; Nath, K.A.; Sethi, S.; Tumlin, J.A.; Mehta, K.; Hogan, M.; et al. A Randomized, Controlled Trial of Rituximab in IgA Nephropathy with Proteinuria and Renal Dysfunction. *J. Am. Soc. Nephrol.* **2017**, *28*, 1306–1313. [CrossRef] [PubMed]
63. Sugiura, H.; Takei, T.; Itabashi, M.; Tsukada, M.; Moriyama, T.; Kojima, C.; Shiohira, T.; Shimizu, A.; Tsuruta, Y.; Amemiya, N.; et al. Effect of single-dose rituximab on primary glomerular diseases. *Nephron Clin. Pract* **2011**, *117*, 98–105. [CrossRef] [PubMed]
64. Coppo, R.; Peruzzi, L.; Loiacono, E.; Bergallo, M.; Krutova, A.; Russo, M.L.; Cocchi, E.; Amore, A.; Lundberg, S.; Maixnerova, D.; et al. Defective gene expression of the membrane complement inhibitor CD46 in patients with progressive immunoglobulin A nephropathy. *Nephrol. Dial Transpl.* **2018**, *34*, 587–596. [CrossRef] [PubMed]
65. Espinosa, M.; Ortega, R.; Sánchez, M.; Segarra, A.; Salcedo, M.T.; González, F.; Camacho, R.; Valdivia, M.A.; Cabrera, R.; López, K.; et al. Association of C4d deposition with clinical outcomes in IgA nephropathy. *Clin. J. Am. Soc. Nephrol.* **2014**, *9*, 897–904. [CrossRef]
66. Zhu, L.; Zhai, Y.L.; Wang, F.M.; Hou, P.; Lv, J.Ch.; Xu, D.M.; Shi, S.F.; Liu, L.J.; Yu, F.; Zhao, M.H.; et al. Variants in complement factor H and complement factor H-related protein genes, CFHR 3 and CFHR1, affect complement activation in IgA nephropathy. *J. Am. Soc. Nephrol.* **2015**, *26*, 1195–1204. [CrossRef]
67. Xie, J.; Kiryluk, K.; Li, Y.; Mladkova, N.; Zhu, L.; Hou, P.; Ren, H.; Wang, W.; Zhang, H.; Chen, N.; et al. Fine mapping implicates a deletion of CFHR1 nad CFHR3 in protection from IgA nephropathy in Han Chinese. *J. Am. Soc. Nephrol.* **2016**, *27*, 3187–3194. [CrossRef]
68. Jullien, P.; Laurent, B.; Claisse, G.; Masson, I.; Dinic, M.; Thibaudin, D.; Berthoux, F.; Alamartine, E.; Mariat, C.; Maillard, N.; et al. Deletion variants of CFHR1 and CFHR3 associate with mesangial immune deposits but not with progression of IgA nephropathy. *J. Am. Soc. Nephrol.* **2018**, *29*, 661–669. [CrossRef]
69. Daha, M.R.; van Kooten, C. Role of complement in IgA nephropathy. *J. Nephrol.* **2016**, *29*, 1–4. [CrossRef]
70. Block, G.A.; Whitaker, S. Maintenance of remission following completion of OMS721 treatment in patients with IgA nephropathy (IGAN). Abstract SA-PO278. *J. Am. Soc. Nephrol.* **2017**, *28*, 749–750.
71. Liu, L.; Zhan, Y.; Duan, X.; Peng, Q.; Liu, Q.; Zhou, Y.; Quan, S.; Xing, G. C3a, C5a renal expression and their receptors are correlated to severity of IgA nephropathy. *J. Clin. Immunol.* **2014**, *34*, 224–232. [CrossRef] [PubMed]
72. ChemoCentryx. Open-Label Study to Evaluate Safety and Efficacy of CCX168 in Subjects With Immunoglobulin A Nephropathy on Stable RAAS Blockade. In *ClinicalTrials.gov [Internet]*; National library of Medicine: Bethesda, MD, USA, 2015. Available online: https://www.clinicaltrials.gov/ct2/show/NCT02384317 (accessed on 20 December 2016).
73. Jayne, D.R.W.; Bruchfeld, A.N.; Harper, L.; Schaier, M.; Venning, M.C.; Hamilton, P.; Burst, V.; Grundmann, F.; Jadoul, M.; Szombati, I.; et al. Randomized trial of C5a receptor inhibitor Avacopan in ANCA-associated vasculitis. *J. Am. Soc. Nephrol.* **2017**, *28*, 2756–2767. [CrossRef] [PubMed]
74. Selvaskandan, H.; Cheung, C.K.; Muto, M.; Barratt, J. New strategies and perspectives on managing IgA nephropathy. *Clin. Exp. Nephrol.* **2019**, *23*, 577–588. [CrossRef]
75. Nakayamada, S.; Tanaka, Y. BAFF- and APRIL targeted therapy in systemic autoimmune diseases. *Inflamm Regen.* **2016**, *36*, 1–6. [CrossRef] [PubMed]
76. Lafayette, R.A.; Kelepouris, E. Immunoglobulin A nephropathy: Advances in understanding of pathogenesis and treatment. *Am. J. Nephrol.* **2018**, *47*, 43–53. [CrossRef] [PubMed]
77. Coppo, R. Biomarkers and targeted new therapies for IgA nephropathy. *Pediatr. Nephrol.* **2017**, *32*, 725–731. [CrossRef]
78. Coppo, R. Proteasome inhibitors in progressive renal diseases. *Nephrol. Dial Transpl.* **2014**, *29*, i25–i30. [CrossRef]

79. Xin, G.; Shi, W.; Xu, L.X.; Su, Y.; Yan, L.J.; Li, K.S. Serum BAFF is elevated in patients with IgA nephropathy and associated with clinical and histopathological features. *J. Nephrol.* **2013**, *26*, 683–690. [CrossRef]
80. Kim, M.J.; McDaid, J.P.; McAdoo, S.P.; Barratt, J.; Molyneux, K.; Masuda, E.S.; Pusey, C.D.; Tam, F.W. Spleen tyrosine kinase is important in the production of proinflammatory cytokines and cell proliferation in human mesangial cells following stimulation with IgA1 isolated from IgA nephropathy patients. *J. Immunol.* **2012**, *189*, 3751–3758. [CrossRef]
81. McAdoo, S.; Tam, F.W.K. Role of the Spleen Tyrosine Kinase Pathway in Driving Inflammation in IgA Nephropathy. *Semin. Nephrol.* **2018**, *38*, 496–503. [CrossRef]
82. Liu, X.W.; Li, D.M.; Xu, G.S.; Sun, S.R. Comparison of the therapeutic effects of leflunomide and mycophenolate mofetil in the treatment of immunoglobulin a nephropathy manifesting with nephrotic syndrome. *Int. J. Clin. Pharmacol. Ther.* **2010**, *48*, 509–513. [CrossRef] [PubMed]
83. Cheng, G.; Liu, D.; Margetts, P.; Liu, L.; Zhao, Z.; Liu, Z.; Tang, L.; Fang, Y.; Li, H.; Guo, Y.; et al. Valsartan combined with clopidogrel and/or leflunomide for the treatment of progressive immunoglobulin A nephropathy. *Nephrology* **2015**, *20*, 77–84. [CrossRef] [PubMed]
84. Samy, E.; Wax, S.; Huard, B.; Hess, H.; Schneider, P. Targeting BAFF and APRIL in systemic lupus erythematosus and oTher. antibody-associated diseases. *Int. Rev. Immunol.* **2017**, *36*, 3–19. [CrossRef] [PubMed]
85. Zhai, Y.; Zhu, L.; Shi, S.; Liu, L.; Lv, J.; Zhang, H. Increased APRIL expression induces IgA1 aberrant glycosylation in IgA nephropathy. *Medicine* **2016**, *95*, e3099. [CrossRef]
86. Isenberg, D.; Gordon, C.; Licu, D.; Copt, S.; Rossi, C.P.; Wofsy, D. Efficacy and safety of atacicept for prevention of flares in patients with moderate-to-severe systemic lupus erythematosus (SLE):52-week data (APRIL-SLE randomised trial). *Ann. Rheum. Dis.* **2015**, *74*, 2006–2015. [CrossRef]
87. Lenert, A.; Niewold, T.B.; Lenert, P. Spotlight on blisibimod and its potential in the treatment of systemic lupus erythematosus:evidenc to date. *Drug Des. Devel Ther.* **2017**, *11*, 747–757. [CrossRef]
88. Richardson, P.G.; Barlogie, B.; Berenson, J.; Singhal, S.; Jagannath, S.; Irwin, D.; Rajkumar, S.V.; Srkalovic, G.; Alsina, M.; Alexanian, R.; et al. A phase 2 study of bortezomib in relapsed, refractory myeloma. *N. Engl. J. Med.* **2003**, *26*, 2609–2617. [CrossRef]
89. Coppo, R.; Camilla, R.; Alfarano, A.; Balegno, S.; Mancuso, D.; Peruzzi, L.; Amore, A.; Canton, A.D.; Sepe, V.; Tovo, P.; et al. Upregulation of the immunoproteasome in peripheral blood mononuclear cells of patients with IgA nephropathy. *Kidney Int.* **2009**, *75*, 536–541. [CrossRef]
90. Bahleda, R.; Le Deley, M.; Bernard, A.; Chaturvedi, S.; Hanley, M.; Poterie, A.; Gazzah, A.; Varga, A.; Touat, M.; Deutsch, E.; et al. Phase I trial of bortezomib daily dose: Safety, pharmacokinetic profile, biological effects and early clinical evaluation in patients with advanced solid tumors. *Investig. New Drugs* **2017**, *5*, 66.
91. Ma, T.K.; McAdoo, S.P.; Tam, F.W.K. Targeting the tyrosine kinase signalling pathways for treatment of immune-mediated glomerulonephritis: From bench to bedside and beyond. *Nephrol. Dial Transpl.* **2017**, *32*, i138. [CrossRef]
92. McAdoo, S.P.; Bhangal, G.; Page, T.; Cook, H.T.; Pusey, C.D.; Tam, F.W.K. Correlation of disease activity in proliferative glomerulonephritis with glomerular spleen tyrosine kinase expression. *Kidney Int.* **2015**, *88*, 52–60. [CrossRef] [PubMed]
93. Taylor, P.C.; Genovese, M.C.; Greenwood, M.; Ho, M.; Nasonov, E.; Oemar, B.; Stoilov, R.; Vencovsky, J.; Weinblatt, M. OSKIRA-4: A phase IIb randomised, placebo-controlled study of the efficacy and safety of fostamatinib monotherapy. *Ann. Rheum. Dis.* **2015**, *74*, 2123–2129. [CrossRef] [PubMed]
94. Simonson, M.S.; Wann, S.; Mene, P.; Dubyak, G.R.; Kester, M.; Nakazato, Y.; Sedor, J.R.; Dunn, M.J. Endothelin stimulates phospholipase C, Na+/H+ exchange, c-Fos expression, and mitogenesis in rat mesangial cells. *J. Clin. Investig.* **1989**, *83*, 708–712. [CrossRef] [PubMed]
95. Ohta, K.; Hirata, Y.; Shichiri, M.; Kanno, K.; Emori, T.; Tomita, K.; Marumo, F. Urinary excretion of endothelin-1 in normal subjects and patients with renal disease. *Kidney Int.* **1991**, *39*, 307–311. [CrossRef] [PubMed]
96. Lehrke, I.; Waldherr, R.; Ritz, E.; Wagner, J. Renal endothelin-1 and endothelin receptor type B expression in glomerular diseases with proteinuria. *J. Am. Soc. Nephrol.* **2001**, *12*, 2321–2329. [PubMed]
97. Maixnerova, D.; Merta, M.; Reiterova, J.; Stekrova, J.; Rysava, R.; Obeidova, H.; Viklicky, O.; Potmesil, P.; Tesar, V. The influence of three endothelin-1 polymorphisms on the progression of IgA nephropathy. *Folia Biol.* **2007**, *53*, 27–32.

98. Tycova, I.; Hruba, P.; Maixnerova, D.; Girmanova, E.; Mrazova, P.; Straňavova, L.; Zachoval, R.; Merta, M.; Slatinska, J.; Kollar, M.; et al. Molecular Profiling in IgA Nephropathy and Focal and Segmental Glomerulosclerosis. *Physiol. Res.* **2018**, *67*, 93–105. [CrossRef]
99. Nakamura, T.; Ebihara, I.; Fukui, M.; Tomino, Y.; Koide, H. Effect of a specific endothelin receptor a antagonist on glomerulonephritis of ddY mice with IgA nephropathy. *Nephron* **1996**, *72*, 454–460. [CrossRef]
100. Trachtman, H.; Nelson, P.; Adler, S.; Campbell, K.N.; Chaudhuri, A.; Derebail, V.K.; Gambaro, G.; Gesualdo, L.; Gipson, D.S.; Hogan, J.; et al. DUET: A Phase 2 Study Evaluating the Efficacy and Safety of Sparsentan in Patients with FSGS. *J. Am. Soc. Nephrol.* **2018**, *29*, 2745–2754. [CrossRef]
101. Komers, R.; Diva, U.; Inrig, J.K.; Loewen, A.; Trachtman, H.; Rote, W.E. Study design of the phase 3 sparsentan versus irbesartan (DUPLEX) study in patients with focal segmental glomerulosclerosis. *Kidney Int. Rep.* **2020**, *5*, 494–502. [CrossRef]
102. Shelton, L.M.; Park, B.K.; Copple, I.M. Role of Nrf2 in protection against acute Kidney injury. *Kidney Int.* **2013**, *84*, 1090–1095. [CrossRef] [PubMed]
103. Pergola, P.E.; Raskin, P.; Toto, R.D.; Meyer, C.J.; Huff, J.W.; Grossman, E.B.; Krauth, M.; Ruiz, S.; Audhya, P.; Christ-Schmidt, H.; et al. Bardoxolone methyl and kidney function in CKD with type 2 diabetes. *N. Engl. J. Med.* **2011**, *365*, 327–336. [CrossRef] [PubMed]
104. Block, G.A. Primary Efficacy Analyses from a Phase 2 Trial of the Safety and Efficacy of Bardoxolone Methyl in Patients with IgA Nephropathy. *ASN Kidney Week* **2018**. poster TH-PO1039. [CrossRef]
105. Rossing, P.; Block, G.A.; Chin, M.P.; Goldsberry, A.; Heerspink, H.J.L.; McCullough, P.A.; Meyer, C.J.; Packham, D.; Pergola, P.E.; Spinowitz, B.; et al. Effect of bardoxolone methyl on the urine albumin-to-creatinine ratio in patients with type 2 diabetes and stage 4 chronic kidney disease. *Kidney Int.* **2019**, *96*, 1030–1036. [CrossRef] [PubMed]

14

The Crucial Role of Xanthine Oxidase in CKD Progression Associated with Hypercholesterolemia

You-Jin Kim [1,2], Se-Hyun Oh [1,2], Ji-Sun Ahn [1], Ju-Min Yook [1], Chan-Duck Kim [1,3], Sun-Hee Park [1,3], Jang-Hee Cho [1,3,*] and Yong-Lim Kim [1,2,3,*]

1 Division of Nephrology, Kyungpook National University Hospital, Daegu 41944, Korea; pinkqic1004@naver.com (Y.-J.K.); ttily@nate.com (S.-H.O.); ggumsuni@hanmail.net (J.-S.A.); jumin18@hanmail.net (J.-M.Y.); drcdkim@mail.knu.ac.kr (C.-D.K.); sh-park@knu.ac.kr (S.-H.P.)

2 Cell and Matrix Research Institute, Kyungpook National University, Daegu 41944, Korea

3 Department of Internal Medicine, School of Medicine, Kyungpook National University, Daegu 41944, Korea

* Correspondence: jh-cho@knu.ac.kr (J.-H.C.); ylkim@knu.ac.kr (Y.-L.K.)

Abstract: In the present study, we investigated the effects of xanthine oxidase (XO) inhibition on cholesterol-induced renal dysfunction in chronic kidney disease (CKD) mice, and in low-density lipoprotein (LDL)-treated human kidney proximal tubule epithelial (HK-2) cells. ApoE knockout (KO) mice underwent uninephrectomy to induce CKD, and were fed a normal diet or high-cholesterol (HC) diet along with the XO inhibitor topiroxostat (1 mg/kg/day). HK-2 cells were treated with LDL (200 μg/mL) and topiroxostat (5 μM) or small interfering RNA against xanthine dehydrogenase (siXDH; 20 nM). In uninephrectomized ApoE KO mice, the HC diet increased cholesterol accumulation, oxidative stress, XO activity, and kidney damage, while topiroxostat attenuated the hypercholesterolemia-associated renal dysfunction. The HC diet induced cholesterol accumulation by regulating the expressions of genes involved in cholesterol efflux (*Nr1h3* and *Abca1*) and synthesis (*Srebf2* and *Hmgcr*), which was reversed by topiroxostat. Topiroxostat suppressed the expressions of genes related to hypercholesterolemia-associated inflammation and fibrosis in the unilateral kidney. LDL stimulation evoked changes in the cholesterol metabolism, nicotinamide adenine dinucleotide phosphate (NADPH) oxidase, and NF-κB pathways in HK-2 cells, which were mitigated by XO inhibition with topiroxostat or siXDH. These findings suggest that XO inhibition exerts renoprotective effects against hypercholesterolemia-associated kidney injury. XO could be a novel therapeutic target for hypercholesterolemia-associated kidney injury in uninephrectomized patients.

Keywords: chronic kidney disease; hypercholesterolemia; xanthine oxidase; inflammation; fibrosis; NF-κB pathway

---

1. Introduction

Compared to people with normal cholesterol levels, those with high cholesterol levels are 1.5 times more likely to develop kidney dysfunction [1,2]. Individuals with metabolic syndrome who serve as kidney donors reportedly show a higher incidence of post-donation kidney disease due to dyslipidemia and obesity compared to normal donors [3,4]. These findings suggest that abnormal cholesterol metabolism independently increases the risk of chronic kidney disease.

Dyslipidemia may directly affect the kidney by causing deleterious renal lipid disturbances, and indirectly affect the kidney through systemic inflammation, oxidative stress and vascular injury [5,6]. We previously reported that high concentrations of uric acid synthesis metabolites lead to the generation of reactive oxygen species (ROS), which promotes hypercholesterolemia with cholesterol accumulation in hepatocytes and incites atherosclerosis in apolipoprotein E (ApoE)-deficient mice [7]. However, the effects of cholesterol on the kidneys have not been confirmed.

In a unilateral kidney, a high-fat diet alters the expressions of genes involved in the cytoskeletal remodeling, fibrosis, and oxidative stress pathways. This suggests that the high-fat diet has synergistic effects that promote gene expression changes related to kidney damage [8]. Additionally, in animal experiments, unilateral kidney dyslipidemia is associated with the exacerbation of kidney damage, characterized by decreased kidney function, vasodilation, fibrosis, oxidative stress, and ER stress, despite normal body weight [9]. These findings suggest that kidney lipid accumulation and lipid toxicity play important roles in the pathogenesis of kidney damage, and are associated with a higher risk of kidney damage in unilateral kidneys.

It has been postulated that oxidative stress—derived from nicotinamide adenine dinucleotide phosphate (NADPH) oxidase, mitochondrial oxidase, and xanthine oxidase (XO)—is involved in renal lipid disturbances [10]. Notably, high cholesterol levels activate XO and lead to excessive ROS formation, resulting in tissue damage, such as inflammation and atherosclerosis [11,12]. Consistently, XO inhibitors exhibit pronounced protective effects against vascular injuries, inflammatory diseases, and tissue damage [13,14]. XO inhibitors can also inhibit the expression of pro-inflammatory proteins. Therefore, XO inhibitors have potential for use as therapeutic drugs that reduce oxidative stress [15]. However, the XO inhibitor allopurinol does not inhibit renal dysfunction in patients with chronic kidney disease (CKD) and high risk of progression [16].Thus, the effect of XO inhibitors in terms of kidney protection remains controversial.

In the present study, we investigated the correlation between cell injury and non-oxidized LDL-induced ROS in vitro, as well as the effects of a high-cholesterol (HC) diet and hypercholesterolemia on lipid accumulation and renal tubule damage in vivo using a unilateral kidney model. We further aimed to identify potential signaling pathways that could be affected by lipid accumulation-induced xanthine oxidase and ROS under a CKD associated with hypercholesterolemia.

2. Results

2.1. Hypercholesterolemia Aggravates Renal Function Through Increased Kidney Lipid Accumulation, Xanthine Oxidase Activity, and Oxidative Stress

PAS staining confirmed that the high-cholesterol (HC) diet led to renal tubular damage in the unilateral kidney (Figure 1A). The HC diet yielded increased serum blood urea nitrogen (BUN) and creatinine, which were highest with HC+uninephrectomy (UN) group (Figure 1B,C). The XO inhibitor topiroxostat (TP) attenuated this kidney dysfunction (Figure 1A–C). Kidney weight was increased in uninephrectomized mice, whereas reduced by TP treatment (Figure 1D). In both sham-operated and UN mice, HC diet yielded increased serum total cholesterol (TC), low-density lipoprotein (LDL), and triglycerides (TG), and TP treatment restored these levels (Figure 1E–G).

Compared to normal control (NC), HC and HC+UN yielded increased lipid droplets in the kidney, showing higher levels with HC+UN versus HC (Figure 1H). Kidney TC was higher with HC and HC+UN versus NC, and was reduced by TP in the HC+UN+TP group (Figure 1I). Free cholesterol did not differ among groups. HC and HC+UN showed trends of increased kidney cholesterol esters (Figure 1J,K). TP decreased kidney cholesterol accumulation, consistent with decreased serum TC, LDL, and TG. The HC diet significantly elevated XO activity, dichlorodihydrofluorescein diacetate (DCFDA), and H_2O_2 excretion in kidney tissue, which were higher with HC+UN versus HC. TP decreased the increased XO activity and intracellular oxidative stress markers (Figure 1L–N).

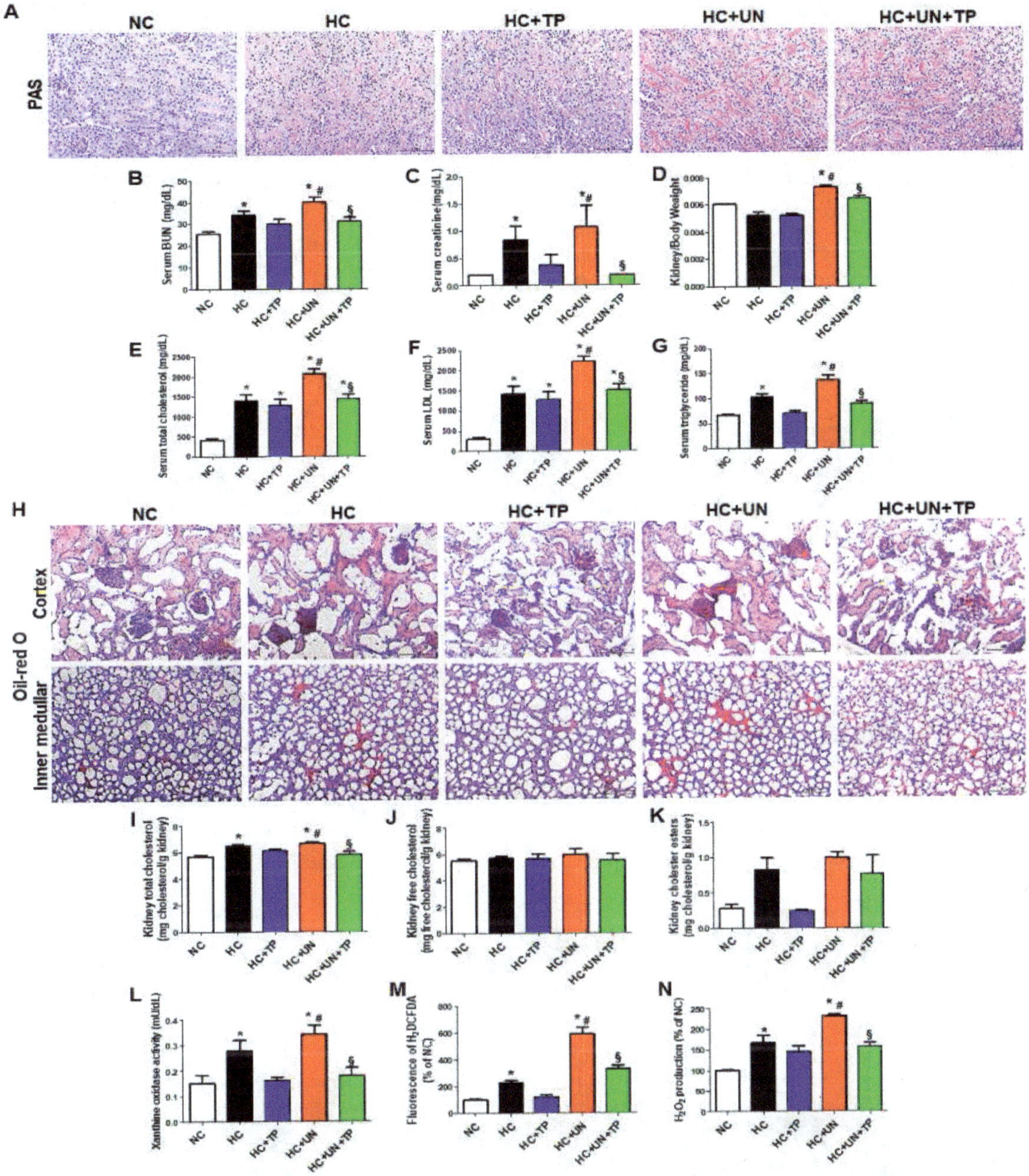

Figure 1. The effects of xanthine oxidase inhibition on high-cholesterol diet-induced cholesterol accumulation, oxidative stress, and damage in the kidney. (**A**) Representative images of periodic acid Schiff (PAS) staining of kidney tissue. Scale bars, 100 μm. (**B–D**) Levels of blood kidney injury factors (BUN and creatinine) and kidney/body weight in mice from different groups. (**E–G**) Serum cholesterol levels in mice from different groups. (**H**) Representative images of Oil red O staining of kidney tissue (upper: cortex, lower: inner-medullar). Scale bars, 100 μm. (**I–K**) Total cholesterol, free cholesterol, and cholesterol ester levels in the kidney. (**L–N**) Xanthine oxidase activity, DCFDA, and H_2O_2 production in kidney tissue. Differences among the groups were analyzed by a one-way non-parametric ANOVA, followed by Tukey's multiple comparison test. Data represent mean and SEM. * $p < 0.05$ vs. NC, # $p < 0.05$ vs. HC, § $p < 0.05$ vs. HC+UN. TP, topiroxostat; UN, uninephrectomy; NC, normal control; HC, high-cholesterol.

2.2. *Effects of Hypercholesterolemia on Genes Related to Cellular Cholesterol Transport and Synthesis in the Unilateral Kidney*

Compared to NC, the HC diet groups exhibited increased mRNA expression of genes related to cholesterol efflux (*Nr1h3* and *Abca1*), LDL and modified LDL uptake (*Ldlr*, *Msr1*, and *Scarb1*),

TG synthesis (*Srebf1*), and cholesterol synthesis (*Srebf2* and *Hmgcr*) (Figure 2A–I). HC+UN yielded decreased *Nr1h3* and *Abca1* (Figure 2A,B), increased *Msr1* and *Scarb1*, and decreased *Ldlr* expression (Figure 2C–E). *Lcat* expression was increased with the HC diet versus normal diet but did not differ between HC and HC+UN (Figure 2F). HC+UN yielded increased *Srebf1*, *Srebf2*, and *Hmgcr* expression (Figure 2G–I). TP treatment (HC+UN+TP) increased *Nr1h3* and *Abca1* expression, and decreased *Srebf1*, *Srebf2*, and *Hmgcr* expression (Figure 2A,B,G–I). The HC diet led to increased ABCA1 and HMGCR protein levels, which were higher with HC+UN versus HC. LXRα protein levels were not altered by HC diet (Figure 2J–L). Overall, TP treatment yielded increased cholesterol efflux gene expression and reduced cholesterol synthesis gene expression (Figure 2).

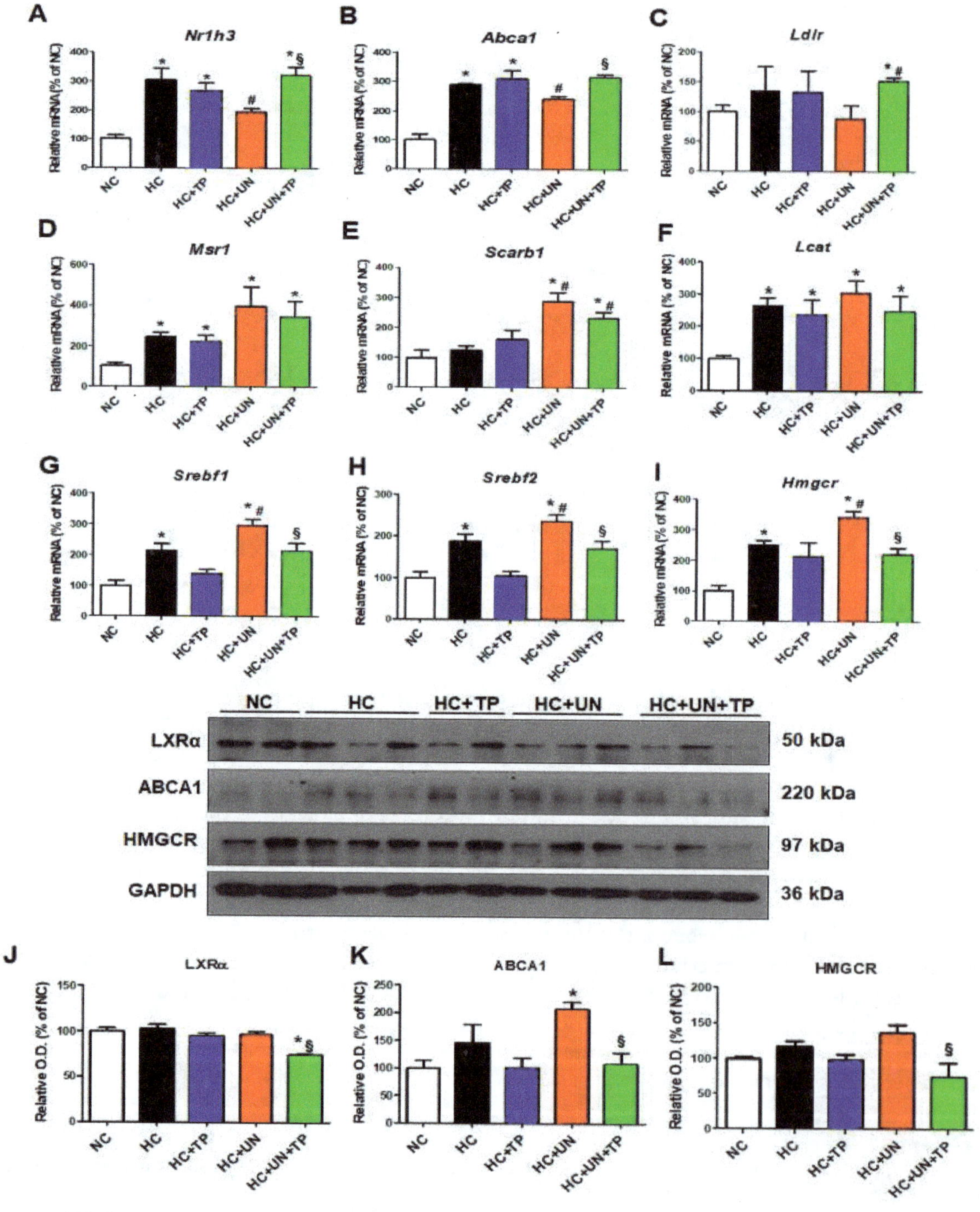

Figure 2. TP decreased cholesterol accumulation in the kidney through regulation of genes involved in cholesterol transport and synthesis. Real-time RT-PCR was performed to determine the expression

levels of genes involved in cholesterol efflux (**A**,**B**), LDL receptor (**C**), modified LDL influx transport (**D**,**E**), cholesterol esterase (**F**), triglyceride synthesis (**G**), and cholesterol synthesis (**H**,**I**). (**J**–**L**) Representative western blot for LXRα, ABCA1, HMGCR, and GAPDH. Relative protein expression was determined using densitometry. Differences among the groups were analyzed by one-way non-parametric ANOVA, followed by Tukey's multiple comparison test. Data represent mean and SEM. * $p < 0.05$ vs. NC, # $p < 0.05$ vs. HC, § $p < 0.05$ vs. HC+UN. LDL, low-density lipoprotein; TP, topiroxostat; UN, uninephrectomy; NC, normal control; HC, high-cholesterol.

2.3. *Effects of LDL on Cholesterol Metabolism and Oxidative Stress in HK-2 Cells*

LDL increased *NR1H3*, *ABCA1*, and *HMGCR* expression in human kidney proximal tubule epithelial (HK-2) cells, without affecting *LDLR*, *SREBF1*, or *SREBF2*. TP decreased only *HMGCR* expression (Figure 3A–F). LDL increased intracellular ROS over the basal level, which peaked at 30 min (Figure 3G), with elevated H_2O_2 level and ROS-dependent DCF fluorescence intensity. TP reduced cellular ROS, similar to the positive control NAC (Figure 3H–I).

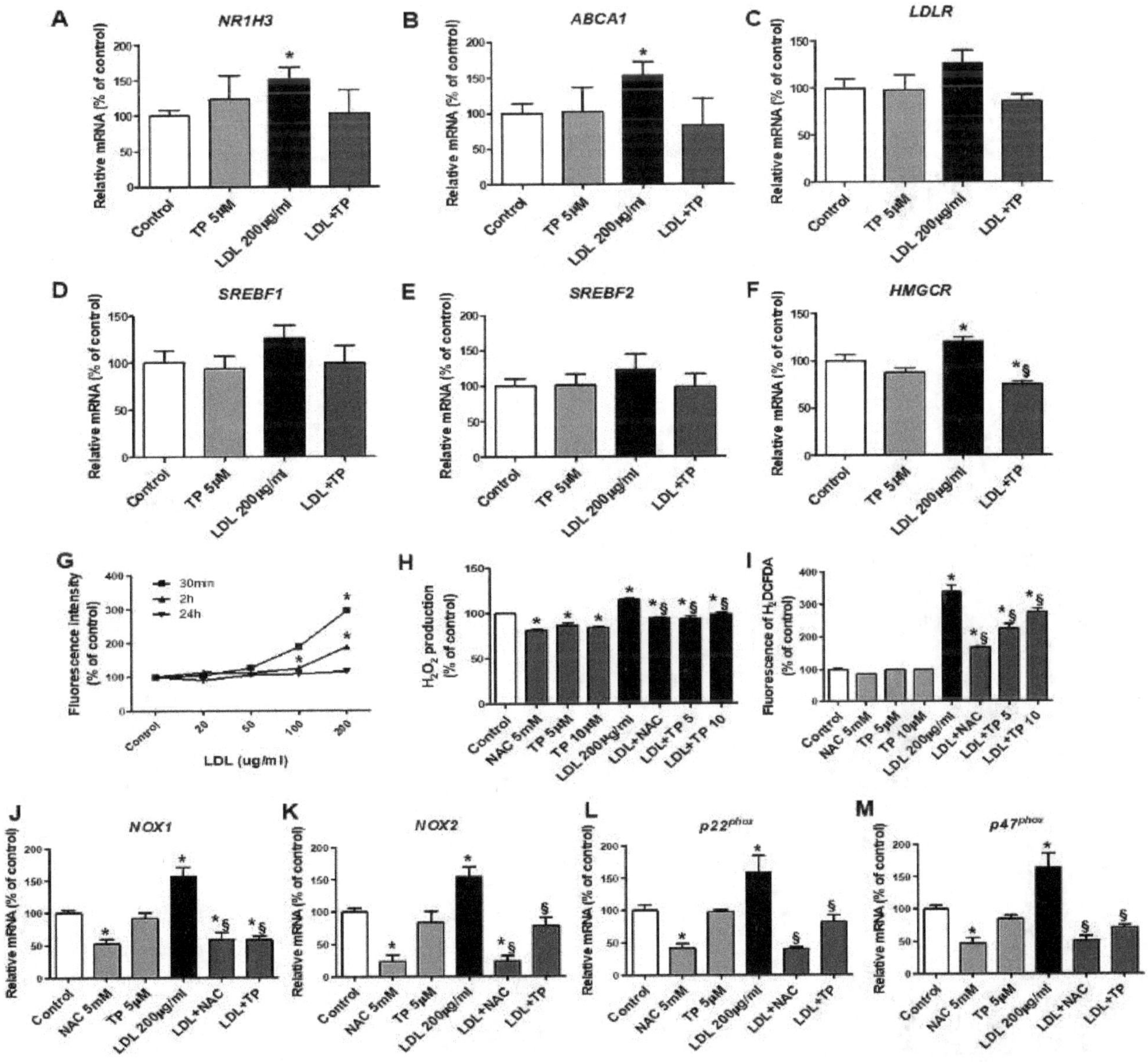

Figure 3. Effects of xanthine oxidase inhibitor on the expression of genes related to cholesterol transport and synthesis and ROS in LDL-stimulated HK-2 cells. Real-time RT-PCR was performed to determine the expression levels of genes related to cholesterol efflux (**A**,**B**), the LDL receptor (**C**), triglyceride synthesis (**D**), and cholesterol synthesis (**E**,**F**). (**G**) After pretreatment with TP (5 or 10 μM) for 1 h,

and stimulation with LDL (200 μg/mL) for 30 min, cellular ROS generation was measured based on the fluorescence intensity of DCF. (**H**,**I**) Measurement of H_2O_2 and DCFDA production. Quantitative PCR was performed to analyze the relative mRNA expression of *NOX1* (**J**), *NOX2* (**K**), and the NADPH oxidase subunits $p22^{phox}$ (**L**), $p47^{phox}$ (**M**). Differences among the groups were analyzed by one-way non-parametric ANOVA, followed by Tukey's multiple comparison test. NAC was used as a positive control. Data represent mean and SEM. * $p < 0.05$ vs. Control, § $p < 0.05$ vs. LDL. TP, topiroxostat; LDL, low-density lipoprotein; DCF, dichlorofluorescein.

Using siXDH, we evaluated how XO knock-down influenced cholesterol-related metabolism. LDL increased *XDH* expression in HK-2 cells (Figure 4G), and induced expression of the cholesterol transport genes *NR1H3* and *ABCA1*, but not *LDLR*. The siXDH reduced transport gene expression in LDL-treated HK-2 cells, to a greater extent than XO inhibitor (Figure 4A–C). XO deficiency regulated cholesterol synthesis genes upon LDL stimulation. LDL stimulation increased expressions of *SREBF1*, *SREBF2*, and *HMGCR*, while siXDH suppressed the increased expressions of *SREBF2* and *HMGCR* (Figure 4D–F).

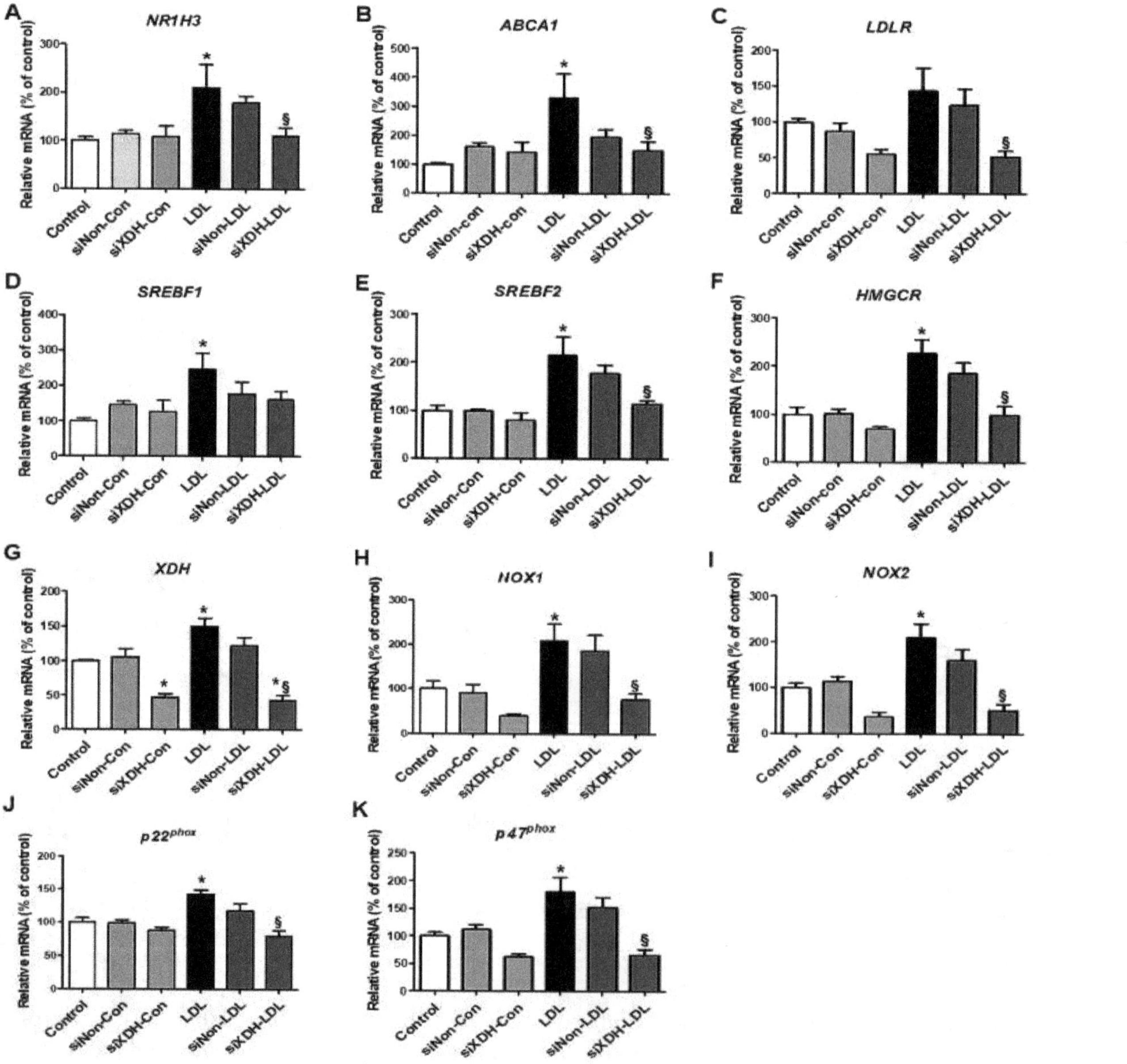

Figure 4. The effects of small interfering RNA against XDH (siXDH) on cholesterol metabolism and oxidative stress in LDL-stimulated HK-2 cells. After transfection with siXDH (20 μM) for 24 h, and

stimulation with LDL (200 μg/mL) for 30 min, real-time RT-PCR was performed to determine expression levels of cholesterol efflux genes (**A**,**B**), LDL receptor (**C**), triglyceride synthesis (**D**), cholesterol synthesis (**E**,**F**), *XDH* (**G**), *NOX1* (**H**), *NOX2* (**I**), and the NADPH oxidase subunits $p22^{phox}$ (**J**) and $p47^{phox}$ (**K**). Differences among the groups were analyzed by one-way non-parametric ANOVA, followed by Tukey's multiple comparison test. Data represent mean and SEM. * $p < 0.05$ vs. control, § $p < 0.05$ vs. LDL. LDL, low-density lipoprotein.

We examined mRNA expressions of subunits of the ROS generation enzyme NADPH oxidase. LDL-treated HK-2 cells exhibited increased mRNA expressions of *NOX1*, *NOX2*, $p22^{phox}$, and $p47^{phox}$. TP inhibited these increased expressions, similar to NAC (Figure 3J–M). siXDH transfection also reduced expression of *NOX1*, *NOX2*, $p22^{phox}$, and $p47^{phox}$ (Figure 4H–K).

2.4. XO Inhibition Reduces Hypercholesterolemia-Associated Kidney Inflammation and Fibrosis in CKD Mice

We evaluated the inflammatory responses to high cholesterol and oxidative stress in the kidney of a CKD model. The HC diet increased inflammation cytokines (e.g., TNF-α) and the macrophage monocyte marker CD68, which were higher with HC+UN versus HC (Figure 5A). Expressions of the inflammation-related genes *Il-1β*, *Il-18*, and *Nlrp3* were also increased with HC+UN versus HC. TP reduced inflammation-related gene expression in uninephrectomized mice (Figure 5B–D). Compared to NC, HC groups showed progression in the fibrosis of glomeruli and interstitium, which was greatest with HC+UN, and was reduced by TP (Figure 5E). Compared to HC, HC+UN yielded increased *Acta2*, *Col1*, and *Fn1* expressions (Figure 5F–I). Fibronectin and α-SMA protein expressions were not significantly increased in the HC+UN group (Figure 5J,K).

Finally, we evaluated the effects of LDL on the NF-κB pathway [17], downstream of TNF-α. LDL-stimulated HK-2 cells showed increased NF-κB p50 and NF-κB p65 levels, which were decreased by TP (Figure 6A,B). We also investigated the NF-κB inhibitors JSH23 and BAY11-7082. In LDL-treated HK-2 cells, JSH23 treatment significantly decreased NF-κB p65, and IL-1β, but did not affect NLRP3 and NF-κB p50 (Figure 6C–F), while BAY11-7082 treatment reduced NF-κB p50, IL-1β, and NLRP3 levels, but did not affect NF-κB p65 (Figure 6G–J).

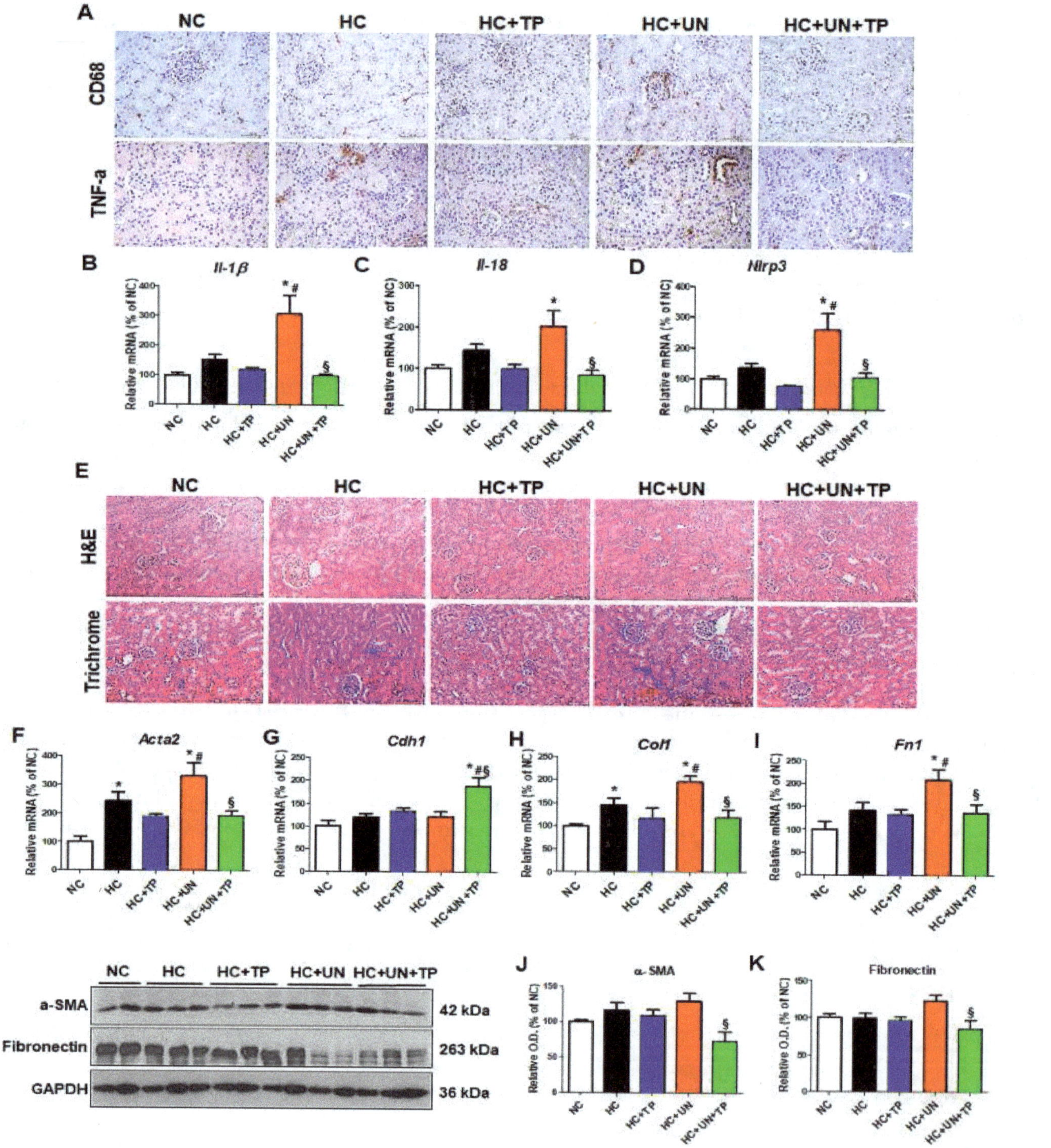

Figure 5. Abnormal lipid metabolism and oxidative stress induced by high-cholesterol diet affect inflammation and fibrosis progression in kidney tissue. (**A**) Representative images of TNF-α and CD68 staining of kidney tissue. Scale bars, 100 μm. (**B**–**D**) Real-time RT-PCR was performed to determine mRNA levels of *Il-1β*, *Il-18*, and *Nlrp3*. (**E**) Representative images of hematoxylin and eosin staining and trichrome staining of kidney tissue. Scale bars, 100 μm. (**F**–**I**) Real-time RT-PCR was performed to determine mRNA levels of *Acta2*, *Cdh1*, *ColI*, and *Fn1*. (**J**,**K**) Representative western blot for α-SMA, fibronectin, and GAPDH. Relative protein expression was determined using densitometry. Differences among the groups were analyzed by one-way non-parametric ANOVA, followed by Tukey's multiple comparison test. Data represent mean and SEM. * $p < 0.05$ vs. NC, # $p < 0.05$ vs. HC, § $p < 0.05$ vs. HC+UN. LDL, low-density lipoprotein; TP, topiroxostat; UN, uninephrectomy; NC, normal control; HC, high-cholesterol.

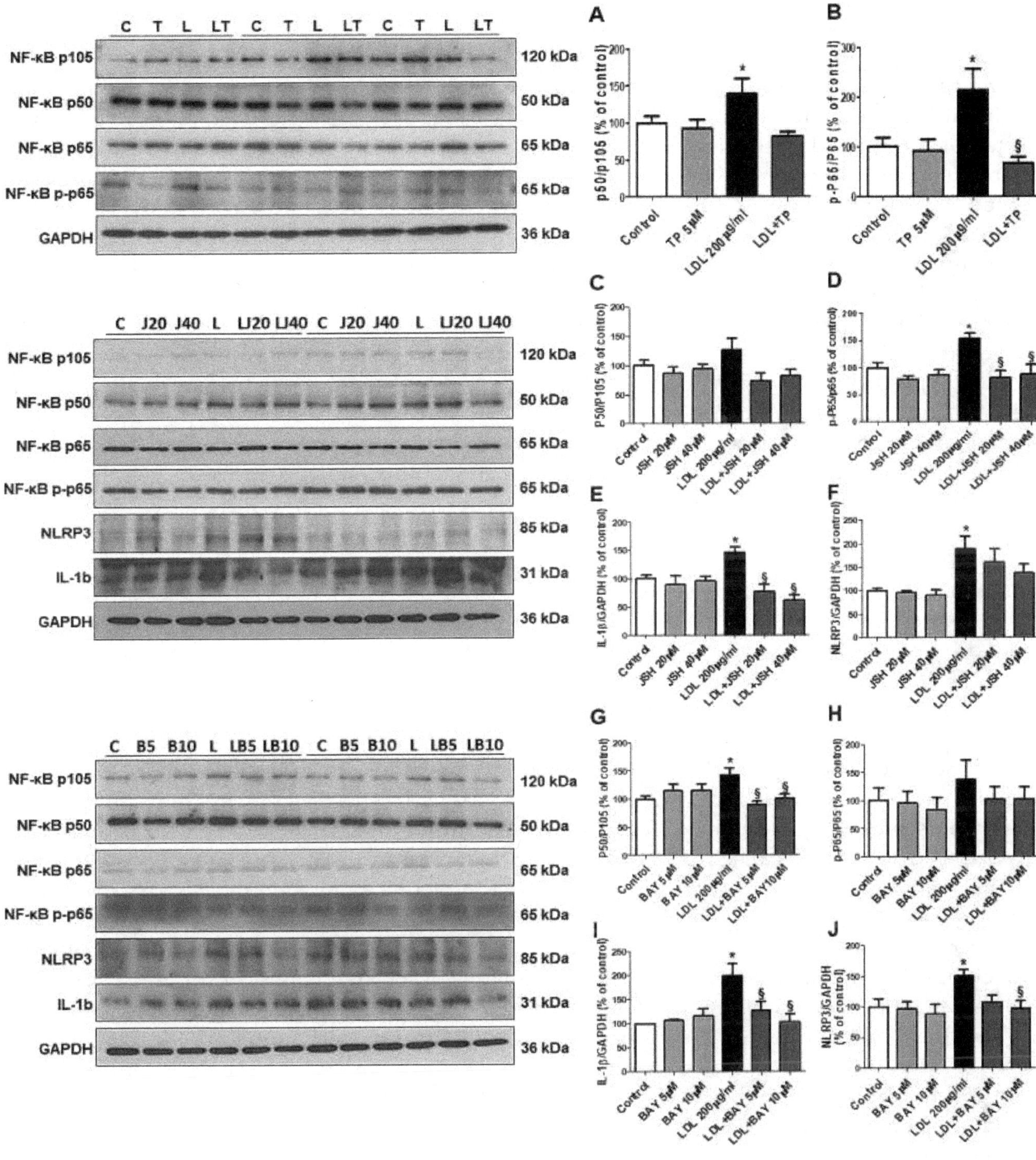

Figure 6. Effects of xanthine oxidase inhibitor on progression of inflammation through the NF-κB pathway in LDL-treated HK-2 cells. (**A**,**B**) Representative western blot for NF-κB p50/p105 ratio, NF-κB p-p65/p65 ratio, and GAPDH in cells that were pretreated with TP (5 μM) for 1 h, and then stimulated with LDL (200 μg/mL) for 30 min. (**C**–**F**) Representative western blot for NF-κB p50/p105 ratio, NF-κB p-p65/p65 ratio, IL-1b, NLRP3, and GAPDH in cells that were pretreated with NF-κB inhibitor (JSH23) for 1 h, and then stimulated with LDL (200 μg/mL) for 30 min. (**G**–**J**) Representative western blot for NF-κB p50/p105 ratio, NF-κB p-p65/p65 ratio, IL-1b, NLRP3, and GAPDH in cells that were pretreated with NF-κB inhibitor (BAY11-7028) for 2 h, and then stimulated with LDL (200 μg/mL) for 30 min. Relative protein expression was determined using densitometry. Differences among the groups were analyzed by a one-way non-parametric ANOVA, followed by Tukey's multiple comparison test. Data represent mean and SEM. * $p < 0.05$ vs. Control, § $p < 0.05$ vs. LDL. LDL, low-density lipoprotein; TP, topiroxostat.

3. Discussion

The present results demonstrated that XO inhibition significantly reduced hypercholesterolemia-associated kidney inflammation and fibrosis in uninephrectomized ApoE KO mice. In vitro experiments revealed that XO inhibition reduced LDL-induced oxidative stress and cholesterol synthesis. The HC diet induced cholesterol accumulation by regulating the expression of genes related to cholesterol efflux and synthesis. Additionally, hypercholesterolemia significantly increased XO activity and NADPH-dependent ROS generation, thus inducing kidney inflammation and fibrosis. LDL stimulation evoked changes in the cholesterol metabolism, NADPH oxidase, and NF-κB pathways in HK-2 cells. XO inhibition modulated the hypercholesterolemia-induced changes in the expression of genes related to cholesterol transport and synthesis. XO inhibition by topiroxostat attenuated inflammation and fibrosis in the unilateral kidney through inhibition of the NF-κB pathway.

Patients with CKD exhibit various lipid abnormalities [18], and abnormal lipid metabolism is associated with kidney disease progression [19,20]. However, the mechanism of lipid-induced kidney damage is not fully understood. In the present study, we used ApoE KO mice with unilateral nephrectomy as a model to evaluate the effects of hypercholesterolemia on CKD progression. Hypercholesterolemia aggravated renal function in the uninephrectomized ApoE KO mice by increasing kidney lipid accumulation. Moreover, these lipid abnormalities were associated with increases of factors mediating kidney injury, such as XO and oxidative stress.

Our results demonstrated that cholesterol accumulation in uninephrectomized mice was induced by upregulation of genes related to cholesterol synthesis, such as *Srebf2* and *Hmgcr,* and downregulation of efflux-related genes, such as *Abca1* and *Nr1h3*, upstream of ABCA1. Cholesterol homeostasis is regulated by multiple pathways, including intracellular cholesterol uptake, synthesis, and efflux actions [21]. Inflammatory stress promotes reduction of cholesterol efflux through the ABCA1 pathway, leading to lipid accumulation in the kidney [22]. ApoE promotes cholesterol efflux through the ABCA1 and ABCG1 cell surface transporters, which facilitate the efflux of phospholipids and cholesterol onto lipid-poor apolipoproteins [23]. The ABCA1 transporter facilitates the efflux of cellular phospholipids and cholesterol to acceptors, such as ApoA-I and ApoE [24]. Selective inactivation of macrophage ABCA1 yields substantially increased cholesterol accumulation in mice [25,26]. Our present results showed that the HC diet caused upregulated expression of both cholesterol synthesis and efflux genes. Furthermore, uninephrectomy plus hypercholesterolemia attenuated the increase of cholesterol efflux genes, while upregulating the increase of cholesterol synthesis genes. It is not yet known why uninephrectomy had different effects on the expression of genes related to cholesterol metabolism. However, our findings suggest that hypercholesterolemia-associated genes contributed to cholesterol accumulation in the kidney, and may potentially play a role in the dysfunction of the unilateral kidney.

The ABCA1 protein level differed from mRNA expression in the unilateral kidney with high cholesterol. The ABCA1 membrane protein rapidly responds to increased cholesterol, and the ABCA1 protein level is independent of its transcription [27]. Cholesterol accumulation inhibits ABCA1 degradation and ubiquitination by decreasing the proteasomal degradation [28]. In our study, the decrease of *Abca1* mRNA may have been associated with the reduced intracellular cholesterol efflux, and thus with the increased cholesterol accumulation in the kidney.

Abnormal lipid metabolism induces monocyte foam cells, and this change is more prominent in patients with kidney dysfunction [29]. Alterations in lipoprotein metabolism promote the production of ROS, such as hydrogen peroxide; however, the effect on intracellular cholesterol has not been clearly demonstrated. Since increased serum LDL level is a representative marker of dyslipidemia, we stimulated renal tubular cells with LDL to examine the molecular changes in cholesterol metabolism and inflammation. LDL stimulation increased the mRNA expression of *NR1H3*, *ABCA1*, *LDLR*, *SREBF2*, and *HMGCR* in HK-2 cells. These changes are consistent with our observations in the animal model, except for the expression of *SREBF1*, which is involved in TG synthesis. These findings suggest that the renal tubular cell damage is also mediated by the lipid accumulation associated with changes in the expression of genes related to cholesterol transport and synthesis.

XO is a key enzyme of the purine pathway, producing uric acid through various oxidized purines [30]. Recent studies demonstrate that XO plays a role as an ROS-producing enzyme, aggravating inflammation, atherosclerosis, and chronic disease [31]. XO activity is increased in obesity, and XO inhibitors regulate the inflammatory process by inhibiting production of ROS and uric acid [32,33]. We previously demonstrated that XO inhibition could decrease cancer cell migration and ROS generation [10]. In our present study, we found that XO activity and gene expression were increased in kidneys with hypercholesterolemia, and in LDL-treated HK-2 cells. This is the first report of cholesterol directly leading to increased XO enzyme activity in the kidney. We further found that XO inhibition improved hypercholesterolemia-associated kidney damage by modulating the expression of genes related to cholesterol metabolism and the progression of inflammation and fibrosis in a unilateral kidney. Overall, our findings suggest that XO is a promising treatment target for hypercholesterolemia-associated kidney injury in uninephrectomized patients.

Expression of NOX1, NOX2, and NOX4 in the kidney mediates oxidative stress and promotes vascular inflammation, dysfunction, and fibrosis in CKD [34]. NADPH oxidases of the kidney exhibit a distinct cellular localization and are activated by various stimuli, including LDL [35]. Our results demonstrated that hypercholesterolemia and LDL increased oxidative stress in kidney tissue and tubule cells, and that XO activity was associated with oxidative stress markers and increased expression of NADPH-related genes. XO inhibition reduced the expression of *NOX1* and *NOX2*, but not *NOX4* (data not shown), showing antioxidant effects similar to with NAC. Transfection with siXDH had the same effect as XO inhibitor in HK-2 cells. These results revealed that XO inhibition controlled NOX activity, thus suppressing oxidative stress and reducing renal damage.

The inflammatory process exacerbates lipid accumulation in the kidney by translocating plasma lipids to the kidney [36]. A high-fat diet activates the inflammatory response by increasing TNF-α expression in the kidney, thus causing kidney damage in obese humans and animal models [37,38]. XO activity is elevated in inflammation, and XO inhibition suppresses inflammation and oxidative stress in macrophages [14]. Treatment with XO inhibitors reportedly attenuates inflammation and fibrosis in animal models of atherosclerosis and nonalcoholic steatohepatitis [39]. Here we found that a HC diet led to increased TNF-α and CD68 in the unilateral kidney, which was downregulated after XO inhibition. These results showed that the mechanism of hypercholesterolemia-associated kidney damage is closely related to inflammation, and that the damage could be suppressed by XO inhibition.

Oxidative stress stimulates inflammatory cells to activate the NF-κB pathway through an intracellular signaling system, thus mediating inflammation [40]. In cells, oxidative stress induces NLRP3 activity, leading to inflammation and apoptosis, along with Caspase-1 activation. Obesity and metabolic syndrome induce NLRP3 inflammatory activation, which weakens phospholipid degradation, leading to kidney damage [41]. In this study, hypercholesterolemia increased NLRP3 and TNF-α, which is one of the most potent inducers of NF-κB. In vitro experiments demonstrated that the NF-κB pathway was an inflammatory mechanism of dyslipidemia-associated kidney damage. LDL stimulation increased the activity of the NF-κB pathway and NLRP3, whereas XO inhibition affected the NF-κB pathway by decreasing phosphorylated NF-κB p65 and NF-κB p50 in HK-2 cells. We further demonstrated that the NF-κB inhibitors JSH23 and BAY11-7028 had effects on NLRP3 similar to those of XO inhibition. This supports the theory that NF-κB is a main pathway of hypercholesterolemia-associated kidney damage.

In conclusion, our present data suggested that XO inhibition has renoprotective effects against hypercholesterolemia-associated kidney injury. This protection from XO inhibition was mediated by regulation of cholesterol metabolism, decreasing NADPH-dependent ROS generation, and reduction of inflammation through the NF-κB pathway. XO could be a novel therapeutic target for hypercholesterolemia-associated kidney disease in uninephrectomized patients.

4. Materials and Methods

4.1. Animals, Diets, and Specimen Collections

Male ApoE KO mice were purchased from Jackson Laboratory (Bar Harbor, ME, USA) at the age of 8 weeks. All animal experiments were approved and performed according to the regulations of the Kyungpook National University Animal Care and Use Committee (KNU-2018-0042, date; 08/03/2018). For 12 weeks, animals were fed normal control diet containing 20.3% protein, 5% fat, and 66% carbohydrate or a high-fat high-cholesterol diet (HC, diet D12336; Research Diets, New Brunswick, NJ, USA) containing 16.0% fat, 1.25% cholesterol, and 0.5% sodium cholic acid.

We randomized the eight-week-old ApoE KO mice into groups that did or did not receive topiroxostat (TP; 1 mg per kg body weight) treatment, and that did or did not undergo uninephrectomy (UN) surgery. There were a total of five groups: NC (n = 5), fed a normal control diet; HC (n = 6), fed a high-cholesterol diet; HC+TP (n = 6), fed a high-cholesterol diet with TP; HC+UN (n = 8), fed a high-cholesterol diet and received uninephrectomy surgery; and HC+UN+TP (n = 8), fed a high-cholesterol diet with TP and received uninephrectomy surgery. All mice that did not undergo uninephrectomy were sham operated. TP was administered by oral gavage for 4 weeks before the end of the experiment.

Uninephrectomy was performed as described previously [42]. For uninephrectomy, after mice were anesthetized with 3–5% isoflurane, the left kidney was surgically removed via a left incision on the back. The adrenal gland was carefully freed from the upper pole of the renal capsule before removed the left kidney. The incision was closed with sutures. In sham surgery, the kidney was manipulated without ablation. At 12 weeks after surgery, all mice were anesthetized and then sacrifice, and kidneys were harvested for the analyses. Half of the kidneys were stored at −80 °C for molecular analysis and the other half was fixed with 4% paraformaldehyde for histological analysis.

4.2. Serum Chemistry

At the end of the experimental period, blood samples from each mouse were collected into tubes by cardiac puncture. The blood was sampled into ethylenediaminetetraacetic acid-free bottles for serum separation. The blood urea nitrogen (BUN), creatinine (Cr), uric acid, total cholesterol (TC), low-density lipoprotein (LDL) and triglycerides level in the serum were measured by GCLabs (Yongin, Korea) using the Cobas 8000 modular analyzer system (Roche, Basel, Switzerland).

4.3. Histopathology

To detect kidney injury, the fixed right kidney was dehydrated in ethanol and embedded in paraffin. Kidney tissue blocks were cut into 2-μm-thick sections and subjected to hematoxylin and eosin (H&E) staining, periodic acid Schiff (PAS) staining, and Masson's trichrome staining. For immunohistochemical analysis of kidney tissues, we used the following antibodies: mouse monoclonal against CD68 (ED1; 1:100; Abcam, Cambridge, MA, USA) and rabbit polyclonal against tumor necrosis factor-α (TNF-α; 1:200; Abcam). Next, secondary antibody was performed using HRP-conjugated polyclonal goat anti-rabbit IgG P0447 or goat anti-mouse IgG p0448 (Dako, Glostrup, Denmark) for 1 h. The sections were visualized using 3,3-diaminobenzidine (DAB; DAKO ChemMate Detection Kit) and counterstained with Mayer's hematoxylin.

4.4. Oil Red O Staining

Fixed frozen kidney tissue was cut into 6-μm-thick sections, and subjected to Oil Red O (Sigma-Aldrich, Saint Louis, MO, USA) staining following the manufacturer's protocol. After the sections were rinsed in distilled water and 60% isopropanol for 1 min, the sections were stained with Oil red O for 15 min. and then rinsed in 60% isopropanol and distilled water each for 1 min. Counterstaining was stained with hematoxylin for 1 min.

4.5. *Cell Treatments*

Human renal proximal tubule epithelial cells (HK-2 cells) were purchased from the Korean Cell Line Bank (KCLB, Seoul, South Korea). The cells were maintained in RPMI-1640 supplemented with 10% fetal bovine serum, and 100 units/mL penicillin and 100 μg/mL streptomycin antibiotic mixture at 37 °C in 5% CO_2 and 95% air. The Cells were pretreated with topiroxostat (TP), xanthine oxidase inhibitor (5 or 10 μM), and 5 mM N-acetylcysteine (NAC) (Sigma-Aldrich) for 1 h, and stimulated with LDL (200 μg/mL) for 30 min to induce lipotoxicity.

4.6. *Hydrogen Peroxide Determination*

H_2O_2 levels were measured using the Amplex Red Hydrogen Peroxide Assay Kit (Molecular Probes, Invitrogen, Eugene, OR, USA), following the manufacturer's protocol. To detect H_2O_2 released from kidney tissue and treated HK cells, cell lysate or culture media were reacted with the Amplex Red Reagent in the presence of horseradish peroxidase to produce the red-fluorescent oxidation product resorufin. The fluorescence of resorufin was determined at 530nm excitation and 590 nm emission using a fluorescence microplate reader (Molecular Devices, Sunnyvale, CA, USA). The concentrations of H_2O_2 were calculated using standard curves. The loading buffer was measured and subtracted from each value in order to exclude background fluorescence.

4.7. *Intracellular ROS Measurement*

Intracellular ROS generation was measured using 2′,7′-dichlorofluorescein diacetate (DCF-DA). HK-2 cells and kidney tissues were stained for 40 min with 10 μM 2′,7′-dichlorodihydrofluorescein diacetate (H_2DCFDA; Molecular Probes) in a black 96-well plate. DCF-DA is hydrolyzed by esterases to dichlorofluorescein (DCF), which is trapped within the cell. Then cellular oxidants oxidize this non-fluorescent molecule to fluorescent dichlorofluorescein (DCF). Fluorescence signal intensity was measured at 480 nm excitation and 520 nm emission using a fluorescence microplate reader (Molecular Devices). The value of the fluorescence signal was expressed as a percentage of the control.

4.8. *Determination of Intracellular Total Cholesterol*

From the kidney tissues of ApoE mice, we extracted cellular lipids by chloroform:methanol extraction (4:2:3, chloroform:methanol:water). Total cholesterol levels were determined using a commercially available kit (Cell Biolabs Inc., San Diego, CA, USA) following the manufacturer's protocol.

4.9. *Transfection of HK-2 with XDH siRNA*

ON-TARGETplus SMARTpool siRNAs used for silencing expression of human XDH genes (ID:7498) and non-targeting (negative control) siRNA were purchased from Dharmacon (Chicago, IL, USA). Four target sequences in human XDH are 5′- AGA GUG AGG UUG ACA AGU U -3′, 5′- GGA GUA ACA UAA CUG GAA U -3′, 5′- UAG AGG AGC UAC ACU AUU C -3′ and 5′- ACA CGG AGA UUG GCA UUG A -3′. siRNAs were used at a concentration of 20 nM. Transfection was performed using Opti-MEM™ transfection medium and Lipofectamine™ (both from Invitrogen, Paisley, UK). One day prior to transfection, HK-2 cells were seeded and cultured to reach 30–40% confluence on the following day. RNAi duplexes for XDH were mixed with Lipofectamine, forming a transfection complex that was added to the plated cells. After 24 h of incubation, the medium was replaced with RPMI, and cells were starved for 6 h. Transfected cells were used for quantitative real-time reverse transcription-polymerase chain reaction (qRT-PCR).

4.10. *Quantitative Real-Time Polymerase Chain Reactions*

Quantitative real-time RT-PCR analysis was performed as described previously [7]. Total RNA was extracted from cell lysates using TRIreagent (Thermo Fisher Scientific, Waltham, MA, USA) according to the provider's instructions. One microgram of total RNA was reverse transcribed to cDNA using the PrimeScript cDNA synthesis kit (TaKaRa, Otsu, Japan). Quantitative real-time RT-PCR was performed on the ABI PRISM 7700 Sequence Detection System (Applied Biosystems, Foster city, CA, USA) using the SYBR green PCR Master Mix (Applied Biosystems, Foster City, CA, USA). The results were analyzed using the comparative Ct method for relative quantification of gene expression. The primer sets used in this study are listed in Table 1.

Table 1. Oligonucleotide primer sequences.

Gene	Forward Primer (5′–3′)	Reverse Primer (5′–3′)
Mouse *Msr1*	CAC GGG ACG CTT CCA GAA T	TGG ACT GAC GAA ATC AAG GAA TT
Mouse *Scarb1*	GGC CTG TTT GTT GGG ATG AA	CGT TCC ATT TGT CCA CCA GAT
Mouse *Lcat*	AGC CTT GGC TGT CTG CAT GT	CCCGAGAGAGATAAAACCATCAA
Mouse *Srebf1*	GGC TAT TCC GTG AAC ATC TCC TA	ATC CAA GGG CAT CTG AGA ACT C
Mouse *Srebf2*	GGT CCT CCA TCA ACG ACA AAA T	TAA TCA ATG GCC TTC CTC AGA AC
Mouse *Nr1h3*	GAG TGT CGA CTT CGC AAA TGC	CCT CTT CTT GCC GCT TCA GT
Mouse *Abca1*	GGC AAT GAG TGT GCC AGA GTT A	TAG TCA CAT GTG GCA CCG TTT T
Mouse *Ldlr*	CCAAATGGCATCACACTAGATCTT	CCGATTGCCCCCATTG
Mouse *Hmgcr*	GGG CCC CAC ATT CAC TCT T	GCC GAA GCA GCA CAT GAT CT
Mouse *Il-1β*	TCG TGC TGT CGG ACC CAT AT	GGTTCTCCTTGTACAAAGCTCATG
Mouse *Nlrp3*	TCTCCCGCATCTCCATTTGTA	CGC GCG TTC CTG TCC TT
Mous *Il-18*	GACAACTTTGGCCGACTTCAC	TCCTCGAACACAGGCTGTCTT
Mouse *Acta2*	CTGACAGAGGCACCACTG	CATCTCCAGAGTCCAGCA
Mouse *Cdh*	GCAGTTCTGCCAGAGAAACC	TGGATCCAAGATGGTGATGA
Mouse *Fn1*	CCA TTC TCC TTC TTC AAG TTT GC	AGG AAT GGC TGT CAG GAT GGT
Mouse *Col1*	ACA ACC GCT TTG CCA CTT CT	CGT AAG TCA CGG GCA CGT T
Mouse *Gapdh*	TAA AGG GCA TCC TGG GCT ACA CT	TTA CTC CTT GGA GGC CAT GTA GG
Human *LDLR*	AGT TGG CTG CGT TAA TGT GAC A	TCT CTA GCC ATG TTG CAG ACT TTG
Human *SREBF1*	GCT CCT CCA TCA ATG ACA AAA TC	TGC AGA AAG CGA ATG TAG TCG AT
Human *SREBF2*	AGG CGG ACA ACC CAT AAT ATC A	CTT GTG CAT CTT GGC GTC TGT
Human *ABCA1*	GAC ATC GTG GCG TTT TTG G	CGA GAT ATG GTC CGG ATT GC
Human *HMGCR*	GGA CAG GAT GCA GCA CAG AA	GCATGGTGCAGCTGATATATAAATCT
Human *NR1H3*	CAC CTA CAT GCG TCG CAA GT	CAG GCG GAT CTG TTC TTC TGA
Human *NOX1*	TGCCTAGAAGGGCTCCAAAC	ACATTCAGCCCTAACCAAACAAC
Human *NOX2*	AGGGTCAAGAACAGGCTAAGGA	TTCTCCACCTCCAACCCTCTTT
Human *p47^phox^*	GGCAGGACCTGTCGGAGAA	ATCGCCCCTGCCTCAATAG
Human *p22^phox^*	ACTTTGGTGCCTACTCCATTGTG	TGTCCCCAGCGCTCCAT
Human *XDH*	GAAGGCCATCTATGCATCGAA	GAAGGCCATCTATGCATCGAA
Human *GAPDH*	TTCACCACCATGGAGAAGGCT	TGGTTCACACCCATGACGAAC

4.11. Immunoblot Analysis

Protein concentration was measured using Bradford's method in lysates of treated HK2 cells and tissues. Total protein (20 µg) was separated by 10% SDS-polyacrylamide gel electrophoresis and transferred to a nitrocellulose membrane. The membrane was blocked with 10% skim milk for 1 h at room temperature, and incubated overnight at 4 °C with primary antibodies. The membrane was incubated with HRP-conjugated polyclonal goat anti-rabbit IgG P0447 or goat anti-mouse IgG p0448 (Dako, Glostrup, Denmark) as the secondary antibody for 1 h and detected using advanced ECL reagents (Amersham Bioscience, Piscataway, NJ, USA). The target protein bands were normalized to that of GAPDH. Expression levels were estimated using Scion Image software (Scion, Frederick, MD, USA). The primary antibodies that detect proteins are listed in Table 2.

Table 2. List of antibodies used in immunohistochemistry and immunoblotting.

Antibodies	Cat. No.	Company
LXRα	Ab176323	abcam
HMGCR	Ab174830	abcam
ABCA1	Ab18180	abcam
α-SMA	Ab5694	abcam
Fibronectin	Ab2413	abcam
IL-1β	12242	Cell signaling
NLRP3	13158	Cell signaling
NF-kappaB p65	8242S	Cell signaling
NF-kappaBphos-p65	3036S	Cell signaling
NF-kappaBp105/p50	3035S	Cell signaling
GAPDH	2118S	Cell signaling

4.12. *Statistical Analysis*

Data are presented as mean ± SEM. Statistical analyses were performed using GraphPad Prism 5.01 (GraphPad Software Inc., La Jolla, CA, USA). The difference among the groups was analyzed using a one-way nonparametric ANOVA followed by Tukey's multiple comparison test. A p value of <0.05 was considered statistically significant.

Author Contributions: Conceptualization, Y.-J.K., J.-H.C. and Y.-L.K.; Formal analysis, Y.-J.K., S.-H.O., C.-D.K., S.-H.P., J.-H.C. and Y.-L.K.; Funding acquisition, Y.-J.K. and Y.-L.K.; Investigation, Y.-J.K., S.-H.O., J.-S.A. and J.-M.Y.; Methodology, Y.-J.K.; Visualization, Y.-J.K. and S.-H.O.; Writing—original draft, Y.-J.K.; Writing—review & editing, J.-H.C. and Y.-L.K. All authors have read and agreed to the published version of the manuscript.

Abbreviations

ABCA1	ATP Binding Cassette Subfamily A Member 1
ABCG1	ATP-binding cassette super-family G Member 1
ApoE KO	Apolipoprotein E Knockout
BUN	Blood urea nitrogen
CD68	Cluster of Differentiation 68
CKD	Chronic kidney disease
DCFDA	Dichlorodihydrofluorescein diacetate
HC	High-cholesterol
HMGCR	3-Hydroxy-3-Methylglutaryl-CoA Reductase
Il-1	Interleukin-1
LCAT	Lecithin-cholesterol acyltransferase
LDL	Low-density lipoprotein
LDLR	Low density lipoprotein receptor
LXRα	Liver X receptor α
MSR1	Macrophage scavenger receptor types I
NR1H3	Nuclear receptor subfamily 1 group H member 3
NADPH	Nicotinamide adenine dinucleotide phosphate
NF-κB	Nuclear Factor-kappaB
NLRP3	NOD-, LRR- and pyrin domain-containing protein 3

NOX	NADPH oxidase
PAS	Periodic acid-Schiff
ROS	Reactive oxygen species
siXDH	Small interfering RNA against XDH
SCARB1	Scavenger receptor class B type 1
SREBF	Sterol regulatory element binding transcription factor
TC	Total cholesterol
TG	Triglyceride
TNF-α	Tumor necrosis factor α
TP	Topiroxostat
XO	Xanthine oxidase
α-SMA	Alpha-smooth muscle actin

References

1. Gelber, R.P.; Kurth, T.; Kausz, A.T.; Manson, J.E.; Buring, J.E.; Levey, A.S.; Gaziano, J.M. Association between body mass index and CKD in apparently healthy men. *Am. J. Kidney Dis.* **2005**, *46*, 871–880. [CrossRef] [PubMed]
2. Reiss, A.B.; Voloshyna, I.; De Leon, J.; Miyawaki, N.; Mattana, J. Cholesterol Metabolism in CKD. *Am. J. Kidney Dis.* **2015**, *66*, 1071–1082. [CrossRef] [PubMed]
3. Locke, J.E.; Reed, R.D.; Massie, A.; MacLennan, P.A.; Sawinski, D.; Kumar, V.; Mehta, S.; Mannon, R.B.; Gaston, R.; Lewis, C.E.; et al. Obesity increases the risk of end-stage renal disease among living kidney donors. *Kidney Int.* **2017**, *91*, 699–703. [CrossRef] [PubMed]
4. Muzaale, A.D.; Massie, A.B.; Wang, M.C.; Montgomery, R.A.; McBride, M.A.; Wainright, J.L.; Segev, D.L. Risk of end-stage renal disease following live kidney donation. *JAMA* **2014**, *311*, 579–586. [CrossRef] [PubMed]
5. Amiya, E. Interaction of hyperlipidemia and reactive oxygen species: Insights from the lipid-raft platform. *World J. Cardiol.* **2016**, *8*, 689–694. [CrossRef] [PubMed]
6. Bobulescu, I.A. Renal lipid metabolism and lipotoxicity. *Curr. Opin. Nephrol. Hypertens.* **2010**, *19*, 393–402. [CrossRef] [PubMed]
7. Ryu, H.M.; Kim, Y.J.; Oh, E.J.; Oh, S.H.; Choi, J.Y.; Cho, J.H.; Kim, C.D.; Park, S.H.; Kim, Y.L. Hypoxanthine induces cholesterol accumulation and incites atherosclerosis in apolipoprotein E-deficient mice and cells. *J. Cell Mol. Med.* **2016**, *20*, 2160–2172. [CrossRef]
8. Gai, Z.; Hiller, C.; Chin, S.H.; Hofstetter, L.; Stieger, B.; Konrad, D.; Kullak-Ublick, G.A. Uninephrectomy augments the effects of high fat diet induced obesity on gene expression in mouse kidney. *Biochim. Biophys. Acta* **2014**, *1842*, 1870–1878. [CrossRef]
9. Bro, S.; Bentzon, J.F.; Falk, E.; Andersen, C.B.; Olgaard, K.; Nielsen, L.B. Chronic renal failure accelerates atherogenesis in apolipoprotein E-deficient mice. *J. Am. Soc. Nephrol.* **2003**, *14*, 2466–2474. [CrossRef]
10. Oh, S.H.; Choi, S.Y.; Choi, H.J.; Ryu, H.M.; Kim, Y.J.; Jung, H.Y.; Cho, J.H.; Kim, C.D.; Park, S.H.; Kwon, T.H.; et al. The emerging role of xanthine oxidase inhibition for suppression of breast cancer cell migration and metastasis associated with hypercholesterolemia. *FASEB J.* **2019**, *33*, 7301–7314. [CrossRef]
11. Gwinner, W.; Scheuer, H.; Haller, H.; Brandes, R.P.; Groene, H.J. Pivotal role of xanthine oxidase in the initiation of tubulointerstitial renal injury in rats with hyperlipidemia. *Kidney Int.* **2006**, *69*, 481–487. [CrossRef] [PubMed]
12. Kataoka, H.; Yang, K.; Rock, K.L. The xanthine oxidase inhibitor Febuxostat reduces tissue uric acid content and inhibits injury-induced inflammation in the liver and lung. *Eur. J. Pharmacol.* **2015**, *746*, 174–179. [CrossRef] [PubMed]
13. Pacher, P.; Nivorozhkin, A.; Szabó, C. Therapeutic effects of xanthine oxidase inhibitors: Renaissance half a century after the discovery of allopurinol. *Pharmacol. Rev.* **2006**, *58*, 87–114. [CrossRef]
14. Nomura, J.; Busso, N.; Ives, A.; Matsui, C.; Tsujimoto, S.; Shirakura, T.; Tamura, M.; Kobayashi, T.; So, A.; Yamanaka, Y. Xanthine oxidase inhibition by febuxostat attenuates experimental atherosclerosis in mice. *Sci. Rep.* **2014**, *4*, 1–9. [CrossRef] [PubMed]
15. Dandona, P.; Ghanim, H.; Brooks, D.P. Antioxidant activity of carvedilol in cardiovascular disease. *J. Hypertens.* **2007**, *25*, 731–741. [CrossRef] [PubMed]

16. Badve, S.V.; Pascoe, E.M.; Tiku, A.; Boudville, N.; Brown, F.G.; Cass, A.; Clarke, P.; Dalbeth, N.; Day, R.O.; de Zoysa, J.R.; et al. Effects of Allopurinol on the Progression of Chronic Kidney Disease. *N. Engl. J. Med.* **2020**, *382*, 2504–2513. [CrossRef] [PubMed]
17. Janabi, M.; Yamashita, S.; Hirano, K.; Sakai, N.; Hiraoka, H.; Matsumoto, K.; Zhang, Z.; Nozaki, S.; Matsuzawa, Y. Oxidized LDL-induced NF-kappa B activation and subsequent expression of proinflammatory genes are defective in monocyte-derived macrophages from CD36-deficient patients. *Arterioscler Thromb Vasc Biol.* **2000**, *20*, 1953–1960. [CrossRef]
18. Cases, A.; Coll, E. Dyslipidemia and the progression of renal disease in chronic renal failure patients. *Kidney Int. Suppl.* **2005**, *68*, S87–S93. [CrossRef]
19. Moorhead, J.; El-Nahas, M.; Chan, M.; Varghese, Z. Lipid nephrotoxicity in chronic progressive glomerular and tubulo-interstitial disease. *Lancet* **1982**, *320*, 1309–1311. [CrossRef]
20. Scarpioni, R.; Ricardi, M.; Albertazzi, V.; Melfa, L. Treatment of dyslipidemia in chronic kidney disease: Effectiveness and safety of statins. *World J. Nephrol.* **2012**, *1*, 184–194. [CrossRef]
21. Afonso, M.S.; Machado, R.M.; Lavrador, M.S.; Quintao, E.C.R.; Moore, K.J.; Lottenberg, A.M. Molecular Pathways Underlying Cholesterol Homeostasis. *Nutrients* **2018**, *10*, 760. [CrossRef] [PubMed]
22. Ruan, X.Z.; Moorhead, J.F.; Fernando, R.Y.; Wheeler, D.C.; Powis, S.H. PPAR agonists protect mesangial cells from interleukin 1β-induced intracellular lipid accumulation by activating the ABCA1 cholesterol efflux pathway. *J. Am. Soc. Nephrol.* **2003**, *14*, 593–600. [CrossRef] [PubMed]
23. Gelissen, I.C.; Harris, M.; Rye, K.A.; Quinn, C.; Brown, A.J.; Kockx, M.; Cartland, S.; Packianathan, M.; Kritharides, L.; Jessup, W. ABCA1 and ABCG1 synergize to mediate cholesterol export to apoA-I. *Arter. Thromb. Vasc. Biol.* **2006**, *26*, 534–540. [CrossRef] [PubMed]
24. Brooks-Wilson, A.; Marcil, M.; Clee, S.M.; Zhang, L.-H.; Roomp, K.; van Dam, M.; Yu, L.; Brewer, C.; Collins, J.A.; Molhuizen, H.O. Mutations in ABC1 in Tangier disease and familial high-density lipoprotein deficiency. *Nat. Genet.* **1999**, *22*, 337. [CrossRef] [PubMed]
25. Zuo, Y.; Yancey, P.; Castro, I.; Khan, W.N.; Motojima, M.; Ichikawa, I.; Fogo, A.B.; Linton, M.F.; Fazio, S.; Kon, V. Renal dysfunction potentiates foam cell formation by repressing ABCA1. *Arter. Thromb. Vasc. Biol.* **2009**, *29*, 1277–1282. [CrossRef]
26. Joyce, C.; Freeman, L.; Brewer, H.B., Jr.; Santamarina-Fojo, S. Study of ABCA1 function in transgenic mice. *Arter. Thromb. Vasc. Biol.* **2003**, *23*, 965–971. [CrossRef]
27. Hsieh, V.; Kim, M.J.; Gelissen, I.C.; Brown, A.J.; Sandoval, C.; Hallab, J.C.; Kockx, M.; Traini, M.; Jessup, W.; Kritharides, L. Cellular cholesterol regulates ubiquitination and degradation of the cholesterol export proteins ABCA1 and ABCG1. *J. Biol. Chem.* **2014**, *289*, 7524–7536. [CrossRef]
28. Wellington, C.L.; Walker, E.K.; Suarez, A.; Kwok, A.; Bissada, N.; Singaraja, R.; Yang, Y.-Z.; Zhang, L.-H.; James, E.; Wilson, J.E. ABCA1 mRNA and Protein Distribution Patterns Predict Multiple Different Roles and Levels of Regulation. *Regulation* **2002**, *82*, 273–283. [CrossRef]
29. Eom, M.; Hudkins, K.L.; Alpers, C.E. Foam cells and the pathogenesis of kidney disease. *Curr. Opin. Nephrol. Hypertens.* **2015**, *24*, 245–251. [CrossRef]
30. Kushiyama, A.; Tanaka, K.; Hara, S.; Kawazu, S. Linking uric acid metabolism to diabetic complications. *World J. Diabetes* **2014**, *5*, 787–795. [CrossRef]
31. Nomura, J.; Busso, N.; Ives, A.; Tsujimoto, S.; Tamura, M.; So, A.; Yamanaka, Y. Febuxostat, an inhibitor of xanthine oxidase, suppresses lipopolysaccharide-induced MCP-1 production via MAPK phosphatase-1-mediated inactivation of JNK. *PLoS ONE* **2013**, *8*, e75527. [CrossRef] [PubMed]
32. Klisic, A.; Kocic, G.; Kavaric, N.; Jovanovic, M.; Stanisic, V.; Ninic, A. Body mass index is independently associated with xanthine oxidase activity in overweight/obese population. *Eat. Weight Disord.* **2020**, *25*, 9–15. [CrossRef] [PubMed]
33. Ives, A.; Nomura, J.; Martinon, F.; Roger, T.; LeRoy, D.; Miner, J.N.; Simon, G.; Busso, N.; So, A. Xanthine oxidoreductase regulates macrophage IL1beta secretion upon NLRP3 inflammasome activation. *Nat. Commun.* **2015**, *6*, 6555. [CrossRef] [PubMed]
34. Honda, T.; Hirakawa, Y.; Nangaku, M. The role of oxidative stress and hypoxia in renal disease. *Kidney Res Clin Pract.* **2019**, *38*, 414–426. [CrossRef]
35. Ratliff, B.B.; Abdulmahdi, W.; Pawar, R.; Wolin, M.S. Oxidant Mechanisms in Renal Injury and Disease. *Antioxid. Redox Signal.* **2016**, *25*, 119–146. [CrossRef]

36. Ruan, X.Z.; Moorhead, J.F.; Varghese, Z. Lipid redistribution in renal dysfunction. *Kidney Int.* **2008**, *74*, 407–409. [CrossRef]
37. Laurencikiene, J.; van Harmelen, V.; Arvidsson Nordstrom, E.; Dicker, A.; Blomqvist, L.; Naslund, E.; Langin, D.; Arner, P.; Ryden, M. NF-kappaB is important for TNF-alpha-induced lipolysis in human adipocytes. *J. Lipid Res.* **2007**, *48*, 1069–1077. [CrossRef]
38. Wang, Z.; Huang, W.; Li, H.; Tang, L.; Sun, H.; Liu, Q.; Zhang, L. Synergistic action of inflammation and lipid dysmetabolism on kidney damage in rats. *Ren. Fail.* **2018**, *40*, 175–182. [CrossRef]
39. Mizuno, Y.; Yamamotoya, T.; Nakatsu, Y.; Ueda, K.; Matsunaga, Y.; Inoue, M.K.; Sakoda, H.; Fujishiro, M.; Ono, H.; Kikuchi, T.; et al. Xanthine Oxidase Inhibitor Febuxostat Exerts an Anti-Inflammatory Action and Protects against Diabetic Nephropathy Development in KK-Ay Obese Diabetic Mice. *Int. J. Mol. Sci.* **2019**, *20*, 4680. [CrossRef]
40. Kim, J.Y. Antioxidants in Sepsis. *Korean J. Crit. Care Med.* **2010**, *25*, 57–60. [CrossRef]
41. Fu, H.; Hu, Z.; Di, X.; Zhang, Q.; Zhou, R.; Du, H. Tenuigenin exhibits protective effects against LPS-induced acute kidney injury via inhibiting TLR4/NF-κB signaling pathway. *Eur. J. Pharmacol.* **2016**, *791*, 229–234. [CrossRef] [PubMed]
42. Arsenijevic, D.; Cajot, J.-F.; Dulloo, A.G.; Montani, J.-P. Uninephrectomy in rats on a fixed food intake results in adipose tissue lipolysis implicating spleen cytokines. *Front. Physiol.* **2015**, *6*, 195. [CrossRef] [PubMed]

15

ND-13, a DJ-1-Derived Peptide, Attenuates the Renal Expression of Fibrotic and Inflammatory Markers Associated with Unilateral Ureter Obstruction

Carmen De Miguel [1,*], Abigayle C. Kraus [1], Mitchell A. Saludes [2], Prasad Konkalmatt [2], Almudena Ruiz Domínguez [3], Laureano D. Asico [2], Patricia S. Latham [4], Daniel Offen [5], Pedro A. Jose [2] and Santiago Cuevas [3,*]

1 Section of Cardio-Renal Physiology and Medicine, Division of Nephrology, Department of Medicine, University of Alabama at Birmingham, AL 35233, USA; abkraus@uab.edu

2 Department of Medicine, Division of Renal Diseases & Hypertension and Pharmacology/Physiology, The George Washington University School of Medicine and Health Sciences, Washington, DC 20052, USA; mtsaludes@live.com (M.A.S.); prk@email.gwu.edu (P.K.); lasico@email.gwu.edu (L.D.A.); pjose@mfa.gwu.edu (P.A.J.)

3 Molecular Inflammation Group, Biomedical Research Institute of Murcia (IMIB), University Clinical Hospital Virgen Arrixaca, 30120 Murcia, Spain; almuruiz_8@hotmail.com

4 Pathology and Internal Medicine The George Washington University School of Medicine and Health Sciences, Washington, DC 20052, USA; pslath@gwu.edu

5 Neuroscience Laboratory, The Felsenstein Medical Research Center, Sackler School of Medicine, Tel-Aviv University, Tel-Aviv 6997801, Israel; danioffen@gmail.com

* Correspondence: cdemigue@uab.edu (C.D.M.); santiago.cuevas@imib.es (S.C.)

Abstract: DJ-1 is a redox-sensitive chaperone with reported antioxidant and anti-inflammatory properties in the kidney. The 20 amino acid (aa) peptide ND-13 consists of 13 highly conserved aas from the DJ-1 sequence and a TAT-derived 7 aa sequence that helps in cell penetration. This study aimed to determine if ND-13 treatment prevents the renal damage and inflammation associated with unilateral ureter obstruction (UUO). Male C57Bl/6 and *DJ-1*$^{-/-}$ mice underwent UUO and were treated with ND-13 or vehicle for 14 days. ND-13 attenuated the renal expression of fibrotic markers *TGF-β* and *collagen1a1* (*Col1a1*) and inflammatory markers *TNF-α* and *IL-6* in C57Bl/6 mice. *DJ-1*$^{-/-}$ mice treated with ND-13 presented similar decreased expression of *TNF-α*, *IL-6* and *TGF-β*. However, in contrast to C57Bl/6 mice, ND-13 failed to prevent renal fibrosis or to ameliorate the expression of *Col1a1* in this genotype. Further, UUO led to elevated urinary levels of the proximal tubular injury marker neutrophil gelatinase-associated lipocalin (NGAL) in *DJ-1*$^{-/-}$ mice, which were blunted by ND-13. Our results suggest that ND-13 protects against UUO-induced renal injury, inflammation and fibrosis. These are all crucial mechanisms in the pathogenesis of kidney injury. Thus, ND-13 may be a new therapeutic approach to prevent renal diseases.

Keywords: renal disease; DJ-1; ND-13; renal inflammation; oxidative stress; UUO; fibrosis

---

1. Introduction

Renal oxidative stress and inflammation are two of the most important factors involved in the pathogenesis of renal diseases and other cardiovascular disease complications [1]. Inflammation, the consequent oxidative stress, and vice versa, are considered major factors triggering fibrosis, and are key components in the development and progression of renal failure [2]. Renal fibrosis is caused, in part, by excess deposition of extracellular matrix, and inflammation is one of the main pathways that trigger this mechanism [3]. The inflammatory response during the initial stages of renal disease is characterized by glomerular and tubulo-interstitial infiltration of immune cells, including neutrophils and macrophages [4]. Furthermore, the activation of neutrophils during these early stages results in the release of proinflammatory and profibrogenic cytokines [4], followed by the infiltration of macrophages and T and B lymphocytes into the tissues. Macrophages are a major source of TGF-β in fibrotic organs [5,6], and recruitment of T and B lymphocytes to the site of injury further facilitates the secretion of fibrogenic cytokines [7,8]. TGF-β is also a potent chemoattractant involved in the recruitment of inflammatory cells [9] and, thereby, facilitates the expansion of the inflammatory process. Renal inflammation plays a central role in the initiation and progression of fibrosis in chronic kidney disease. Therefore, attenuation of the inflammatory response may be a critical step for the restoration of the proper balance between pro and antifibrotic signaling pathways [10,11] in the kidney and other organs.

DJ-1, also known as Park 7, is a multifunctional oxidative stress response protein. *DJ-1* was initially identified as an autosomal recessive gene associated with Parkinson's disease, and it has been shown to be expressed in the brain, heart, kidney, liver, pancreas, and skeletal muscle in rodents as well as in humans [12]. DJ-1 functions as a redox-sensitive chaperone with intrinsic antioxidant properties, especially in the mitochondria, and it regulates the expression of several antioxidant genes such as glutathione and heat shock protein 70 in dopaminergic neurons [13,14]. DJ-1 is mainly present in the cytoplasm and, to a lesser extent, in the mitochondria. However, upon an oxidant challenge, DJ-1 translocates from the cytoplasm to the mitochondria where it protects mitochondrial function [15]. In a previous report, our group demonstrated that renal DJ-1 plays a critical role in the regulation of oxidative stress-dependent hypertension in mice [16].

Nrf2 (nuclear factor erythroid 2-related factor 2) is a transcription factor that regulates the expression of several antioxidant genes and also inhibits the development and progression of acute kidney injury caused by heavy metals, ischemia and xenobiotics such as cyclosporin A and cisplatin [17]. Nrf2 attenuates the NFκB-inflammatory pathway and suppresses proinflammatory cell signaling [18,19]. We previously reported that the kidney-selective silencing of *DJ-1* in mice leads to impairment of the antioxidant response mediated by the dopamine receptor 2 and increases in blood pressure associated with decreased Nrf2 expression and activity in the kidney [16,20]. In addition, mice with *DJ-1* selectively silenced in the kidney, and mice with germline deletion of *DJ-1* (*DJ-1*$^{-/-}$ mice), develop high blood pressure, renal damage and decreased kidney expression and activity of Nrf2 [20], suggesting that DJ-1 inhibits the production of renal reactive oxygen species (ROS), at least in part, via the activation of Nrf2-controlled antioxidant genes. We also recently demonstrated the important role of the antioxidant protein UCP2 in hypertension associated with the depletion of DJ-1 [21]. Moreover, other reports also implicated the DJ-1/Nrf2 pathway in the pathogenesis of several renal diseases, such as diabetic nephropathy in rats [22].

Dr. Daniel Offen's laboratory, at the University of Tel Aviv, developed a 13 aa-long peptide derived from the most conserved sequence of DJ-1 [23]. To achieve cell permeability, this 13 aa chain was fused to a 7 aa TAT sequence (YGRKKRR). The resulting 20 amino acid compound was named ND-13 and was demonstrated to be effective in protecting neuronal cultures from the effects of relevant neurotoxins in the setting of Parkinson's disease, amyotrophic lateral sclerosis or multiple system atrophy [23–25]. ND-13 exerts these protective effects by reducing apoptosis and by inactivating the proapoptotic protein caspase-3 in neuronal cell lines exposed to these neurotoxic insults. In those studies, ND-13 treatment led to the activation of the Nrf2 pathway and the consequent increased expression of Nrf2-induced antioxidant genes [23], similar observations to our previous findings in the kidney of *DJ-1*$^{-/-}$ mice [20]. However, the potential protective effects of ND-13 against the development of renal disease remain unknown. Therefore, the goal of these studies was to determine if ND-13 prevents the renal damage and inflammation associated with an animal model of progressive kidney fibrosis, the unilateral ureter obstruction (UUO) model, and if this protection is mediated by the activation of the DJ-1/Nrf2 pathway.

2. Results

2.1. *ND-13 Treatment Reduces UUO-Induced Renal Fibrosis in WT Mice, but Not in $DJ\text{-}1^{-/-}$ Mice*

Because UUO is a classical model of progressive renal fibrosis, we evaluated by RT-PCR the expression levels of markers of fibrosis in the cortex of wild type (WT) mice that underwent sham or UUO surgery and were treated with ND-13 or vehicle for 14 days. We found that after UUO surgery, WT mice treated with vehicle presented a significant upregulation of the markers of fibrosis *Col1a1* and *TGF-β* (~70-fold increase for *Col1a1* and ~7-fold increase for *TGF-β* $p < 0.05$; Figure 1) in the renal cortex. Importantly, daily treatment with ND-13 significantly decreased the cortical expression of both markers of fibrosis, suggesting a protective effect of this peptide against the development of the cortical fibrosis typically induced by UUO.

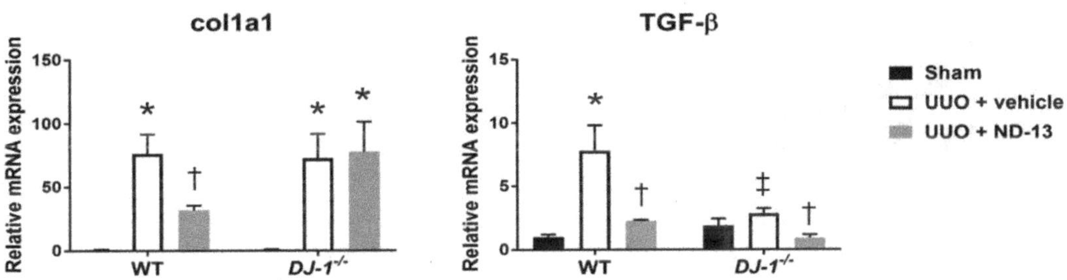

Figure 1. Treatment with ND-13 reduces the unilateral ureter obstruction (UUO)-induced renal expression of fibrotic markers in wild type (WT) mice, but not in $DJ\text{-}1^{-/-}$ mice. Relative mRNA expression of markers of fibrosis *col1a1* and *TGF-β* in renal cortex of WT and $DJ\text{-}1^{-/-}$ mice that underwent sham surgery, UUO and vehicle treatment or UUO and ND-13 treatment. N = 4–5/group; * $p < 0.05$ vs. same genotype sham, † $p < 0.05$ vs. same genotype UUO + vehicle, ‡ $p < 0.05$ vs. WT UUO + vehicle; two-way ANOVA with Tukey's post-hoc test.

In order to characterize the role of DJ-1 in the development of the renal fibrosis associated with UUO, we performed similar studies using the *DJ-1* global knockout ($DJ\text{-}1^{-/-}$) mouse. In response to UUO, and similar to our findings in the WT mice, $DJ\text{-}1^{-/-}$ mice significantly upregulated the mRNA expression of the marker of fibrosis *Col1a1* compared to the levels that the sham group presented (Figure 1). However, and contrary to the results found in WT mice, treatment of $DJ\text{-}1^{-/-}$ mice with ND-13 failed to prevent the elevation of *Col1a1* in the cortex after UUO. In contrast, the cortical levels of *TGF-β* after UUO did not significantly increase in the $DJ\text{-}1^{-/-}$ mice compared to sham controls, but interestingly, treatment with ND-13 was efficient in decreasing the mRNA expression of *TGF-β* in the renal cortex (Figure 1).

Similar to the results obtained by RT-PCR, Masson's blue trichrome histological staining demonstrated extensive interstitial fibrosis in the cortex, outer and inner medulla in WT mice treated with vehicle, as indicated by the homogeneous presence of blue staining in Figure 2A. Although deposition of fibrotic material was also apparent in the WT mice treated with ND-13, examination of the tissue at higher magnification revealed that the cortical fibrosis was not as homogenously distributed, and tended to be localized to certain areas of the cortex while other areas appeared fibrosis-free (Figures 2A and 3A), suggesting that treatment with ND-13 may be blunting the accumulation of fibrotic material in the renal cortex. Despite these observations of the extension of fibrosis and the clear trend of the results, no significant difference in the cortical fibrosis quantification was found among the WT groups (relative fibrosis: sham: 1 ± 0.4, UUO + vehicle: 2.1 ± 0.3 and UUO + ND-13: 1.0 ± 0.4, $p > 0.05$, n = 4–5/group, Figure 2B).

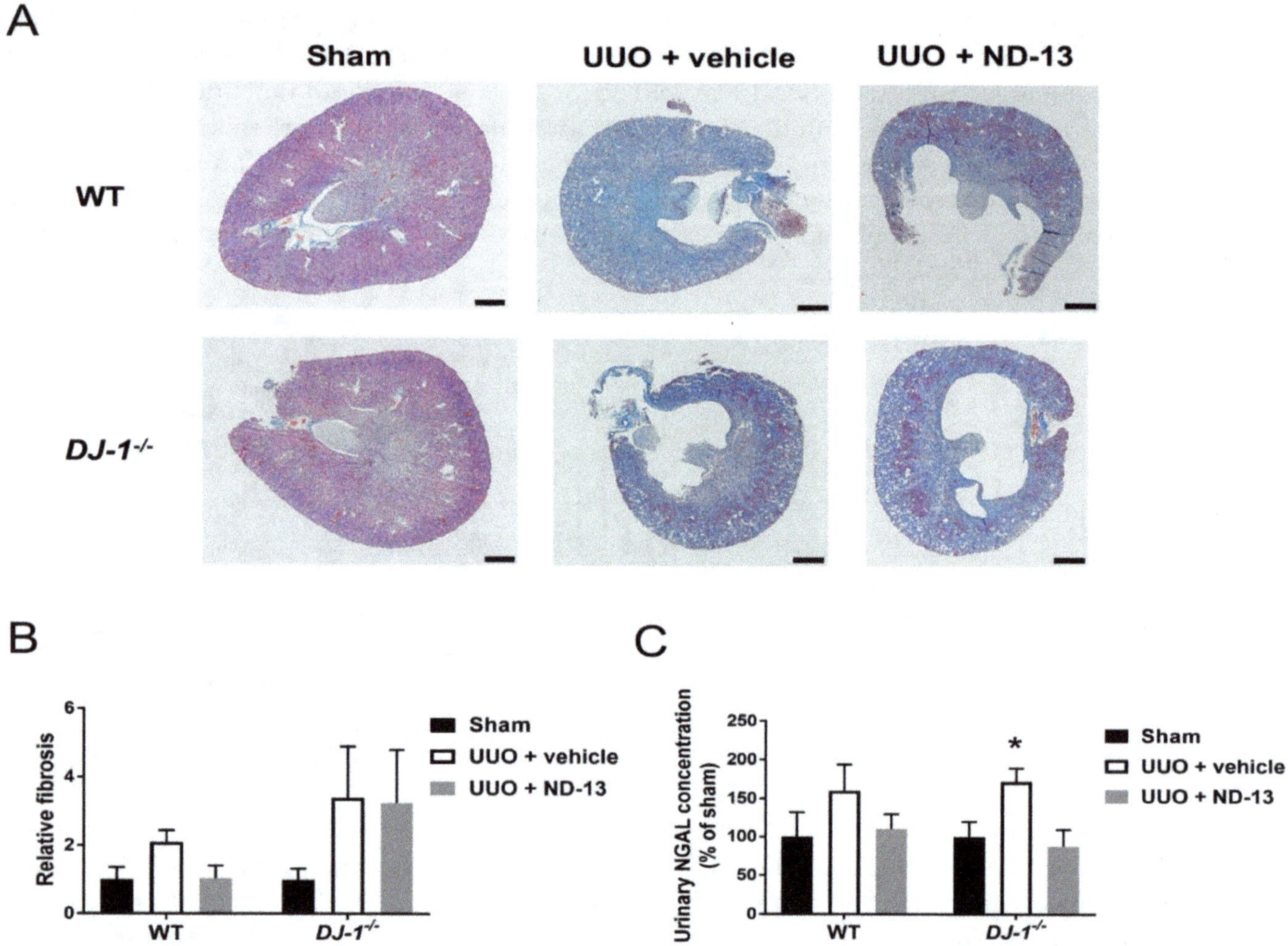

Figure 2. Treatment with ND-13 reduces UUO-induced renal fibrosis in WT mice. (**A**) Representative full scan images of Masson's blue trichrome-stained kidneys obtained from WT and $DJ\text{-}1^{-/-}$ mice that underwent sham surgery, UUO and vehicle treatment or UUO and ND-13 treatment (scale bar = 500 μm). (**B**) Quantification of collagen deposition in renal cortex of WT and $DJ\text{-}1^{-/-}$ mice that underwent sham surgery, UUO and vehicle treatment or UUO and ND-13 treatment. (**C**) Urinary concentration of the proximal tubule marker NGAL in WT and $DJ\text{-}1^{-/-}$ mice that underwent sham surgery, UUO and vehicle treatment or UUO and ND-13 treatment. n = 4–5/group; * $p < 0.05$ vs. same genotype sham, two-way ANOVA with Tukey's post hoc test.

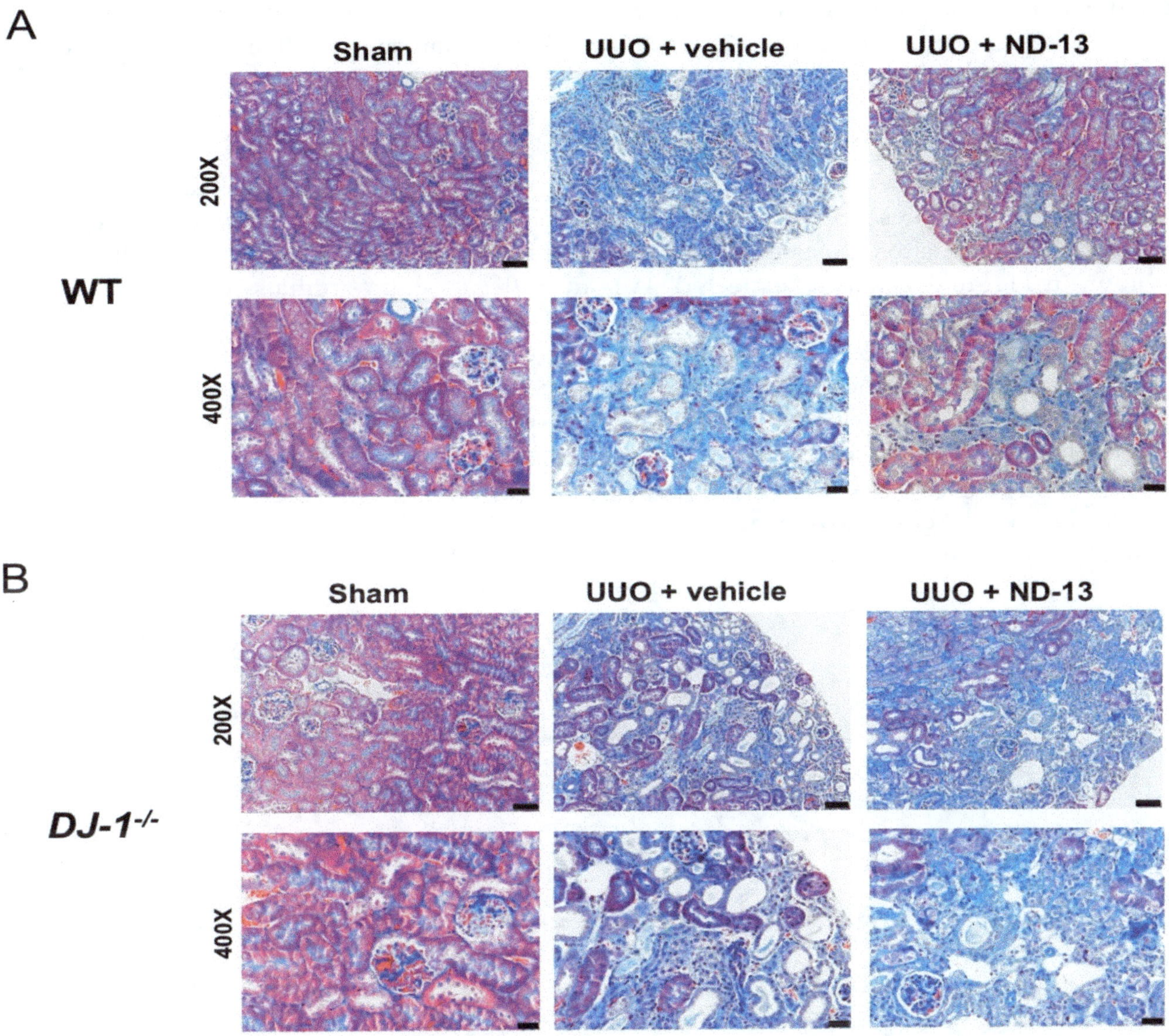

Figure 3. Treatment with ND-13 seems to blunt the spread of UUO-induced fibrosis accumulation in the cortex of WT mice but fails to do so in *DJ-1*$^{-/-}$ mice. (**A**) Representative Masson's blue trichrome images of renal cortex of WT mice that underwent sham surgery, UUO and vehicle treatment or UUO and ND-13 treatment: 200× (upper panels; scale bar = 50 μm) and 400× magnification (bottom panels; scale bar = 20 μm). (**B**) Representative Masson's blue trichrome images of renal cortex of *DJ-1*$^{-/-}$ mice that underwent sham surgery, UUO and vehicle treatment or UUO and ND-13 treatment: 200× (upper panels; scale bar = 50 μm) and 400× magnification (bottom panels; scale bar = 20 μm).

Likewise, histological evaluation of cortical tissue obtained from *DJ-1*$^{-/-}$ mice after the UUO protocol supported the molecular findings in this genotype, as ND-13 treatment had no effect on the amount of collagen deposition detected by trichrome blue staining in this region of the kidney (relative fibrosis, UUO + vehicle vs. UUO + ND-13: 3.4 ± 1.5 vs. 3.3 ± 1.5; Figure 2A,B and Figure 3B). The renal fibrosis in *DJ-1*$^{-/-}$ mice was found to be evenly distributed across the cortical region (Figure 3B).

To determine the extent of renal damage, the concentration of neutrophil gelatinase-associated lipocalin (NGAL), a marker of proximal tubule damage, was measured in urine. We found that the urinary concentrations of NGAL were similar among the three experimental groups of WT mice, suggesting that these groups presented similar levels of renal damage (Figure 2C). On the other hand, fourteen days after UUO, *DJ-1*$^{-/-}$ mice presented significantly greater amounts of urinary NGAL compared to *DJ-1*$^{-/-}$ mice that underwent sham surgery, and daily treatment of these mice with ND-13 resulted in a normalization of these urinary values to sham levels (Figure 2C). These results suggest that *DJ-1*$^{-/-}$ mice are more sensitive to UUO-induced kidney damage, and that ND-13 ameliorates the damage inflicted to the proximal tubules by UUO.

2.2. Treatment with ND-13 Does Not Prevent UUO-Induced Cell Death in the Kidney

To determine if treatment with ND-13 effectively protected against kidney cell death in response to the UUO protocol, the presence of Terminal Deoxynucleotidyl Transferase-Mediated dUTP Nick-End Labeling (TUNEL)-positive areas in kidney cortex and medulla was quantified in both genotypes. As shown in Figure 4A, and as expected, WT and *DJ-1*$^{-/-}$ sham animals hardly presented any TUNEL-positive cells in the kidney cortex. UUO induced cell death in mice of both genotypes treated with vehicle, although the elevation in the percentage area of the kidney that stained positive for TUNEL only reached significance in the *DJ-1*$^{-/-}$ mice, and appeared to be greater than in WT mice ($p > 0.05$, Figure 4B). Upon closer examination, the cortical TUNEL-positive stain was observed in glomeruli, tubular cells and interstitial cells in both genotypes. Treatment with ND-13 was unable to prevent cortical cell death in either genotype, as the percentage area of the kidney stained for TUNEL remained elevated in both. No differences between the treatments and genotypes were observed in the renal medulla (Figure 4B).

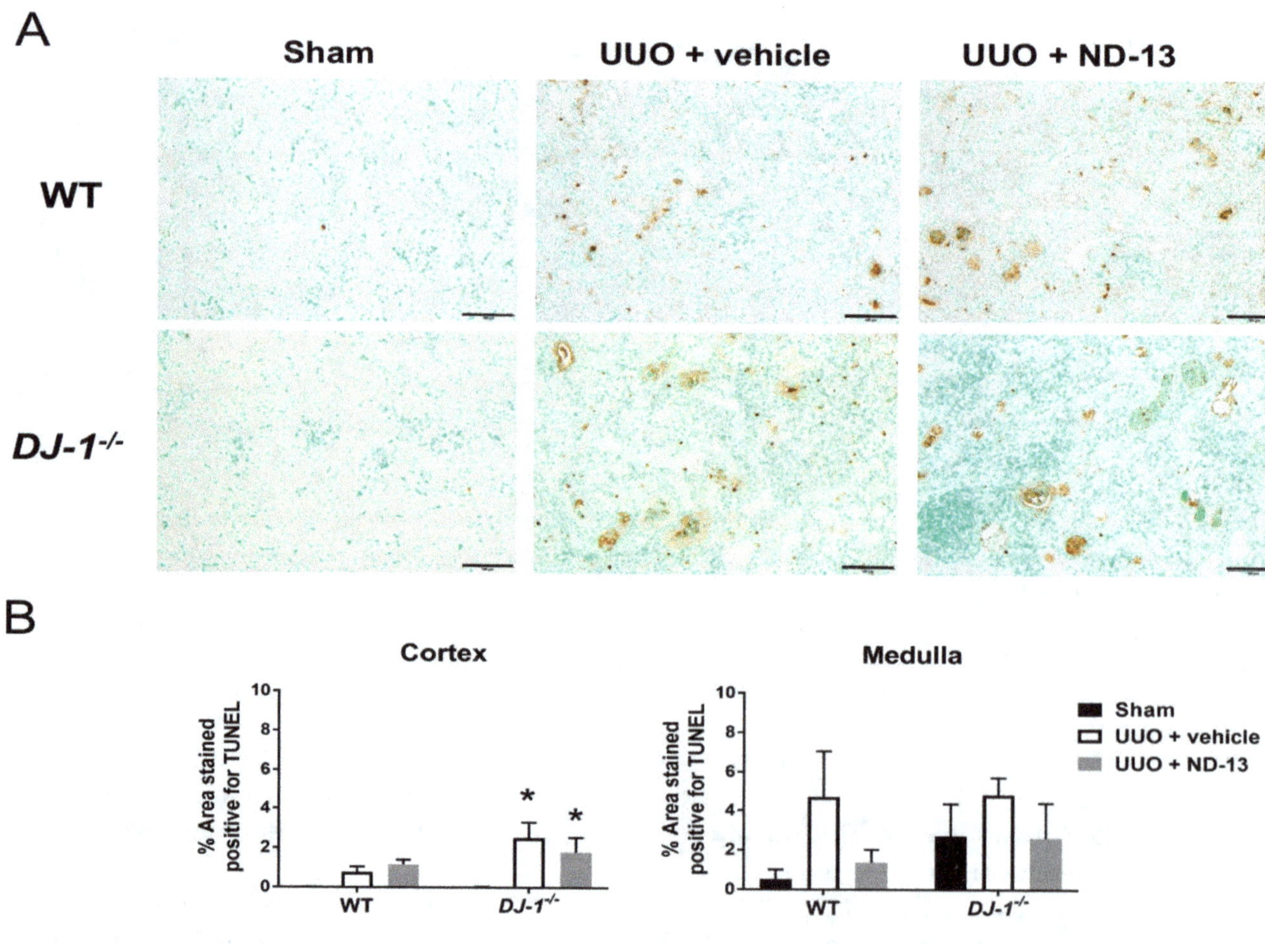

Figure 4. ND-13 does not protect against UUO-induced cell death. (**A**) Representative images of TUNEL stained (brown color) kidney cortex from WT (upper panels) and *DJ-1*$^{-/-}$ mice that underwent sham surgery, UUO and vehicle treatment or UUO and ND-13 treatment (scale bar = 100 μm). (**B**) Quantification of cell death (% TUNEL-positive area) in kidney cortex and medulla of WT and *DJ-1*$^{-/-}$ mice that underwent sham surgery, UUO and vehicle treatment or UUO and ND-13 treatment. n = 4–5/group; * $p < 0.05$ vs. same genotype sham, two-way ANOVA with Tukey's post-hoc test.

2.3. *Renal Expression of Cytokine and Chemokine Genes Associated with UUO Is Ameliorated in Mice Treated with ND-13*

Renal inflammation has been proven to be intimately associated with the development of kidney damage [2]. Therefore, we evaluated the level of kidney inflammation in our experimental animals and found that WT mice that underwent UUO, and were treated with vehicle, had significantly upregulated expression of cytokines *TNF-α* and *IL-6* and chemokine *CCL25* in the renal cortex (Figure 5). Interestingly, daily treatment with ND-13 led to a significant attenuation in the expression of these markers of inflammation, bringing their expression levels to values similar to those found in the sham WT group.

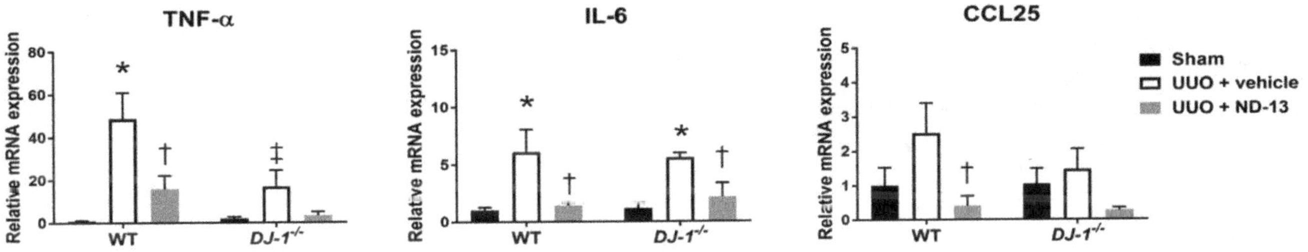

Figure 5. Expression of cytokine and chemokine genes associated with UUO is attenuated in kidneys obtained from WT mice treated with ND-13. Relative mRNA expression of cytokines *TNF-α* and *IL-6* and chemokine *CCL25* in renal cortex of WT mice and *DJ-1*$^{-/-}$ mice that underwent sham surgery, UUO and vehicle treatment or UUO and ND-13 treatment. $n = 4$–5/group; * $p < 0.05$ vs. same genotype sham, † $p < 0.05$ vs. same genotype UUO + vehicle, ‡ $p < 0.05$ vs. WT UUO + vehicle; two-way ANOVA with Tukey's post-hoc test.

Similar to the trends found in WT mice, ND-13 had anti-inflammatory effects on *DJ-1*$^{-/-}$ mice that underwent UUO surgery, as indicated by the blunted expression of *TNF-α*, *CCL25* and *IL-6* in the renal cortex compared to the values observed in the vehicle-treated group (Figure 5). Of note, the *TNF-α* response to UUO was significantly smaller in *DJ-1*$^{-/-}$ mice treated with vehicle than the response observed in WT mice treated with vehicle (Figure 5).

2.4. *ND-13 Treatment Attenuates the UUO-Induced Cortical Macrophage Inflammation in WT Mice, but Not in DJ-1*$^{-/-}$ *Mice, While Not Preventing the Infiltration of T-Lymphocytes in Either Genotype*

As expected, the population of T-lymphocytes ($CD3^+$ cells) in the cortex was elevated in WT mice after UUO, although it did not reach statistical significance from the levels shown in mice that underwent sham surgery (sham vs. UUO + vehicle: 4.6 ± 0.7 vs. 14.9 ± 4.6 cells/field, $p > 0.05$, $n = 4$–5/group). Daily treatment with ND-13 failed to normalize the kidney T-cell inflammation in WT mice (16.1 ± 2.8 cells/field; Figure 6). Similarly, *DJ-1*$^{-/-}$ mice showed an increased infiltration of T-lymphocytes in the renal cortex (Figure 6) in response to UUO (sham vs. UUO + vehicle: 3.7 ± 0.3 vs. 24.9 ± 2.2 cells/field, $p < 0.05$, $n = 4$–5/group). However, the magnitude of T cell accumulation in the cortex of *DJ-1*$^{-/-}$ mice was greater than in WT mice (WT mice vs. *DJ-1*$^{-/-}$ mice: 14.9 ± 4.6 vs. 24.9 ± 2.2 cells/field), and it remained elevated despite the ND-13 treatment (26.0 ± 8.3 cells/field). Raw data for the T cell numbers in each of the 10 fields evaluated per animal, as well as the mean and SEM per animal, are provided in Supplementary Table S1.

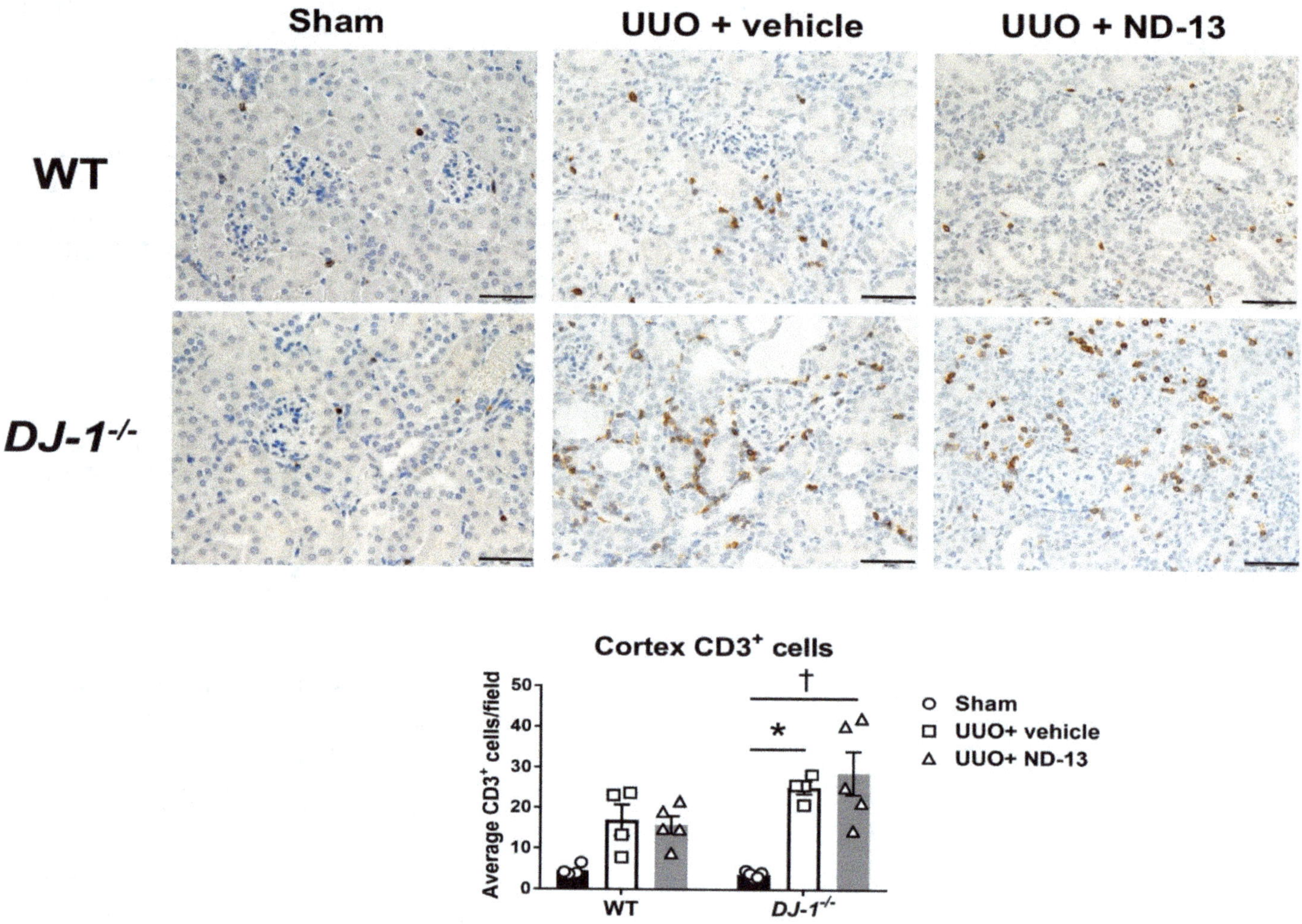

Figure 6. Treatment with ND-13 does not prevent the UUO-induced infiltration of T cells into the kidney cortex of mice that underwent UUO. Representative images and quantification of T cell (CD3+ cells) infiltration in renal cortex of WT (upper panels) and *DJ-1*$^{-/-}$ (bottom panels) mice that underwent sham surgery, UUO and vehicle treatment or UUO and ND-13 treatment (scale bar = 20 μm). * $p < 0.05$ vs. same genotype sham, † $p < 0.05$ vs. same genotype UUO + vehicle; two-way ANOVA with Tukey's post hoc test.

Similar to what was found with T cells, the number of macrophages infiltrating the cortex was elevated fourteen days after UUO surgery (sham vs. UUO + vehicle: 0.1 ± 0.0 vs. 2.4 ± 1.1 % area stained positive for F4/80, $p > 0.05$, n = 4–5/group). However, treatment with ND-13 only tended to attenuate those numbers (0.7 ± 0.3 % area stained positive; Figure 7). Evaluation of the macrophage population in the renal cortex of *DJ-1*$^{-/-}$ mice also revealed elevated numbers of these immune cells after UUO (sham vs. UUO + vehicle: 0.2 ± 0.1 vs. 6.5 ± 1.2 % area stained positive for F4/80, $p < 0.05$, n = 4–5/group); however, in contrast to WT mice, treatment with ND-13 failed to prevent macrophage infiltration in these mice, and the numbers of macrophages were similar to those found in mice treated with vehicle (7.0 ± 2.0 % area stained positive) (Figure 7). Of note, the magnitude of the cortical infiltration of macrophages after UUO was significantly worse in the case of the *DJ-1*$^{-/-}$ mice compared to WT mice (UUO + vehicle, WT mice vs. *DJ-1*$^{-/-}$ mice: 2.4 ± 1.1 vs. 6.5 ± 1.2 % area stained positive, $p < 0.05$, n = 4–5/group). Raw data for the percentage area stained positive for F4/80 quantified in each of the 10 fields/animal, as well as the mean and SEM per animal, are provided in Supplementary Table S2.

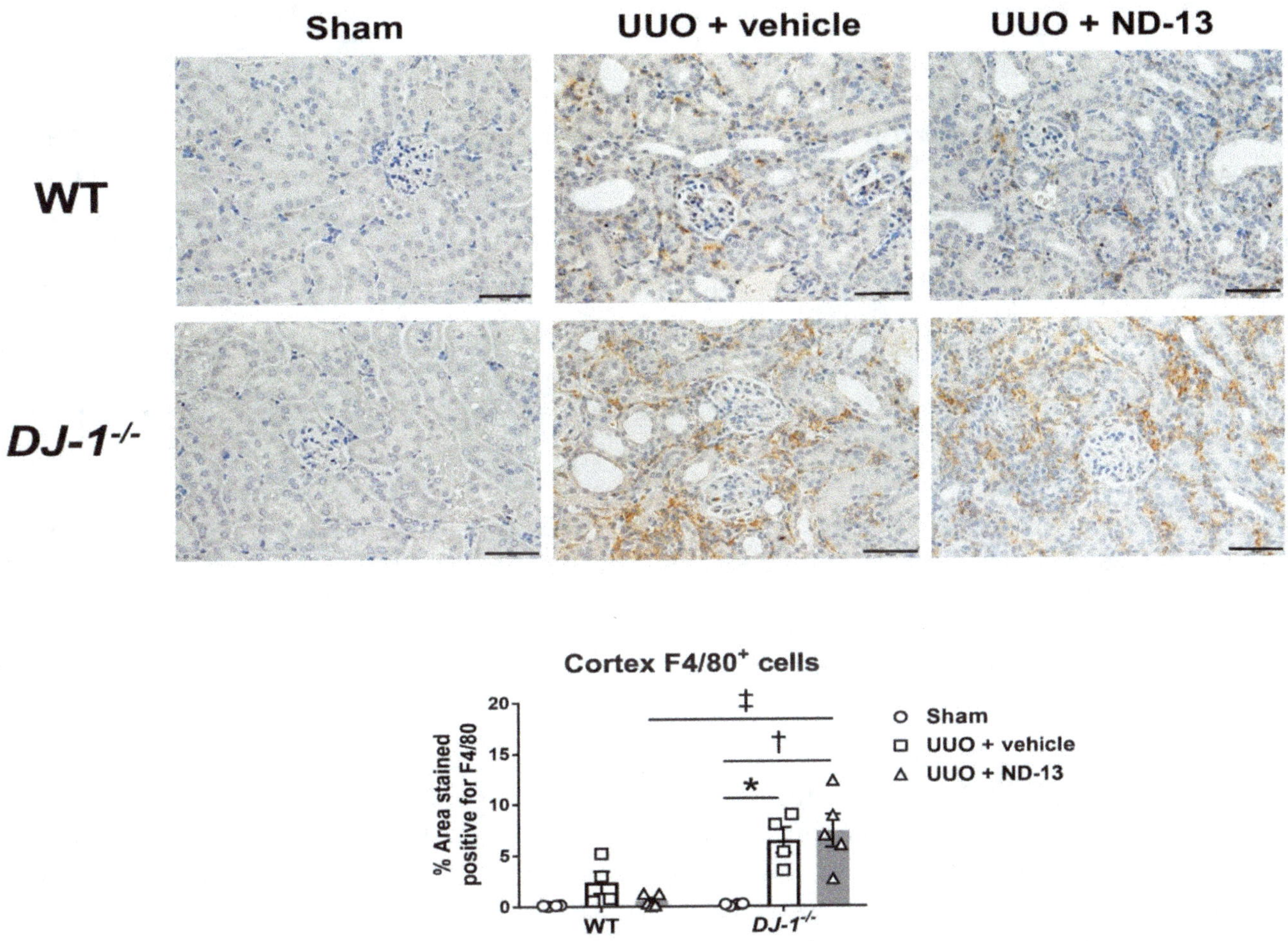

Figure 7. Treatment with ND-13 tends to decrease the UUO-induced macrophage infiltration into the renal cortex of WT mice that underwent UUO but fails to prevent this inflammation in *DJ-1*$^{-/-}$ mice that underwent UUO. Representative images and quantification of macrophage infiltration (% area stained for F4/80) in renal cortex of WT mice that underwent sham surgery, UUO and vehicle treatment or UUO and ND-13 treatment (scale bar = 20 μm). * $p < 0.05$ vs. same genotype sham, † $p < 0.05$ vs. same genotype UUO + vehicle, ‡ $p < 0.05$ vs. WT UUO + vehicle; two-way ANOVA with Tukey's post hoc test.

2.5. *ND-13 Does Not Improve the Renal Damage Score in UUO Mice*

The tubular damage and neutrophilic infiltrates present in the kidneys obtained from the experimental mice were evaluated using hematoxylin and eosin (H&E) stained sections and given a combined renal damage score. Kidneys obtained from UUO mice showed epithelial flattening and focally dilated tubules, with moderate proteinaceous contents and casts, and showed no difference between genetic backgrounds or treatment conditions. The glomerular morphology presented unremarkable changes in all groups. The renal damage score based on H&E staining showed a very small, insignificant protective effect of ND-13 on the extent of the neutrophilic infiltrate in the cortex. The means and standard errors of these inflammation scores, adjusted by density, are the following: C57BL/6 mice with UU0 + vehicle: 1.45 ± 0.83 vs. UU0 + N-13: 1.15 ± 0.81; *DJ-1*$^{-/-}$ mice with UU0 + vehicle: 3.13 ± 1.04 vs UU0 + N-13: 2.31 ± 1.14. Significant differences were not found between the groups. No inflammation was found in the control mice and no apparent morphological changes were found in the contralateral kidneys.

3. Discussion

The major finding of this study is that treatment with ND-13 is effective in preventing the exaggerated expression of kidney fibrotic and inflammatory markers that normally develop as consequences of UUO. We demonstrated that ND-13 significantly reduced the expression of fibrotic markers col1a1 and TGF-β and prevented the accumulation of macrophages in the kidney of C57Bl/6J mice after UUO. The fact that ND-13 did not protect *DJ-1*$^{-/-}$ mice against the UUO-induced renal damage highlights the critical role of DJ-1 as an important mediator of this protective mechanism. To our knowledge, this is the first report to evaluate the protective effects of ND-13 in renal diseases.

According to the Center for Disease Control, 37 million Americans suffered from chronic kidney disease in 2019, with associated health costs of about $114 billion to care for these patients [26]. Current therapies are not effective in preventing the development of renal disease [27]. Thus, new therapeutic alternatives are urgently needed. There is abundant evidence in the literature that demonstrates that renal inflammation and renal fibrosis precede the development of chronic kidney disease [28], highlighting the critical involvement of these two factors in the pathogenesis of renal damage. Among other kidney diseases, inflammation and fibrosis are involved in the progression of glomerulonephritis [29], acute kidney injury [7], polycystic kidney disease [30], renal artery stenosis [31], lupus nephritis [32] and diabetic nephropathy [33]. Accordingly, pharmacological therapies aimed at the attenuation of inflammatory and fibrotic processes may be an appropriate approach in the prevention of these renal pathologies.

UUO is a model of progressive kidney fibrosis and inflammation that is characterized by tubular dilation, loss of proximal tubular mass, interstitial expansion, hypertrophy, hydronephrosis and tubular epithelial cell death [34]. The mechanical stretching induced by the tying of the ureter stimulates a massive production of reactive oxygen species (ROS) and cellular apoptosis in the affected kidney that, in turn, result in alterations of the hemodynamic status and significant inflammation and fibrosis [34]. Therefore, UUO is an ideal experimental model to evaluate the putative preventive effects of ND-13 against renal damage and, particularly, on kidney fibrosis.

To examine DJ-1 as a possible novel therapeutic target for renal diseases, we used the 20 aa peptide known as ND-13 [23]. Treatment of WT mice with ND-13 blunted the UUO-induced upregulation in the kidney expression of *TGF-β* and *Col1a1*, and also decreased the kidney expression of inflammatory markers *TNF-α*, *IL-6* and *CCL25*. Interestingly, the ND-13-mediated decrease in fibrotic marker expression was not accompanied by a significant improvement in the deposition of collagen in the kidney. These seemingly contradictory findings could be due to the long timeline in our studies, where the animals were examined a full two weeks after the UUO protocol. This timeline, compared to shorter postsurgical times, is known to induce severe injury to the kidney and stimulate extreme deposition of collagen in this organ [34–36]. The protective effects of ND-13 against collagen deposition may have been hindered by starting the treatment at the same time as the UUO pathology. Interestingly, and although it did not reach statistical significance, we observed that the cortical fibrosis in the WT mice treated with ND-13 was not as generalized as it was in mice treated with vehicle, possibly suggesting that treatment with ND-13 may have slightly slowed down the fibrotic deposition. Considering the profound reduction in kidney fibrotic marker expression induced by ND-13, it is likely that its effects on kidney fibrosis would have been different if the animals were treated with this peptide for a period of time prior to the UUO protocol. This is a research avenue that our group will investigate in the future. Similarly, the protective effects of ND-13 did not extend to the renal T cell infiltration, which remained elevated. However, it seemed to prevent the macrophage influx into this organ. It is possible that ND-13 shifted the phenotype of the T cell and macrophage populations present in the kidney from a proinflammatory type to an anti-inflammatory type (i.e., Tregs vs. Th17 cells, or M1 vs. M2 macrophages) attenuating the inflammatory response and renal damage. Future follow-up studies will focus on the further evaluation of immune cell subtypes present in the kidneys of these animals in order to completely understand the effects of ND-13 in proinflammatory versus anti-inflammatory immune populations in the kidney after UUO. Moreover, these results suggest promising protective effects of ND-13 that could be more evident in less aggressive animal models of kidney disease with pathogenic mechanisms more similar to human renal disease.

On the other hand, and despite the attenuation in the expression of inflammatory cytokines that we observed in $DJ\text{-}1^{-/-}$ mice that underwent UUO and were treated with ND-13, we did not find differences in kidney fibrosis nor collagen deposition in these mice when compared with the shams. The fact that treatment with ND-13 did not decrease kidney fibrosis in $DJ\text{-}1^{-/-}$ mice, but it did in WT mice, strongly underlines the essential role of renal DJ-1 in the prevention of renal damage.

Our group previously reported the effects that deletion of *DJ-1* has on renal oxidative stress and injury as well as on blood pressure [16,20,21] and a protective role of DJ-1 in endotoxin-induced acute kidney injury was recently described [36]. We demonstrated that silencing *DJ-1* expression in mouse kidneys, and in mouse proximal tubule cells specifically, attenuates the expression and activity of Nrf2 and results in increased ROS production [20]. Nrf2 is a master regulator of antioxidant and anti-inflammatory factors [19], and its activity and expression is regulated by ROS production [37]. Moreover, genetic deletion of *DJ-1* leads to increased ubiquitination of Nrf2, suggesting that the renal protection exerted by DJ-1 is mediated by preventing the degradation of Nrf2 [20]. Interestingly, both DJ-1 and Nrf2 are activated in acute kidney injury [38], and Nrf2 has been proven to inhibit the development and progression of several diseases affecting the kidney [17,39]. In previous studies, we also demonstrated that DJ-1 increases Nrf2 expression and activity only under pathological conditions and has no effects on Nrf2 in the physiological setting.

Consistent with our results, previous studies demonstrated that DJ-1 stabilized Nrf2 by preventing binding to Keap1 and Nrf2's subsequent ubiquitination [40]. DJ-1 may amplify Nrf2 activity by avoiding its degradation. However, the ability of DJ-1 to stimulate directly the Nrf2 pathway has not been demonstrated [41]. We speculate that ND-13 prevents the undesirable consequences of chronic Nrf2 activation. Thereby, ND-13 may be an appropriate therapeutic approach to enhance the actions of Nrf2, and it could be used to minimize the side effects associated with treatment of chronic Nrf2 activation by other Nrf2 inducers i.e., bardoxolone [42,43] in humans. Our working hypothesis is that the ROS and inflammation that are induced by UUO lead to increased levels of interleukins and chemokines and, in turn, to the activation of the immune response in the kidney. This inflammatory and oxidative milieu creates a vicious cycle that leads to fibrosis and promotes kidney damage and kidney dysfunction. In this setting, DJ-1 prevents the ubiquitination of Nrf2, amplifying this molecule's antioxidant response. We speculate that Nrf2 would attenuate oxidative stress and inflammation in the kidney, leading to reduced cytokine expression and thereby preventing inflammation and preserving renal function (Figure 8).

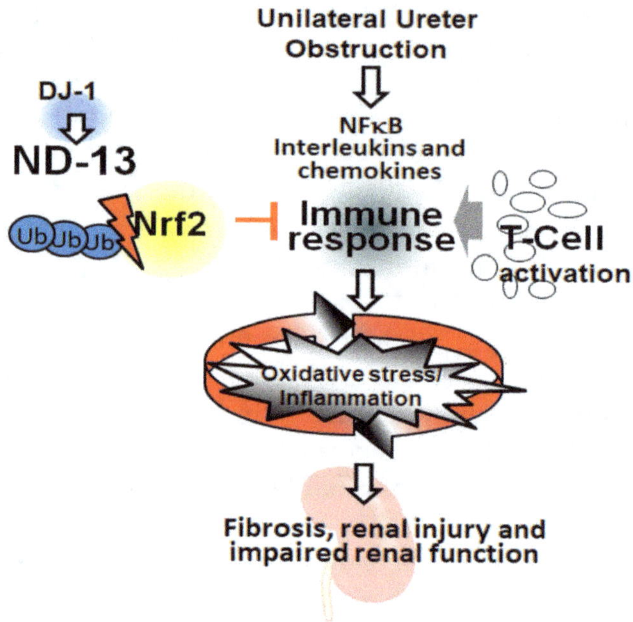

Figure 8. Working hypothesis. ROS and inflammation induced by unilateral ureter obstruction increase interleukin and chemokine expression activating the immune response. This inflammatory/oxidative environment leads to a vicious cycle, which may produce fibrosis and induce renal damage and kidney dysfunction. DJ-1 prevents the ubiquitination of Nrf2 and amplifies its response. Nrf2 may be acting by attenuating the oxidative stress and inflammation, leading to a reduced cytokine expression and preventing inflammation, resulting in protection of the renal function.

In summary, these data suggest that ND-13 prevents the renal inflammation and fibrosis associated with the acute renal damage induced by UUO. Further studies are needed to confirm if ND-13 treatment may be a new therapeutic approach for the prevention of renal injury, fibrosis and inflammation in human renal disease.

4. Materials and Methods

4.1. Animal Studies

All protocols were conducted in accordance with the Guide for the Care and Use of Laboratory Animals, and were approved by the Institutional Animal Care and Use Committee of the George Washington University (project identification numbers A353 and A412, approved on 26 February 2019 and 21 February 2019, respectively). Eight to nine-week old male C57Bl/6J (Jax Labs, Bar Harbor, ME) or *DJ-1*$^{-/-}$ mice (from our in-house colony) were used in these studies. Mice of each genotype underwent sham or unilateral ureter obstruction (UUO) surgery. In short, mice were anesthetized, the lower abdomen was opened and the left ureter was completely tied off using suture [44]. In those mice in the sham group, the abdomen was opened, the left ureter touched with a cotton tipped applicator and the abdomen was then sutured. The mice that underwent UUO surgery received either ND-13 (3 mg/kg/day, s.c.) or vehicle (scrambled peptide; 3 mg/kg/day, s.c.) starting from the day after surgery until the end of the study. Twelve days into the study, mice were placed in metabolic cages, acclimated to the cages for one day, and 24 h-urine was collected on the second day on the metabolic cages. On day 14 of the study, the mice were sacrificed, and kidneys harvested. One of the kidneys was snap-frozen in liquid nitrogen, while the other was placed in formalin for histological studies. No significant differences were found among the experimental groups regarding body weight, food intake, water intake or urine production (Table 1).

Table 1. Physical characteristics of the experimental groups.

	Body Weight (g)					
	Pre		Post		Gain/Loss	
	Mean	SEM	Mean	SEM	Mean	SEM
WT sham	28.75	3.22	28.85	2.90	0.10	0.38
DJ-1$^{-/-}$ sham	25.38	1.58	25.74	1.62	0.36	0.09
WT vehicle	23.30	2.05	23.94	2.00	0.64	0.31
DJ-1$^{-/-}$ vehicle	26.20	3.12	26.40	3.18	0.20	0.16
WT ND-13	28.72	2.89	29.26	2.76	0.54	0.76
DJ-1$^{-/-}$ ND-13	24.80	3.40	25.02	4.01	0.22	0.34
	Food Intake (g)					
	Pre		Post		Net	
	Mean	SEM	Mean	SEM	Mean	SEM
WT sham	75.85	0.57	72.40	2.95	3.45	2.57
DJ-1$^{-/-}$ sham	74.00	3.74	70.84	2.99	3.16	1.14
WT vehicle	70.66	3.89	64.80	3.87	5.86	1.88
DJ-1$^{-/-}$ vehicle	74.50	4.08	71.70	4.16	2.80	0.12
WT ND-13	71.06	3.14	65.56	3.76	5.50	1.29
DJ-1$^{-/-}$ ND-13	71.78	3.02	68.53	3.21	3.25	1.41
	Water Intake (mL)					
	Pre		Post		Net	
	Mean	SEM	Mean	SEM	Mean	SEM
WT sham	53.43	6.34	50.73	7.44	2.70	1.31
DJ-1$^{-/-}$ sham	55.44	4.97	51.48	3.90	3.96	1.60
WT vehicle	55.08	2.22	49.98	3.89	5.10	1.82
DJ-1$^{-/-}$ vehicle	57.90	6.12	54.25	6.02	3.65	0.53
WT ND-13	56.08	1.93	50.34	2.28	5.74	0.57
DJ-1$^{-/-}$ ND-13	59.58	2.75	55.45	2.22	4.13	1.97
			Urine (mL)			
			Mean	SEM		
WT sham			0.63	0.28		
DJ-1$^{-/-}$ sham			0.69	0.32		
WT vehicle			1.10	0.36		
DJ-1$^{-/-}$ vehicle			1.18	0.28		
WT ND-13			1.86	0.65		
DJ-1$^{-/-}$ ND-13			1.38	0.51		

M: mean; SEM: standard error of the mean.

4.2. Quantitative RT-PCR

RNeasy mini kit (Qiagen, Valencia, CA, USA) was used to extract RNA from the kidney cortex. The amount of extracted RNA was quantified by spectrophotometry (NanoDrop ND-1000, Thermo Scientific, Waltham, MA, USA). RNA reverse transcription was performed using Quantitect Reverse Transcription kit (Qiagen) and following manufacturer's instructions. Primers were purchased from QuantiTect (Qiagen): *Col1a1* (QT00371308), *TGF-β* QT00371308), *TNF-α*QT00371308), *CCL25* (QT00371308) and *IL-6* (QT00371308). GAPDH was used as housekeeping gene (QT01658692). RNA expression was detected by the Quantitect SYBR green kit (Qiagen) and using a CFX96 Touch RT-PCR detection system (Bio-Rad, Hercules, CA, USA).

4.3. *Histology and Fibrosis Quantification*

Kidneys were fixed overnight in 4% buffered formalin solution at room temperature, transferred to 70% ethanol for 24 h, and paraffin-embedded. Tissues were cut longitudinally into 4 μm-thick sections and mounted on Superfrost slides. Masson's trichrome blue staining was used to visualize renal fibrosis using bright-field microscopy (Olympus BX40 with 10× eyepiece lens; Olympus America, Melville, NY, USA). Full scans of the kidneys were obtained using a microscope fitted with a motorized XY stage and a digital camera (Olympus DP71), with sequential 20× images of each kidney taken and digitally stitched together with CellSense imaging software (Olympus). The cortical area of each full kidney scan was outlined and the percentage of blue fibrotic deposition within the outlined area was quantified using MetaMorph software (Molecular Devices LLC., San Jose, CA, USA). The average percentage fibrotic area for each experimental group was calculated and then normalized to the sham group. Data are presented as relative fibrosis compared to sham group.

4.4. *Immunohistochemistry and Quantification of Immune Cell Infiltration in the Kidney*

Tissue sections were stained with primary antibodies specific for CD3 (1:600; Abcam, Cambridge, MA, USA) and F4/80 (1:200; Bio-Rad, Hercules, CA, USA) and detected with polymer conjugated secondary antibody (Biocare Medical, Concord, CA, USA). Quantification of renal T-lymphocyte ($CD3^+$ cells) infiltration was performed by blindly counting 10 microscopic fields (200 × 200 μm, 400× magnification) in each renal cortex. Infiltrating T cell numbers are reported as the average of the counts in the 10 fields per renal cortex. Quantification of renal macrophages ($F4/80^+$ cells) was performed by taking 10 cortical images from each animal at 400× magnification. The percentage of cortical area stained positive for F4/80 was quantified in each image using MetaMorph software and the average expression per animal was calculated. The data are reported as the average percentage area that stained positively for F4/80 per experimental group.

4.5. *Terminal Deoxynucleotidyl Transferase-Mediated dUTP Nick-End Labeling (TUNEL) Assay and Quantification*

Tissue sections were stained using the Apoptag® Plus Peroxidase In Situ Apoptosis Kit (S7101, MP Biomedicals, Santa Ana, CA, USA) in order to detect dead cells. Ten microscopy images were taken of each kidney cortex and medulla (400 × 400 μm fields at 200× magnification) and the area stained positively with TUNEL in each image was quantified using Metamorph software and averaged per kidney region and animal. The data are reported as the average percentage area that stained positive for TUNEL in cortex and medulla per experimental group.

4.6. *Urinary NGAL Measurements*

Urine collected on day two of the metabolic cage study was analyzed for concentration levels of the proximal tubular injury marker neutrophil gelatinase-associated lipocalin (NGAL) using an ELISA kit (Abcam). Average concentration per experiment group was calculated and the data are presented as percentage of sham group.

4.7. *Renal Damage Evaluation*

Five images per mouse kidney section stained with H&E were evaluated by a blinded pathologist and each mouse was assigned a renal damage score based on the following criteria: inflammatory involvement (1 = <25%, 2 = 25–50%, 3 = 50–75%, 4 = >75%), inflammatory density (1 = mild, 2 = mild-moderate, 3 = moderate-severe, 4 = severe), dilation of tubules and tubular injury with neutrophilic infiltrates (PMNs) (1 = <2, 2 = 2–4, 3 = several, 4 = many) and casts (1 = <3, 2 = easily found; 3 = many).

4.8. Statistical Analysis

All data are expressed as mean ± SEM. Differences between groups were analyzed by two-way analysis of variance with a Tukey's post hoc test. A $p < 0.05$ was considered statistically significant. All statistical analyses were conducted using SigmaPlot 11 (Systat Software, Inc., San Jose, CA, USA).

Author Contributions: Conceptualization, C.D.M. and S.C.; methodology, C.D.M., S.C. and D.O.; formal analysis, C.D.M. and S.C.; investigation, C.D.M., A.C.K., M.A.S., P.K., A.R.D., L.D.A., P.S.L. and S.C.; resources, C.D.M. and P.A.J.; writing—original draft preparation, C.D.M. and S.C.; writing—review and editing, C.D.M., S.C., P.A.J., P.S.L. and D.O.; visualization, C.D.M. and S.C.; supervision, C.D.M. and S.C.; funding acquisition, C.D.M., S.C. and P.A.J. All authors have read and agreed to the published version of the manuscript.

Acknowledgments: The authors thank the Histology Services at the George Washington University Research Pathology Core Lab for their expertise.

Abbreviations

UUO	Unilateral ureter obstruction
Col1a1	Collagen 1a1
Nrf2	Nuclear factor erythroid 2-related factor 2

References

1. Giacco, F.; Brownlee, M. Oxidative stress and diabetic complications. *Circ. Res.* **2010**, *107*, 1058–1070. [CrossRef] [PubMed]
2. Navarro-Gonzalez, J.F.; Mora-Fernandez, C. The role of inflammatory cytokines in diabetic nephropathy. *J. Am. Soc. Nephrol.* **2008**, *19*, 433–442. [CrossRef] [PubMed]
3. Lee, S.B.; Kalluri, R. Mechanistic connection between inflammation and fibrosis. *Kidney Int.* **2010**, *78*, S22–S26. [CrossRef] [PubMed]
4. Imig, J.D.; Ryan, M.J. Immune and inflammatory role in renal disease. *Compr. Physiol.* **2013**, *3*, 957–976. [CrossRef]
5. Anders, H.J.; Ryu, M. Renal microenvironments and macrophage phenotypes determine progression or resolution of renal inflammation and fibrosis. *Kidney Int.* **2011**, *80*, 915–925. [CrossRef] [PubMed]
6. Duffield, J.S. Macrophages and immunologic inflammation of the kidney. *Semin. Nephrol.* **2010**, *30*, 234–254. [CrossRef]
7. Cao, Q.; Harris, D.C.; Wang, Y. Macrophages in kidney injury, inflammation, and fibrosis. *Physiology* **2015**, *30*, 183–194. [CrossRef] [PubMed]
8. Kisseleva, T.; Brenner, D.A. Fibrogenesis of parenchymal organs. *Proc. Am. Thorac. Soc.* **2008**, *5*, 338–342. [CrossRef]
9. Brenmoehl, J.; Miller, S.N.; Hofmann, C.; Vogl, D.; Falk, W.; Scholmerich, J.; Rogler, G. Transforming growth factor-beta 1 induces intestinal myofibroblast differentiation and modulates their migration. *World J. Gastroenterol.* **2009**, *15*, 1431–1442. [CrossRef]
10. Meng, X.M.; Nikolic-Paterson, D.J.; Lan, H.Y. Inflammatory processes in renal fibrosis. *Nat. Rev. Nephrol.* **2014**, *10*, 493–503. [CrossRef]
11. Lv, W.; Booz, G.W.; Wang, Y.; Fan, F.; Roman, R.J. Inflammation and renal fibrosis: Recent developments on key signaling molecules as potential therapeutic targets. *Eur. J. Pharmacol.* **2018**, *820*, 65–76. [CrossRef] [PubMed]
12. Nagakubo, D.; Taira, T.; Kitaura, H.; Ikeda, M.; Tamai, K.; Iguchi-Ariga, S.M.; Ariga, H. DJ-1, a novel oncogene which transforms mouse NIH3T3 cells in cooperation with ras. *Biochem. Biophys. Res. Commun.* **1997**, *231*, 509–513. [CrossRef] [PubMed]

13. Liu, F.; Nguyen, J.L.; Hulleman, J.D.; Li, L.; Rochet, J.C. Mechanisms of DJ-1 neuroprotection in a cellular model of Parkinson's disease. *J. Neurochem.* **2008**, *105*, 2435–2453. [CrossRef] [PubMed]
14. Zhou, W.; Freed, C.R. DJ-1 up-regulates glutathione synthesis during oxidative stress and inhibits A53T alpha-synuclein toxicity. *J. Biol. Chem.* **2005**, *280*, 43150–43158. [CrossRef] [PubMed]
15. Junn, E.; Jang, W.H.; Zhao, X.; Jeong, B.S.; Mouradian, M.M. Mitochondrial localization of DJ-1 leads to enhanced neuroprotection. *J. Neurosci. Res.* **2009**, *87*, 123–129. [CrossRef]
16. Cuevas, S.; Zhang, Y.; Yang, Y.; Escano, C.; Asico, L.; Jones, J.E.; Armando, I.; Jose, P.A. Role of renal DJ-1 in the pathogenesis of hypertension associated with increased reactive oxygen species production. *Hypertension* **2012**, *59*, 446–452. [CrossRef]
17. Shelton, L.M.; Park, B.K.; Copple, I.M. Role of Nrf2 in protection against acute kidney injury. *Kidney Int.* **2013**, *84*, 1090–1095. [CrossRef]
18. Li, W.; Khor, T.O.; Xu, C.; Shen, G.; Jeong, W.S.; Yu, S.; Kong, A.N. Activation of Nrf2-antioxidant signaling attenuates NFkappaB-inflammatory response and elicits apoptosis. *Biochem. Pharmacol.* **2008**, *76*, 1485–1489. [CrossRef]
19. Kobayashi, E.H.; Suzuki, T.; Funayama, R.; Nagashima, T.; Hayashi, M.; Sekine, H.; Tanaka, N.; Moriguchi, T.; Motohashi, H.; Nakayama, K.; et al. Nrf2 suppresses macrophage inflammatory response by blocking proinflammatory cytokine transcription. *Nat. Commun.* **2016**, *7*, 11624. [CrossRef]
20. Cuevas, S.; Yang, Y.; Konkalmatt, P.; Asico, L.D.; Feranil, J.; Jones, J.; Villar, V.A.; Armando, I.; Jose, P.A. Role of nuclear factor erythroid 2-related factor 2 in the oxidative stress-dependent hypertension associated with the depletion of DJ-1. *Hypertension* **2015**, *65*, 1251–1257. [CrossRef]
21. De Miguel, C.; Hamrick, W.C.; Sedaka, R.; Jagarlamudi, S.; Asico, L.D.; Jose, P.A.; Cuevas, S. Uncoupling Protein 2 Increases Blood Pressure in DJ -1 Knockout Mice. *J. Am. Heart Assoc.* **2019**, *8*, e011856. [CrossRef] [PubMed]
22. Sun, Q.; Shen, Z.Y.; Meng, Q.T.; Liu, H.Z.; Duan, W.N.; Xia, Z.Y. The role of DJ-1/Nrf2 pathway in the pathogenesis of diabetic nephropathy in rats. *Renal Fail.* **2016**, *38*, 294–304. [CrossRef] [PubMed]
23. Lev, N.; Barhum, Y.; Ben-Zur, T.; Aharony, I.; Trifonov, L.; Regev, N.; Melamed, E.; Gruzman, A.; Offen, D. A DJ-1 Based Peptide Attenuates Dopaminergic Degeneration in Mice Models of Parkinson's Disease via Enhancing Nrf2. *PLoS ONE* **2015**, *10*, e0127549. [CrossRef] [PubMed]
24. Glat, M.J.; Ben-Zur, T.; Barhum, Y.; Offen, D. Neuroprotective Effect of a DJ-1 Based Peptide in a Toxin Induced Mouse Model of Multiple System Atrophy. *PLoS ONE* **2016**, *11*, e0148170. [CrossRef] [PubMed]
25. Lev, N.; Barhum, Y.; Lotan, I.; Steiner, I.; Offen, D. DJ-1 knockout augments disease severity and shortens survival in a mouse model of ALS. *PLoS ONE* **2015**, *10*, e0117190. [CrossRef]
26. Centers for Disease Control and Prevention. *Chronic Kidney Disease in the United States, 2019*; US Department of Health and Human Services, Centers for Disease Control and Prevention: Atlanta, GA, USA, 2019.
27. Higgins, G.C.; Coughlan, M.T. Mitochondrial dysfunction and mitophagy: The beginning and end to diabetic nephropathy? *Br. J. Pharmacol.* **2014**, *171*, 1917–1942. [CrossRef]
28. Mihai, S.; Codrici, E.; Popescu, I.D.; Enciu, A.M.; Albulescu, L.; Necula, L.G.; Mambet, C.; Anton, G.; Tanase, C. Inflammation-Related Mechanisms in Chronic Kidney Disease Prediction, Progression, and Outcome. *J. Immunol. Res.* **2018**, *2018*, 2180373. [CrossRef]
29. Han, Y.; Ma, F.Y.; Tesch, G.H.; Manthey, C.L.; Nikolic-Paterson, D.J. Role of macrophages in the fibrotic phase of rat crescentic glomerulonephritis. *Am. J. Physiol. Renal Physiol.* **2013**, *304*, F1043–F1053. [CrossRef]
30. Song, C.J.; Zimmerman, K.A.; Henke, S.J.; Yoder, B.K. Inflammation and Fibrosis in Polycystic Kidney Disease. *Results Probl. Cell Differ.* **2017**, *60*, 323–344. [CrossRef]
31. Ma, Z.; Jin, X.; He, L.; Wang, Y. CXCL16 regulates renal injury and fibrosis in experimental renal artery stenosis. *Am. J. Physiol. Heart Circ. Physiol.* **2016**, *311*, H815–H821. [CrossRef]
32. Hill, G.S.; Delahousse, M.; Nochy, D.; Thervet, E.; Vrtovsnik, F.; Remy, P.; Glotz, D.; Bariety, J. Outcome of relapse in lupus nephritis: Roles of reversal of renal fibrosis and response of inflammation to therapy. *Kidney Int.* **2002**, *61*, 2176–2186. [CrossRef] [PubMed]
33. Brennan, E.P.; Cacace, A.; Godson, C. Specialized pro-resolving mediators in renal fibrosis. *Mol. Asp. Med.* **2017**, *58*, 102–113. [CrossRef] [PubMed]
34. Martinez-Klimova, E.; Aparicio-Trejo, O.E.; Tapia, E.; Pedraza-Chaverri, J. Unilateral Ureteral Obstruction as a Model to Investigate Fibrosis-Attenuating Treatments. *Biomolecules* **2019**, *9*. [CrossRef] [PubMed]

35. Chevalier, R.L.; Forbes, M.S.; Thornhill, B.A. Ureteral obstruction as a model of renal interstitial fibrosis and obstructive nephropathy. *Kidney Int.* **2009**, *75*, 1145–1152. [CrossRef]
36. Leeds, J.; Scindia, Y.; Loi, V.; Wlazlo, E.; Ghias, E.; Cechova, S.; Portilla, D.; Ledesma, J.; Swaminathan, S. Protective Role of DJ-1 in Endotoxin-induced Acute Kidney Injury. *Am. J. Physiol. Renal Physiol.* **2020**. [CrossRef]
37. Niture, S.K.; Khatri, R.; Jaiswal, A.K. Regulation of Nrf2-an update. *Free Rad. Biol. Med.* **2014**, *66*, 36–44. [CrossRef]
38. Sun, Q.; Shen, Z.Y.; Duan, W.N.; Meng, Q.T.; Xia, Z.Y. Mechanism of myocardial ischemia/reperfusion-induced acute kidney injury through DJ-1/Nrf2 pathway in diabetic rats. *Exp. Ther. Med.* **2017**, *14*, 4201–4207. [CrossRef]
39. Schmidlin, C.J.; Dodson, M.B.; Zhang, D.D. Filtering through the role of NRF2 in kidney disease. *Arch. Pharm. Res.* **2019**. [CrossRef]
40. Clements, C.M.; McNally, R.S.; Conti, B.J.; Mak, T.W.; Ting, J.P. DJ-1, a cancer- and Parkinson's disease-associated protein, stabilizes the antioxidant transcriptional master regulator Nrf2. *Proc. Natl. Acad. Sci. USA* **2006**, *103*, 15091–15096. [CrossRef]
41. Gan, L.; Johnson, D.A.; Johnson, J.A. Keap1-Nrf2 activation in the presence and absence of DJ-1. *Eur. J. Neurosci.* **2010**, *31*, 967–977. [CrossRef]
42. Himmelfarb, J.; Tuttle, K.R. New therapies for diabetic kidney disease. *N. Engl. J. Med.* **2013**, *369*, 2549–2550. [CrossRef] [PubMed]
43. Rossing, P. Diabetic nephropathy: Could problems with bardoxolone methyl have been predicted? *Nat. Rev. Nephrol.* **2013**, *9*, 128–130. [CrossRef] [PubMed]
44. Li, Z.; Xie, W.B.; Escano, C.S.; Asico, L.D.; Xie, Q.; Jose, P.A.; Chen, S.Y. Response gene to complement 32 is essential for fibroblast activation in renal fibrosis. *J. Biol. Chem.* **2011**, *286*, 41323–41330. [CrossRef] [PubMed]

Permissions

All chapters in this book were first published by MDPI; hereby published with permission under the Creative Commons Attribution License or equivalent. Every chapter published in this book has been scrutinized by our experts. Their significance has been extensively debated. The topics covered herein carry significant findings which will fuel the growth of the discipline. They may even be implemented as practical applications or may be referred to as a beginning point for another development.

The contributors of this book come from diverse backgrounds, making this book a truly international effort. This book will bring forth new frontiers with its revolutionizing research information and detailed analysis of the nascent developments around the world.

We would like to thank all the contributing authors for lending their expertise to make the book truly unique. They have played a crucial role in the development of this book. Without their invaluable contributions this book wouldn't have been possible. They have made vital efforts to compile up to date information on the varied aspects of this subject to make this book a valuable addition to the collection of many professionals and students.

This book was conceptualized with the vision of imparting up-to-date information and advanced data in this field. To ensure the same, a matchless editorial board was set up. Every individual on the board went through rigorous rounds of assessment to prove their worth. After which they invested a large part of their time researching and compiling the most relevant data for our readers.

The editorial board has been involved in producing this book since its inception. They have spent rigorous hours researching and exploring the diverse topics which have resulted in the successful publishing of this book. They have passed on their knowledge of decades through this book. To expedite this challenging task, the publisher supported the team at every step. A small team of assistant editors was also appointed to further simplify the editing procedure and attain best results for the readers.

Apart from the editorial board, the designing team has also invested a significant amount of their time in understanding the subject and creating the most relevant covers. They scrutinized every image to scout for the most suitable representation of the subject and create an appropriate cover for the book.

The publishing team has been an ardent support to the editorial, designing and production team. Their endless efforts to recruit the best for this project, has resulted in the accomplishment of this book. They are a veteran in the field of academics and their pool of knowledge is as vast as their experience in printing. Their expertise and guidance has proved useful at every step. Their uncompromising quality standards have made this book an exceptional effort. Their encouragement from time to time has been an inspiration for everyone.

The publisher and the editorial board hope that this book will prove to be a valuable piece of knowledge for researchers, students, practitioners and scholars across the globe.

List of Contributors

Ya-Lien Cheng, George Kuo and Ya-Chung Tian
Kidney Research Center, Department of Nephrology, Chang Gung Memorial Hospital, College of Medicine, Chang Gung University, Taoyuan 333, Taiwan

Cheng-Chia Lee, Chih-Hsiang Chang and Yi-Jung Li
Kidney Research Center, Department of Nephrology, Chang Gung Memorial Hospital, College of Medicine, Chang Gung University, Taoyuan 333, Taiwan
Graduate Institute of Clinical Medical Sciences, College of Medicine, Chang Gung University, Taoyuan 333, Taiwan

Shao-Wei Chen
Graduate Institute of Clinical Medical Sciences, College of Medicine, Chang Gung University, Taoyuan 333, Taiwan
Department of Cardiothoracic and Vascular Surgery, Chang Gung Memorial Hospital, Linkou branch, College of Medicine, Chang Gung University, Taoyuan 333, Taiwan

Yi-Ting Chen
Department of Biomedical Sciences, College of Medicine, Chang Gung University, Taoyuan 333, Taiwan

Pedro Rojas-Morales, Jessica Granados-Pineda and José Pedraza-Chaverri
Departamento de Biología, Facultad de Química, Universidad Nacional Autónoma de México, Ciudad de México 04510, Mexico

Edilia Tapia, Laura Gabriela Sánchez-Lozada and Horacio Osorio-Alonso
Departamento de Fisiopatología Cardio-Renal, Instituto Nacional de Cardiología Ignacio Chávez, Ciudad de México 14080, Mexico

Juan Carlos León-Contreras and Rogelio Hernández-Pando
Departamento de Patología, Instituto Nacional de Ciencias Médicas y Nutrición Salvador Zubirán, Ciudad de México 14080, Mexico

Susana González-Reyes
Laboratorio de Bioquímica, Facultad de Medicina y Psicología, Universidad Nacional Autónoma de Baja California, Tijuana 22390, Mexico

Angélica Saraí Jiménez-Osorio
Laboratorio de Medicina Genómica, Hospital Regional Lic. Adolfo López Mateos, ISSSTE, Ciudad de México 01030, Mexico

Joyce Trujillo
Consejo Nacional de Ciencia y Tecnología-Consorcio de Investigación, Innovación y Desarrollo para las Zonas Áridas- Instituto Potosino de Investigación Científica y Tecnológica, San Luis Potosí 78216, Mexico

Natalia Pavón
Departamento de Farmacología, Instituto Nacional de Cardiología Ignacio Chávez, Ciudad de México 14080, Mexico

Panupong Hansrivijit
Department of Internal Medicine, University of Pittsburgh Medical Center Pinnacle, Harrisburg, PA 17105, USA

Ploypin Lertjitbanjong and Kanramon Watthanasuntorn
Department of Internal Medicine, Bassett Medical Center, Cooperstown, NY 13326, USA

Charat Thongprayoon and Api Chewcharat
Division of Nephrology and Hypertension, Mayo Clinic, Rochester, MN 55905, USA

Wisit Cheungpasitporn and Sohail Abdul Salim
Division of Nephrology, University of Mississippi Medical Center, Jackson, MS 39216, USA

Narothama Reddy Aeddula
Department of Internal Medicine, Deaconess Health System, Evansville, IN 47747, USA

Narat Srivali
Division of Pulmonary and Critical Care Medicine, St. Agnes Hospital, Baltimore, MD 21229, USA

Michael A. Mao and Karn Wijarnpreecha
Department of Medicine, Mayo Clinic, Jacksonville, FL 32224, USA

Patompong Ungprasert
Department of Rheumatic and Immunologic Diseases, Cleveland Clinic, Cleveland Clinic Lerner College of Medicine of Case Western Reserve University, Cleveland, OH 44106, USA

Wisit Kaewput
Department of Military and Community Medicine, Phramongkutklao College of Medicine, Bangkok 10400, Thailand

Tarun Bathini
Department of Internal Medicine, University of Arizona, Tucson, AZ 85721, USA

Jan Wysocki and Daniel Batlle
Department of Medicine, Division of Nephrology and Hypertension, Feinberg School of Medicine, Northwestern University, Chicago, IL 60611-3008, USA

Arndt Schulze
Department of Medicine, Division of Nephrology and Hypertension, Feinberg School of Medicine, Northwestern University, Chicago, IL 60611-3008, USA
Department of Medicine, Charité-Universitätsmedizin, D-10117 Berlin, Germany

Lana Nežić and Ranko Škrbić
Department of Pharmacology, Toxicology and Clinical Pharmacology, School of Medicine, University of Banja Luka, 14 Save Mrkalja St, 78000 Banja Luka, Bosnia and Herzegovina

Ljiljana Amidžić
Center for Biomedical Research, School of Medicine, University of Banja Luka, 14 Save Mrkalja St, 78000 Banja Luka, Bosnia and Herzegovina

Radoslav Gajanin
Institute of Pathology, University Clinical Center of Republic of Srpska, School of Medicine, University of Banja Luka, 12 Beba St, 78000 Banja Luka, Bosnia and Herzegovina

Zoran Milovanović
Special Police Unit, Police Department of the City of Belgrade, Ministry of Interior, Trebevićka 12/A, 11030 Belgrade, Serbia

Eugenie Nepovimova
Department of Chemistry, Faculty of Science, University of Hradec Kralove, Rokitanského 62, 500 03 Hradec Králové, Czech Republic

Kamil Kuča
Department of Chemistry, Faculty of Science, University of Hradec Kralove, Rokitanského 62, 500 03 Hradec Králové, Czech Republic
Biomedical Research Center, University Hospital Hradec Kralove, 500 02 Hradec Kralove, Czech Republic

Vesna Jaćević
Department of Chemistry, Faculty of Science, University of Hradec Kralove, Rokitanského 62, 500 03 Hradec Králové, Czech Republic
Department for Experimental Toxicology and Pharmacology, National Poison Control Centre, Military Medical Academy, 11 Crnotravska St, 11000 Belgrade, Serbia
Department of Pharmacological Sciences, Medical Faculty of the Military Medical Academy, the University of Defence in Belgrade, 17 Crnotravska St, 11000 Belgrade, Serbia

Foteini Moschovaki-Filippidou, Stefanie Steiger, Andrea Ribeiro, Ekaterina von Rauchhaupt, Clemens D. Cohen, Hans-Joachim Anders and Maciej Lech
LMU Klinikum, Medizinische Klinik und Poliklinik IV, Ludwig-Maximilians-Universität Munich, 80336 München, Germany

Georg Lorenz and Christoph Schmaderer
Klinikum rechts der Isar, Department of Nephrology, Technical University Munich, 81675 München, Germany

Maja Lindenmeyer
Department of Medicine, University Medical Center Hamburg-Eppendorf, 20246 Hamburg, Germany

Ewa Kwiatkowska
Clinical Department of Nephrology, Transplantology and Internal Medicine, Pomeranian Medical University, 70-111 Szczecin, Poland

Katarzyna Stefańska
Department of Obstetrics, Medical University of Gdańsk, 80-210 Gdańsk, Poland

Maciej Zieliński, Justyna Sakowska, Martyna Jankowiak and Piotr Trzonkowski
Department of Medical Immunology, Medical University of Gdańsk, 80-210 Gdańsk, Poland

Natalia Marek-Trzonkowska
International Centre for Cancer Vaccine Science Cancer Immunology Group, University of Gdansk, 80-822 Gdańsk, Poland
Laboratory of Immunoregulation and Cellular Therapies, Department of Family Medicine, Medical University of Gdańsk, 80-210 Gdańsk, Poland

Sebastian Kwiatkowski
Department of Obstetrics and Gynecology, Pomeranian Medical University, 70-111 Szczecin, Poland

Jean-Paul Decuypere, Shawn Hutchinson, Diethard Monbaliu, Jacques Pirenne and Ina Jochmans
Laboratory of Abdominal Transplantation, Transplantation Research Group, Department of Microbiology and Immunology, KU Leuven, B-3000 Leuven, Belgium
Department of Abdominal Transplant Surgery, University Hospitals Leuven, B-3000 Leuven, Belgium

Wim Martinet
Department of Pharmaceutical Sciences, University of Antwerp, B-2610 Antwerp, Belgium

Hee-Yeon Jung, Se-Hyun Oh, Eun-Joo Oh, You-Jin Kim, Chan-Duck Kim, Sun-Hee Park and Jang-Hee Cho
Division of Nephrology, Department of Internal Medicine, School of Medicine, Kyungpook National University, Kyungpook National University Hospital, Daegu 41944, Korea

Yu Ah Hong and Cheol Whee Park
Division of Nephrology, Department of Internal Medicine, The Catholic University of Korea, Seoul 06591, Korea

So Young Jung and Keum Jin Yang
Clinical Research Institute, Daejeon St. Mary's Hospital, Daejeon 34943, Korea

Dai Sig Im
Department of Chemistry, College of Natural Sciences, Soonchunhyang University, Asan 31538, Korea
SH Company, 507, SCH BIT Business Incubator B/D, 22 Soonchunhyang-ro, Shinchang, Asan, Chungnam 31538, Korea

Kyung Hwan Jeong and Hyeon Seok Hwang
Division of Nephrology, Department of Internal Medicine, College of Medicine, Kyung Hee University, Seoul 02447, Korea

Louisa Steines, Helen Poth, Marlene Herrmann, Antonia Schuster, Bernhard Banas and Tobias Bergler
Department of Nephrology, University Hospital Regensburg, 93042 Regensburg, Germany

Sebastian Mertowski, Izabela Morawska, Ewelina Grywalska and Jacek Roliński
Department of Clinical Immunology and Immunotherapy, Medical University of Lublin, 20-093 Lublin, Poland

Paulina Lipa
Department of Genetics and Microbiology, Institute of Microbiology and Biotechnology, Faculty of Biology and Biotechnology, Maria Curie-Skłodowska University, Akademicka 19 St., 20-033 Lublin, Poland

Paulina Niedźwiedzka-Rystwej, Dominika Bębnowska and Rafał Hrynkiewicz
Institute of Biology, University of Szczecin, Felczaka 3c, 71-412 Szczecin, Poland

Wojciech Załuska
Department of Nephrology, Medical University of Lublin, 20-954 Lublin, Poland

Dita Maixnerova and Vladimir Tesar
1st Faculty of Medicine, General University Hospital, Department of Nephrology, Charles University, 128 08 Prague, Czech Republic

Ji-Sun Ahn and Ju-Min Yook
Division of Nephrology, Kyungpook National University Hospital, Daegu 41944, Korea

Yong-Lim Kim
Division of Nephrology, Kyungpook National University Hospital, Daegu 41944, Korea
Cell and Matrix Research Institute, Kyungpook National University, Daegu 41944, Korea
Department of Internal Medicine, School of Medicine, Kyungpook National University, Daegu 41944, Korea

Carmen De Miguel and Abigayle C. Kraus
Section of Cardio-Renal Physiology and Medicine, Division of Nephrology, Department of Medicine, University of Alabama at Birmingham, AL 35233, USA

Mitchell A. Saludes, Prasad Konkalmatt, Laureano D. Asico and Pedro A. Jose
Department of Medicine, Division of Renal Diseases & Hypertension and Pharmacology/Physiology, The GeorgeWashington University School of Medicine and Health Sciences,Washington, DC 20052, USA

Almudena Ruiz Domínguez and Santiago Cuevas
Molecular Inflammation Group, Biomedical Research Institute of Murcia (IMIB), University Clinical Hospital Virgen Arrixaca, 30120 Murcia, Spain

Patricia S. Latham
Pathology and Internal Medicine The George Washington University School of Medicine and Health Sciences, Washington, DC 20052, USA

Daniel Offen
Neuroscience Laboratory, The Felsenstein Medical Research Center, Sackler School of Medicine, Tel-Aviv University, Tel-Aviv 6997801, Israel

Index

www.ingramcontent.com/pod-product-compliance
Lightning Source LLC
LaVergne TN
LVHW081021210926
848485LV00004B/920